MW00379125

PARASITOLOGY

MEDICAL PARASITOLOGY

J. WALTER BECK, B.S., M.S., Ph.D., M.P.H.

Adjunct Professor, Department of Epidemiology and Public Health,
University of Miami School of Medicine; formerly Professor of
Community Health and Microbiology, Medical Center Campus,
Miami-Dade Community College; Consultant, Mount Sinai Hospital,
Jackson Memorial Hospital, and Veterans Administration Hospital,
Miami, Florida

JOHN E. DAVIES, M.B.B.S., L.R.C.P. (London), M.D., M.P.H.

Chairman and Professor of the Department of Epidemiology and Public
Health, University of Miami School of Medicine; Consultant, World Health
Organization, National Academy of Sciences, U.S. Environmental
Protection Agency, UC/US Aid for International Development Program,
Jackson Memorial Hospital, Miami, Florida

THIRD EDITION

with 399 *illustrations, including 7 color plates*

The C. V. Mosby Company

ST. LOUIS • TORONTO • LONDON   1981

THIRD EDITION

Copyright © 1981 by The C. V. Mosby Company

All rights reserved. No part of this book may be reproduced in any manner without written permission of the publisher.

Previous editions copyrighted 1971, 1976

Printed in the United States of America

The C. V. Mosby Company
11830 Westline Industrial Drive, St. Louis, Missouri 63141

Library of Congress Cataloging in Publication Data

Beck, J   Walter, 1913-
    Medical parasitology.

    Bibliography: p.
    Includes index.
    1. Medical parasitology. I. Davies, John E.,
joint author. II. Title. [DNLM: 1. Parasites.
2. Parasitic diseases. WC 695 B393m]
RC119.B36 1981   616.9´6   80-25201
ISBN 0-8016-0552-0

GW/VH/VH 9 8 7 6 5 4   01/C/056

Preface

As indicated in previous editions, this text is an outgrowth of a manual that, supplemented with lectures and laboratory instruction, is used in the teaching of medical parasitology. The format of presentation has been essentially unchanged. The use of questions at the ends of chapters has been maintained and expanded. References have been significantly increased and updated. Treatment, in many instances, has been presented in tabular form including both adult and pediatric dosages. Numerous illustrations from the skillful pen of Joan Davies have been added along with photographs drawn from the resources of fellow scientists and the Armed Forces Institute of Pathology. Ronald Fayer and J. K. Frenkel have contributed significantly to the sections on Coccidia and *Pneumocystis*. Advances in the immunology and serology of the parasitic diseases are included. Several parasitic diseases, not previously discussed, are added and others are updated. The section on medical arthropodology has been enlarged to include recent developments in the area of pest control, kindly made available to us by the World Health Organization, and the expanding field of pesticide management and agromedicine. Grateful appreciation is expressed to The Medical Letter, Inc., 56 Harrison Street, New Rochelle, New York, for permission to use their recent information on drugs for parasitic infections and infestations; to Charles M. Bailey, Department of Biomedical Communications, University of Miami School of Medicine, for the reproduction of many photographs; and to Ronna Schneider for her skill and patience in typing the many drafts of the manuscript.

J. Walter Beck
John E. Davies

Contents

MEDICAL
PARASITOLOGY

CHAPTER 1

Introduction to medical parasitology

Medical parasitology is that branch of the medical sciences dealing with the members of the animal kingdom living in and on the body of humans and with aspects of this host-parasite relationship having medical significance. This science includes the study of vectors, reservoirs, definitive and intermediate hosts, and all factors of an ecologic and epidemiologic nature associated with disease transmission and prevention.

The parasites of medical importance may be divided into the following three major groups for convenience of study:

Protozoa—one-celled organisms
Helminths—worms
Arthropods—insects and their allies

As with most disciplines, parasitology also uses many terms unique unto itself. It is not advisable to learn all these terms at one sitting since their use in context, in most instances, will convey their meaning with greater clarity and impact. It is desirable, nevertheless, to become familiar with basic terms for purposes of early orientation. The *parasite* is the animal agent that parasitizes man, the *host*. Other parasitized animals that may serve as a source of infection for humans are called *reservoir hosts*. Some parasites are *obligatory* guests unable to survive outside a host, whereas others are *facultative* and capable of an independent existence outside the host. Those causing harm to the host are *pathogens*, whereas the harmless (nonpathogenic) species are known as *commensals*. The arthropods, living on the body surface no matter how brief

a period of time, are called *ectoparasites*, whereas the protozoa and helminths living within the body are called *endoparasites*. The former cause *infestations* and the latter, *infections*. Confusion in terminology may exist in some instances wherein arthropods actually become endoparasitic. Fly larvae, for example, may live in the gastrointestinal tract in the same environment with the protozoa and helminths. In the opinion of some authors, such parasites cause an infection and are truly endoparasites.

Although parasites, in general, are more common in the tropics and subtropics than elsewhere in the world, they are by no means confined to these areas. Two chief reasons accounting for their prevalence in tropical climes are (1) the increased density of population as opposed to that in the temperate and frigid regions and (2) poor sanitation and public health practice. The ability of suitable vectors, when involved in transmission, to propagate more readily and sometimes exclusively in such areas is also involved. In countries where malnutrition is widespread, the debilitated condition of large populations further enhances the indifference to sanitation. Thus, in an environment with very few factors detrimental to the survival and dissemination of parasites, the low level of sanitation ensures the widespread prevalence of the parasitic diseases.

In addition to poor sanitation and public health practice, the prevalence of many parasitic diseases is aided and abetted by the customs, taboos, and habits of the people. This fact is especially pertinent for those disease agents transmitted in food and drink and by hand-to-mouth contamination. Thus, amebiasis, which is particularly prevalent wherever night soil (human feces) is used as fertilizer or where sewage contaminates drinking water, occurs not only in the tropics but also within the Arctic Circle. In areas where the schistosomes prevail, the habits of the natives, who use the same irrigation ditches or freshwater streams for the washing of clothes, bathing, and, all too frequently, urination and defecation, serve to keep infected the appropriate snail inhabitants that constitute a perennial source of reinfection for man. Trichinosis would no longer be a health menace in the United States (where it is not uncommon) if uncooked garbage was not fed to hogs, or if inadequately cooked pork products were no longer consumed.

Parasites that are well adjusted to their hosts live more or less in a state of "armed truce," benefiting from their association with a minimum of damage to their keepers. Tissue repair may keep pace with tissue damage, and in an otherwise healthy well-nourished person, no symptoms may be discernible. Some parasites may live as commensals at times, whereas under different circumstances they may become pathogenic, causing severe damage, even death, to the parasitized individual. Variations from host to host occur for a given parasite. Some parasites are harmless at all times, but their similarity in morphology to the pathogens makes their recognition imperative so that errors in diagnosis are avoided.

The adaptation of parasites to their hosts sometimes results in complicated pathways, both within and outside the human body. The route or course of a parasite followed from any one stage of development throughout its life history back to that same stage is known as its life cycle. The life cycle of a parasite consists of two essential parts, each important in its own right. Through an understanding of the route followed by a para-

site within the human body from the time and site of entry until it makes its exit from the host we are led to an understanding of the symptomatology and pathology of the disease it causes. Frequently the method of diagnosis and route of medication to be employed may be suggested. Knowing the whereabouts of the parasite outside the body is essential to an understanding of the epidemiology of disease and its prevention.

In medical parasitology, probably more than in the other medical sciences, the diagnosis of a disease will almost always depend on the laboratory findings. The incubation period, the time from infection to the first clinical manifestations of disease, is of concern to the physician; the prepatent period, the time when parasites can be first observed, is of importance to the laboratory diagnostician. Clinical signs and symptoms will, at best, be only suggestive of the cause of infection. Thus the laboratory diagnosis of the parasitic diseases of humans becomes, in reality, the chief and frequently the only method of diagnosis available. It has been said that the famous French police, the Sûreté Nationale, have as their motto *Cherchez la femme*—"Search for the woman"—and you will solve the crime. We may well paraphrase that by saying: "Search for the parasite" and you will diagnose the case. Parasites can and do occur in nearly every part of the human body and techniques specific to their particular location must be employed for their recovery. Less often, when recovery is impossible, other procedures must be resorted to in order to make a diagnosis.

The ultimate goal of the physician is to make the patient well. This task usually involves either complete eradication of the parasite or a reduction in its number. Unfortunately, most antiparasitic drugs effective against the parasite are also toxic to the host. Therefore the physician must carefully weigh the disease entity against the treatment. Since the protozoa multiply within the host much as bacteria do, their complete eradication is usually necessary and treatment to this end must be employed. The worms, in contrast, usually do not increase their numbers per se, and symptoms and signs can frequently be controlled by a reduction in number so that unnecessary drug therapy is avoided. For example, one should distinguish between hookworm disease requiring medical treatment and hookworm infection that can be managed by diet rich in protein. During World War II many a G.I. was hospitalized and treated because hookworm eggs were found in his stool. He suffered unduly from the toxic drugs used in an attempt to rid him of every last worm, when, in fact, his military environment with its good diet and the wearing of shoes would have adequately resolved the problem.

REVIEW QUESTIONS

1. What are the three major branches of medical parasitology?
2. Give a broad definition of a parasite.
3. Why is the laboratory diagnosis of most parasitic diseases of humans so important?
4. What two factors determine the geographic distribution of parasites?
5. What is the significance of the life cycle of a parasite from a medical point of view?
6. What is the rationale behind the treatment of protozoa? Of helminths?

REFERENCES

Ash, J. E., and S. Spitz. 1945. Pathology of tropical diseases: an atlas. W. B. Saunders Co., Philadelphia.

Belding, D. L. 1965. Textbook of clinical parasitology. Ed. 2. Appleton-Century-Crofts, New York.

Binford, C. H., and D. H. Connor. 1976. Pathology of tropical and extraordinary diseases: an atlas. Vols. I and II. Armed Forces Institute of Pathology, Washington, D.C.

Brown, H. W. 1975. Basic clinical parasitology. Ed. 4. Appleton-Century-Crofts, New York.

Chandler, A. C., and C. P. Reed. 1961. Introduction to parasitology. Ed. 10. John Wiley & Sons, Inc., New York.

Faust, E. C., P. C. Beaver, and R. C. Jung. 1968. Animal agents and vectors of human disease. Ed. 3. Lea & Febiger, Philadelphia.

Faust, E. C., P. F. Russell, and R. C. Jung. 1970. Clinical parasitology. Ed. 8. Lea & Febiger, Philadelphia.

Garcia, L. S., and L. R. Ash. 1979. Diagnostic parasitology: clinical laboratory manual. Ed. 2. The C. V. Mosby Co., St. Louis.

Hunter III, G. W., J. C. Swartzwelder, and D. F. Clyde, Editors. 1976. Tropical medicine. Ed. 5. W. B. Saunders Co., Philadelphia.

Kean, B. H., K. E. Mott, and A. J. Russel, Editors. 1978. Tropical medicine and parasitology: classical investigations. Vols. I and II. Cornell University Press, New York.

Knight, R., M. G. Schultz, D. W. Hoskins, and P. D. Marsden. 1973. Progress report—intestinal parasites. Gut **14**:145-168.

Maegraith, B. G. 1980. Adams and Maegraith: clinical tropical diseases. Ed. 7. Blackwell, Oxford and Edinburgh.

Maegraith, B. G., and H. M. Gilles, Editors. 1971. Management and treatment of tropical diseases. Blackwell, Oxford and Edinburgh.

Marcial-Rojas, R. A., Editor. 1971. Pathology of protozoal and helminthic diseases with clinical correlation. Churchill Livingstone, Edinburgh.

Medical protozoology and helminthology. 1965. Rev. ed. U.S. Naval Medical School, Bethesda, Maryland.

Read, C. P. 1970. Parasitism and symbiology. The Ronald Press Co., New York.

Russel, P. F., L. S. West, R. D. Manwell, and G. Macdonald. 1963. Practical malariology. Ed. 2. Oxford University Press, London.

Schmidt, G. D., and L. S. Roberts. 1977. Foundations of parasitology. The C. V. Mosby Co., St. Louis.

Spencer, F. M., and L. S. Monroe. 1975. The color atlas of intestinal parasites. Charles C Thomas, Publisher, Springfield, Ill.

Spencer, H., and others. 1973. Tropical pathology. Springer-Verlag, New York.

Sterky, G. 1977. SAREC report: challenges in research on tropical diseases. No. R:1—Swedish Agency for Research Cooperation with Developing Countries.

Wilcocks, C., and P. E. C. Manson-Bahr, Editors. 1972. Manson's tropical diseases. Baillière, Tindall, and Cox, London.

Woodruff, A. W., Editor. 1974. Medicine in the tropics. Churchill Livingstone, Edinburgh.

PART ONE

Medical protozoology

CHAPTER 2

Introduction to the protozoa

The protozoa are single-celled animals comparable in function to multicellular animals and not to isolated cells from such organisms. Beneath the cell membrane lies the ectoplasm, which is more gelatinous in contrast to the relatively fluid inner endoplasm. Both are colloidal states of the cytoplasm, however, and are reversible. The nucleus or nuclei may be vesicular or compact, depending on the species. Vesicular nuclei contain nucleoplasm and one or more densely staining bodies called endosomes or karyosomes. Chromatin material may or may not be present adjacent to the inner wall of the nuclear membrane. Compact nuclei have solid chromatin material. Organelles may be present in protozoa in such forms as cilia, flagella, pseudopodia, undulating membranes, and kinetoplasts and function in various ways.

Protozoa vary in size, shape, and morphologic details and on these bases are divided into classes, orders, families, genera, and species.

The classes of medical importance are as follows:

Sarcodina—amebas
Mastigophora—flagellates
Ciliata—ciliates
Sporozoa—sporozoa

Parasites are also categorized according to the areas of the body invaded. Thus those found in the intestinal tract are known as intestinal protozoa; those found in the mouth, vagina, and urethra are known as atrial or, more specifically, oral and urogenital; those found in the blood and body tissues are blood and tissue protozoa.

GEOGRAPHIC DISTRIBUTION

Protozoa, in general, have a cosmopolitan distribution and may be found wherever humans make their homes. This range extends from the arctic wastelands to the torrid tropics. The majority of the species are found, and the greatest intensity of infection occurs, in the tropics and subtropics. Where vectors are involved, distribution may be quite restricted, as in the case of tsetses in the transmission of African sleeping sickness.

HOST-PARASITE RELATIONSHIP

The pathogenic protozoa are somewhat like bacteria in that they multiply within the host and, unless stopped by the defense mechanisms of the patient or by artificial means such as chemotherapy, they may eventually destroy the host. The onset of infection may be acute and fulminating, with sudden death, or never more than subclinical. A chronic state may follow clinical manifestations and may sometimes persist throughout the life of the host, being interrupted with exacerbations of the disease. The chronic state represents a kind of "armed truce" between host and parasite, each waiting for the opportunity to take advantage of a favorable situation. When the balance of power tips one way or the other, one becomes the victor, the other the vanquished, unless equilibrium is again reached. Thus, the protozoa vary in their pathogenicity from host to host and within a given host from time to time. The majority of the intestinal protozoa live a benign existence, although some may, at times, produce a very severe disease and death. The blood and tissue parasites are pathogenic to a varying degree. Dissemination of the protozoa throughout the body is not uncommon, with foci of infections being established in various organs and tissues of the host. Some show no tissue specificity at all, whereas others tend to settle in certain organs or cells to the exclusion of others. Thus, symptomatology and pathology, in some instances, may be highly suggestive of the etiologic agent. The invasion of the posterior cervical lymph nodes by the African trypanosomes, for example, has given rise to "Winterbottom's sign," a sign of diagnostic value in African sleeping sickness.

Tissue response of the host varies among the protozoa. For example, little or no cellular reaction occurs with extraintestinal amebiasis, whereas hyperplasia of the reticuloendothelial system is seen in the leishmaniases. In contrast with the helminths, there is no eosinophilic response, though the number of circulating leukocytes may be changed; a leukopenia, for instance, is typical in kala-azar, whereas in extraintestinal amebiasis a leukocytosis may occur.

The nature of the immune response is varied and, in many instances, poorly understood. Both cell-mediated and humoral antibodies are involved. There appears to be a stronger natural immunity in blacks as compared with whites. This is exemplified in benign tertian malaria in which paroxysms, when present, are usually much milder. Immunity, in many instances, also seems to increase with age, the greater pathogenicity occurring in infants and children. Since protozoa multiply within the host and may remain present for as long as the life span of the host, it is difficult to distinguish premunition (immunity resulting from the presence of parasites) from a sustained, acquired immunity resulting from an old infection. Some healthy individuals appear to be completely refractory to infection, as evidenced, for example, by the inability to establish *Entamoeba histolytica* by the oral feeding of

viable cysts. In most, however, patency can be demonstrated even though the host response may vary from a subclinical infection to a fulminating case terminating in death. The state of health of the host has a marked effect on the immune response. Such factors as malnutrition, alcoholism, and debilitating diseases contribute to a breakdown in the immune mechanisms and greatly enhance the chances for successful establishment of infection. *Balantidium coli*, a parasite to which healthy individuals are highly immune, is almost nonexistent in the United States, where the general level of nutrition is high among those exposed to this parasite, whereas in many of the undeveloped countries of the world balantidiasis is more common.

LIFE CYCLES

Among the protozoa, life cycles are quite simple, with few exceptions. The intestinal and atrial protozoa multiply asexually by binary fission in the active feeding, growing, trophozoite stage. Encystation, when present, occurs by the extrusion of undigested food particles, loss of organelles such as flagella and cilia, and the secretion of a cyst wall, which protects the organism against adverse environmental influences. Various factors, such as a change in pH, oxygen tension, degree of dehydration, and inherent determinants, have been suggested as the cause of this phenomenon. Nuclear division may or may not take place in the cyst stage. Transmission to humans of the intestinal parasites occurs chiefly through the ingestion of contaminated food and drink; of the atrial forms, transmission occurs by droplet contamination and sexual intercourse. When present in the life cycle, cysts are the transmissible stage, being able to withstand adverse environmental changes outside the host as well as gastric acidity within the host.

The hemoflagellates are members of the same family and bear a close relationship to one another. Of the four morphologic forms or stages that may be present, all species have at least one stage in an arthropod and another stage in human beings and reservoir vertebrate hosts, asexual reproduction by longitudinal division occurring in both. In one species, all four morphologic forms are present in the life cycle. The arthropod serves as the vector or carrier to human beings and other animals. Geographic distribution is thus determined by the ecology of the arthropod hosts.

The sporozoa are unique among the parasitic protozoa in that both asexual and sexual reproduction occurs. The definitive or final host harbors the sexual stages, and the asexual forms are found in the intermediate host. Various stages of growth are appropriately designated. Man may serve as both hosts, as in some coccidia, or only the intermediate host, as in malaria.

REVIEW QUESTIONS

1. What is a vesicular nucleus? A compact nucleus? An organelle? Give examples of each.
2. What are the classes of protozoa of medical importance?
3. Discuss the nature of the host-parasite relationship of the protozoa in human beings.
4. How are most intestinal protozoa transmitted? Atrial protozoa? Hemoflagellates?
5. What is a definitive host? An intermediate host? Give an example of each.
6. What is the significance of the immune response?

REFERENCES

Belding, D. L. 1965. Textbook of clinical parasitology. Ed. 2. Appleton-Century-Crofts, New York.

Binford, C. H., and D. H. Conner. 1976. Pathology of tropical and extraordinary diseases: an atlas. Vol. I. Armed Forces Institute of Pathology, Washington, D.C.

Brown, H. W. 1975. Basic clinical parasitology. Ed. 4. Appleton-Century-Crofts, New York.

Faust, E. C., P. C. Beaver, and R. C. Jung. 1975. Animal agents and vectors of human disease. Ed. 4. Lea & Febiger, Philadelphia.

Faust, E. C., P. F. Russell, and R. C. Jung. 1970. Clinical parasitology. Ed. 8. Lea & Febiger, Philadelphia.

Garcia, L. S., and L. R. Ash. 1979. Diagnostic parasitology: clinical laboratory manual. Ed. 2. The C. V. Mosby Co., St. Louis.

Hoare, C. A. 1949. Handbook of medical protozoology. Baillière, Tindall and Cox, London.

Kean, B. H., K. E. Mott, and A. J. Russel, Editors. 1978. Tropical medicine and parasitology: classic investigations. Vols. I and II. Cornell University Press, Ithaca, New York.

Knight, R., and others. 1973. Progress report—intestinal parasites. Gut 14:145-168.

Kouri, P. J., G. Basnuevo, and F. Sotolongo. 1947. Protozoología médica. Ed. 2. In Lecciones de parasitología y medicina tropical. Vol. 3. A. Muñiz y Hno., Havana.

Kudo, R. R. 1960. Protozoology. Ed. 4. Charles C Thomas, Publisher, Springfield, Ill.

Maegraith, B. G., and H. M. Gilles, Editors. 1971. Management and treatment of tropical diseases. Blackwell, Oxford and Edinburgh.

Marcial-Rojas, R. A., Editor. 1971. Pathology of protozoal and helminthic diseases with clinical correlation. Churchill Livingstone, Edinburgh.

Melvin, D. H., and M. M. Brooke. 1974. Laboratory procedures for the diagnosis of intestinal parasites. U.S. Department of Health, Education, and Welfare, Center for Disease Control, Atlanta, Ga.

Spencer, F. M., and L. S. Monroe. 1975. The color atlas of intestinal parasites. Charles C Thomas, Publisher, Springfield, Ill.

Steck, E. A. 1972. The chemotherapy of protozoan diseases. Vols. 1 to 4. Walter Reed Army Institute of Research, Washington, D.C.

Wilcocks, C., and P. E. C. Manson-Bahr. 1972. Manson's tropical diseases. Baillière, Tindall, and Cox, London.

CHAPTER 3

The amebas (Sarcodina)

The following amebas are parasitic in humans:

Atrial (oral)
    Entamoeba gingivalis
Intestinal
    Entamoeba histolytica
    Entamoeba hartmanni
    Entamoeba coli
    Entamoeba polecki
    Endolimax nana
    Iodamoeba bütschlii

The amebas have often been described as naked bits of protoplasm. By means of protoplasmic extensions called pseudopodia the trophozoites are able to move on a substrate and engulf food. The nature of this movement, as in *Entamoeba histolytica*, is, at times, of diagnostic significance. Reproduction occurs by binary fission. When pathogenicity is associated with the organisms, it is only the trophozoite stage that is involved. They are all cosmopolitan in distribution.

The trophozoite is a delicate, fragile organism readily destroyed by the gastric juice of the stomach and, among the intestinal forms, not transmissible to humans. When seen in the feces, it occurs most commonly in soft, mushy, poorly formed, or watery stools. Flushing of the cecum by catharsis may result in the passage of these stages, when only cysts are seen in formed stool.

In a fresh saline mount, trophozoites are usually difficult to identify. Nuclei are not readily discernible without stains, and though motility characteristics and pseudopod formation are described in the literature as being of diagnostic value, many times there is an overlapping of characteristics among the species, making identification difficult (Table 3-1).

During the process of encystation the amebas pass through a period when many identifying characteristics of the trophozoite stage are lost and the diagnostic features of the cyst have not as yet made an appearance. These precyst forms are best identified after staining with iron-hematoxylin, trichrome, or other stains when nuclear detail may be studied.

Cysts are formed by shrinkage of the trophozoites as they assume the characteristic shape for that species. Inclusion bodies, such as undigested food particles, are extruded from the cytoplasm, and a protective cyst wall is secreted by the organism. Unorganized chromatoidal material in some young cysts may, as the cyst matures, become organized into bars of diagnostic significance. The number and morphology of nuclei formed as a result of nuclear division, in some instances, will aid also in the identification of cysts.

With the exception of *Entamoeba gingivalis*, which occurs in the mouth, the amebas are intestinal in habitat. Except for this ameba, which is known only in the trophozoite form, all have trophozoite and cyst stages in their life cycles.

Excystation takes place in the ileocecal region of the intestine. The young trophozoites multiply rapidly and become established in the cecum. Eventually encystation takes place and a colony of both trophozoites and cysts is established. The amebas occur

Table 3-1. Differential characteristics of trophozoites and cysts

	Entamoeba histolytica	Entamoeba coli	Endolimax nana	Iodamoeba bütschlii	Entamoeba hartmanni
Trophozoites					
Size	Small race, average 8 μm Large race, average 15 μm Dysentery, average 25 μm	Average 20 μm (12 to 30 μm)	Average 8 μm (6 to 12 μm)	Average 10 μm (6 to 20 μm)	Averages 10 μm
Motility	Actively progressive and directional; sluglike forms (galloping ameba)	Sluggish, rarely progressive, nondirectional; rare, sluglike forms	Similar to E. coli	Similar to E. coli	Similar to E. histolytica
Pseudopodia	Fingerlike, explosive, clear and glasslike. In old specimens, similar to those of E. coli	Short, blunt, broad, slow, less glasslike	Similar to E. coli	Similar to E. coli	Similar to E. histolytica
Red blood cells	May be present	Never present	Never present	Never present	Never present
Cytoplasm	Clean appearance	Dirty appearance; bacteria, vacuoles, crystals, etc. present	Similar to E. coli	Similar to E. coli	Similar to E. histolytica
Nucleus (unstained)	Usually invisible in saline solution	Visible in saline, grayish to black ring	Similar to E. histolytica	Similar to E. histolytica	Similar to E. histolytica
Nucleus (stained)	Delicate nuclear membrane; discrete, delicate chromatin granules on periphery; karyosome delicate, usually central	Thick, coarse nuclear membrane; thick, coarse coalescing chromatin granules on periphery; karyosome coarse, thick, usually eccentric	Nuclear membrane intermedial between E. histolytica and E. coli; no chromatin granules on periphery; karyosome large, central, or eccentric on periphery	Similar to Endolimax nana; karyosome surrounded by achromatic granules	Similar to E. histolytica
Cysts					
Size	Small race, average 8 μm Large race, average 12 μm	Average 18 μm	Average 8 μm	Average 10 μm	Average 8 μm
Shape	Spherical, sometimes oval	Similar to E. histolytica	Oval, sometimes spherical	Typically varied; round, oval elliptical, rhomboidal, etc.	Similar to E. histolytica
Glycogen	Diffuse mass in center of young cysts; not heavy	Dense, large, well-defined mass in center of young binucleated cysts	None visible	Well-defined glycogen mass persistent throughout life of cyst	Similar to E. histolytica

Volutin granules	None	None	None	Black granules in clusters usually present	None
Nuclei	1 to 4 present; not visible in saline; same as trophozoites when stained but smaller	1 to 8 present; often visible in saline; same as trophozoite when stained but smaller	1 to 4 present; usually visible in saline; same as trophozoite when stained but smaller	1 present; not visible in saline usually; same as trophozoite when stained but small and karyosome is eccentric, near nuclear membrane	Similar to *E. histolytica*
Chromatoid	Unorganized in young cysts; later formed into bars with rounded ends in older cysts; present in over 50% of cysts	Unorganized in young cysts; later formed into splinterlike sticks with ragged edges in old cysts; present in less than 10% of cysts	None diagnostic	None diagnostic	Similar to *E. histolytica*

most abundantly in the cecum, next in the rectosigmoid area. Trophozoites, once passed in the feces, do not undergo encystation but perish rapidly outside the body (except in culture). Cysts, likewise, do not excyst after passage in the stool (except in culture) but only after ingestion and passage into the small intestine.

Entamoeba gingivalis

Entamoeba gingivalis is a nonpathogen found only in the trophozoite stage (Fig. 3-1). The average size varies from 10 to 20 μm. The organism closely resembles *E. histolytica*, even in the ingestion of red blood cells. A striking feature of the trophozoite is the large number of food vacuoles, frequently containing degenerated nuclei from endothelial cells, lymphocytes, and polymorphonuclear leukocytes. A small proportion may contain bacteria.

The organism, which lives around the gumline of the teeth in the tartar and gingival pockets, is essentially a scavenger of disintegrated cells. This accounts for its greater prevalence in pyorrhea, dental caries, and inflammatory lesions. Active amebas may be demonstrated by micropscopically examining scrapings smeared in saline on a glass slide.

Transmission occurs most probably by mouth-to-mouth contact through kissing and droplet contamination. The organisms do not survive passage through the stomach.

Entamoeba histolytica

Life cycle and morphology. *Entamoeba histolytica* has two stages in its life cycle, the trophozoite and the cyst. Intestinal infections occur through the ingestion of the latter stage chiefly in contaminated food and drink but also by hand-to-mouth contact.

Trophozoites may be identifiable in freshly passed, unstained stools by characteristic progressive, directional motility (galloping amebas), explosive pseudopodia showing a marked delineation between ectoplasm and

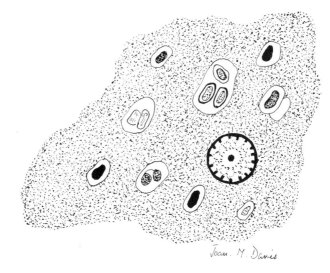

Fig. 3-1. *Entamoeba gingivalis* trophozoite. Note the ingested red blood cells and numerous food vacuoles.

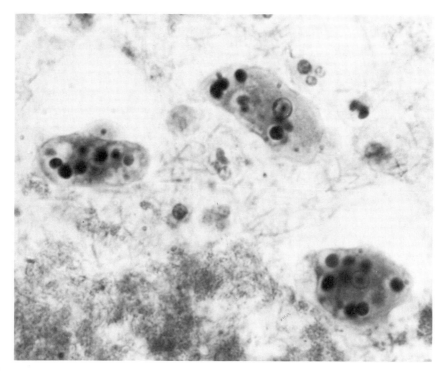

Fig. 3-2. *Entamoeba histolytica* trophozoites showing ingested red blood cells and directional motility. (Photograph by Charles M. Bailey.)

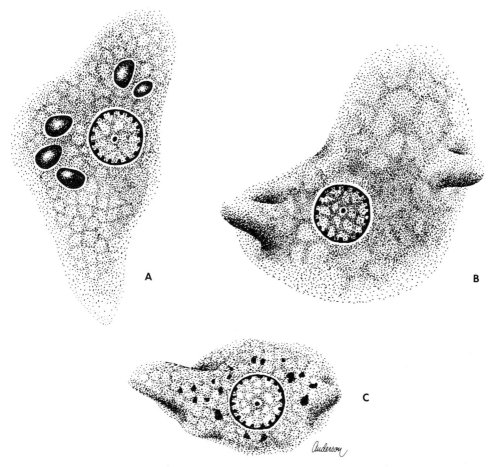

Fig. 3-3. *Entamoeba histolytica* trophozoites showing **A,** ingested red blood cells; **B,** explosive pseudopodia; and **C,** ingested bacteria. Note the typical nucleus in each.

endoplasm, and the presence, at times, of red blood cells in the cytoplasm (Fig. 3-2). The nucleus is usually invisible in saline, and the cytoplasm presents a "clean" appearance, unless it contains ingested bacteria. Size varies, depending on the race, from about 8 to 30 μm in diameter. When stained, the nucleus reveals a delicate nuclear membrane with discrete, delicate chromatin granules on the inner surface and a delicate karyosome, usually centrally located (Fig. 3-3).

Encystation occurs in the cecum and colon through the rounding up of the trophozoite, extrusion of undigested food particles,

shrinkage in size, and the secretion of a cyst wall. Young cysts appear first as uninucleated forms with a diffuse, usually centrally located, glycogen mass easily discernible with iodine. Unorganized chromatoidal material is also frequently present and later becomes organized into bars with rounded or squared ends. Both the stored glycogen and the chromatoidal bars, which probably represent stored food, eventually disappear, leaving a mature, quadrinucleated cyst. The latter is the transmissible stage to humans.

For some time two races were differentiated on the basis of cyst size, the larger averaging 12 μm in diameter and the smaller averaging 8 μm. The general opinion now is that the small race constitutes a distinct species, *Entamoeba hartmanni*, which is considered by most to be nonpathogenic in humans. Overlapping in size of the two races may occur in some instances, conditioned no doubt in part by nutritional status of the organism, thus rendering differentiation difficult at best, if not impossible at times.

Other nonpathogenic *E. histolytica*–like amebas have also been reported, which differ immunologically and physiologically from the common DKB strain. The Laredo strain grows at room temperature as well as at 37° C. Other strains from man demonstrating this characteristic suggest to some that these organisms may well constitute a group distinct from the commonly accepted *E. histolytica* and that *Entamoeba invadens*, pathogenic in snakes and *E. histolytica* from humans, may have evolved from a common ancestor of the Laredo type (parasitic in snakes but not in humans). A further evolutionary relationship to *Entamoeba moskovskii*, isolated from sewage in several countries and experimentally infective for hamsters, is suggested.

Ingested mature cysts undergo excystation in the ileocecal region of the intestine. Multiplication by binary fission results in the establishment of a colony in the cecum and later throughout the colon. Cyst formation follows as part of the normal course of the life cycle. Dehydration of the fecal mass as it moves down the colon toward the anus probably plays a role in inducing cyst formation. Whenever cysts are seen in the stool, trophozoites must be present somewhere in the colon (Fig. 3-4).

Penetration of the intestinal mucosa by trophozoites results in lesions in the intestine, most commonly in the cecum, and flexures of the colon and rectosigmoid area. Invasion of the bloodstream may occur with metastases to various organs of the body. The liver is the most common site of extraintestinal disease with or without secondary spread to the lungs via the diaphragm, but the trophozoites may become established anywhere in the body.

Epidemiology. The use of night soil for fertilizer, flies carrying contaminated feces on the proboscis and sticky feet to the dining room table and other places of food display, unclean food handlers, and contaminated soil washing into wells and onto vegetable gardens are all means whereby the cysts (Fig. 3-5) of *E. histolytica* can eventually reach the gastrointestinal tract of humans. Even sophisticated water-supply systems may become contaminated and result in urban epidemics of amebiasis; such an outbreak at the Chicago World's Fair during the 1930s resulted in approximately 100 deaths. Most of these epidemics are brought about by the fecal contamination of a faulty water-supply system, since routine chlorination as employed in modern city waterworks does not destroy the cysts of *E. histolytica*.

In South Bend, Indiana, in the 1950s a serious outbreak occurred in a commercial plant because of the juxtaposition of faulty connections in the sewage and fresh water lines, resulting in a back siphonage into the drinking water system. Several deaths occurred among the employees.

The high incidence of amebiasis in the tropics is attributable chiefly to poor sanitation. In addition to the use of night soil for fertilizer, promiscuous defecation habits, particularly of children, result in the seeding of the soil with cysts and the pollution of the local water supply. Children playing in the area contaminate their hands, and their fingers inevitably end up in the mouth. The simple habit of defecation into a deep hole in the ground when toilets are not available and the avoidance of using feces for fertilizer would help greatly in reducing the incidence of this disease.

Quite erroneously, many think of amebiasis as a disease confined to the tropics and otherwise found only in those northern wayfarers who venture into the tropics on

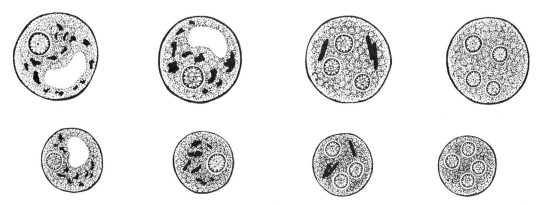

Fig. 3-4. *Entamoeba histolytica* cysts. *Top row:* large race. *Bottom row:* small race, designated by some as *Entamoeba hartmanni.* Note the typical nuclei (maximum of four) and the chromatoidal bodies later becoming bars.

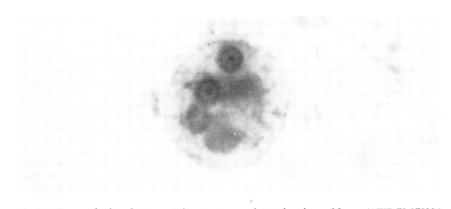

Fig. 3-5. *Entamoeba histolytica* cyst showing two nuclei in the plane of focus. (AFIP 72-17636.)

business or pleasure. In reality, it is surprisingly common in the more highly sanitized and cultured areas of the temperate regions as an endemic disease.

In the United States the majority of exposures in the general population are probably light and only repeated exposures result in infection. Conservative estimates give an incidence of up to 5%. Variations in virulence of strains of the organism, plus the high degree of resistance resulting from a good nutritional state and general good health of the people, may account for the higher prevalence of asymptomatic carriers or of only

mildly disturbed individuals who go unnoticed in better-developed countries.

On the other hand, in mental institutions, where crowding occurs and personal hygiene is often poor, heavy infections may account for epidemics of considerable proportion. Such conditions also may account for epidemics among the Eskimos. The infection rate of 25% some years ago in the industrial population of the island of Aruba, whose source of food and water was ameba free and who were serviced by a modern sewage treatment plant, dropped 90% when the Chinese foodhandlers with an infection rate

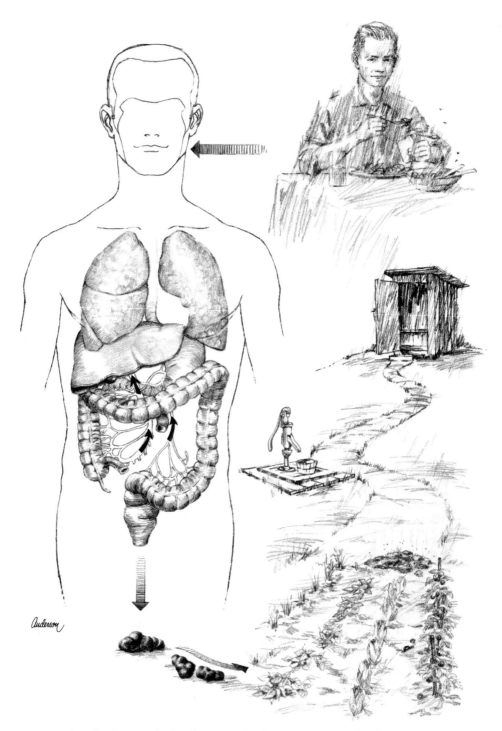

Fig. 3-6. Life cycle of *Entamoeba histolytica*. Food and water contaminated with infective cysts are ingested. Excystation in the ileocecal region results in a colony of trophozoites and cysts becoming established in the cecum and colon. Penetration of the mucosa by trophozoites, with subsequent invasion of the portal circulation, may result in extraintestinal amebiasis. Cysts passed in the feces contaminate food and water, which, in turn, are ingested by humans.

of 33% were successfully treated for *E. histo-lytica*, thus attesting to the important role of foodhandlers in the transmission of this disease. The possible role of animal reservoirs cannot be overlooked. Many species of monkeys throughout the world are infected with an ameba morphologically resembling *E. histolytica*. In many tropical villages close to the forest habitats of monkeys where contact is apparent, polluted surroundings afford the opportunity for human exposure. Considerable evidence suggests that diets high in carbohydrates and low in protein support infections, a condition common in the tropics where hypoproteinemia is common and starches dominate in the diet. Such diets, although favoring infection, apparently reduce tissue invasion. There is no evidence of protective immunity in man although protection has been shown in guinea pigs following injection of amebic antigen.

Though the cysts of *E. histolytica* succumb readily to desiccation and high temperature, in a moist environment the survival rate increases markedly as the temperature drops below 50° C, reaching a peak survival of 90 days in water at 0° C. Even undiluted feces at 37° C, with its high rate of bacterial growth that is destructive to cysts, allow survival for 1 to 2 weeks (Fig. 3-6).

Intestinal amebiasis

Symptomatology. Symptoms associated with intestinal amebiasis are various and rarely, if ever, pathognomonic of the disease. Some workers believe that *E. histolytica*, for the most part, lives as a commensal (avirulent minuta form) feeding on such elements as bacteria and fungi and doing no harm to the intestinal mucosa. For reasons as yet not clearly understood, apparently some trophozoites from this large race may, at times, develop into larger than normal organisms (virulent magna forms) and become tissue invaders. Under optimal conditions of pH and ionic concentrations the evidence suggests that commensal forms may become virulent when they contain a certain ratio of

starch to cholesterol. These forms, according to the proponents of this theory, are the organisms associated with mucosal damage and eventual invasion of the bloodstream. Such trophozoites with ingested red blood cells and increased pseudopod activity are the ones seen in bloody diarrheal stools. If tissue damage is slight and repair keeps pace with it, symptoms may be mild or absent. Thus, according to this theory, an explanation is available for the varied symptoms that may be present in intestinal amebiasis, from the asymptomatic carrier to the amebic dysentery patient. On the other hand, others maintain that the large race is always pathogenic, and tissue invasion, therefore, is always in progress, although repair may keep pace with damage. Support for this concept is afforded by the demonstration of lesions by sigmoidoscopy in many asymptomatic carriers. Lesions in these patients frequently differ only in degree from lesions seen in persons with clinical manifestations. The degree of tissue invasion and damage may vary, thus accounting for the varied degree of symptoms produced (Fig. 3-7). Most workers believe that the small race *E. hartmanni*, is nonpathogenic. Confusion is added to the picture by the report of the transformation, in culture, of one race to another.

In otherwise healthy individuals many infections may occur without symptoms or with only mild vague gastrointestinal disturbances attributable to a wide variety of causes. In others, slight nausea, abdominal discomfort, mild constipation alternating with mild diarrhea, or one without the other, may be present. When tissue invasion becomes more extensive, sharp abdominal pain may occur referable to the right lower quadrant and suggestive of appendicitis. Nausea and vomiting may be pronounced, and marked constipation with or without diarrhea may occur. Symptoms may increase until the amebic dysentery syndrome may be present, characterized by severe diarrhea with 10 to 20 or more bloody mucous stools a day and marked tenesmus. Severe dysen-

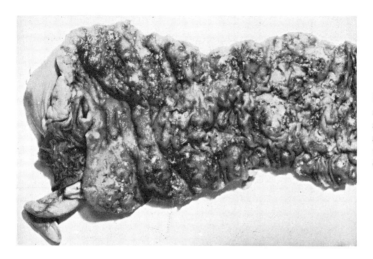

Fig. 3-7. Amebic colitis. Note the shaggy and irregular areas of ulceration. (From Anderson, W. A. D., and Scotti, T. M.: Synopsis of pathology, ed. 9, St. Louis, 1976, The C. V. Mosby Co.)

tery, unlike other forms of intestinal amebiasis, may be associated with fever and leukocytosis, suggestive of concomitant bacterial invasion. Extensive ulceration of the colon is present in these cases, frequently in the rectosigmoid area.

Variations in virulence of different strains of the organism and host susceptibility, influenced by temperate and intemperate habits, undoubtedly play significant roles in determining symptoms and the degree of tissue invasion. However, it must be kept in mind that the symptoms present in the patient may bear little or no relationship to the presence of E. histolytica in the stool and other causes for symptomatology must be considered.

The invasion of intact mucosa by trophozoites may pave the way for invasion of pathogenic bacteria such as the salmonellas or shigellas. Typhoid fever, for example, may be the dominant disease for consideration under such circumstances. An asymptomatic carrier may have blood in the stool and abdominal discomfort because of a carcinoma of the colon.

Pathology. Normal motility of the cecum, proper establishment of metabolic requirements, low oxygen tension, and adequate bacterial flora allow trophozoites to multiply and colonize in the glandular crypts, where

penetration of the mucosa occurs. Hypermotility will decrease the colonization and diminish the chances for penetration. Tiny pinpoint lesions occur at the site of entry. Electron microscopy reveals that the trophozoites cause contact-dependent lysis of epithelial cells and are chemotactic to neutrophils, the latter being killed on contact. Degranulation of the neutrophils, however, probably contributes to local tissue damage. The resulting endothelial damage leads to thrombosis of capillaries and venules in the lamina propria. The relation of virus particles found in E. histolytica to the virulence of the organism is, at present, uncertain. Multiple lesions characteristically show normal mucosa between sites of invasion (Fig. 3-8), a feature differentiating amebic dysentery from bacillary dysentery in which hyperemia is uniform throughout. Elevated necrotic lesions reveal active trophozoites. By means of their proteolytic enzymes the organisms, feeding on living cells, reach the muscular mucosa. Lesions may be confined to the mucosa with resultant resolution and repair. Proponents of the theory that E. histolytica is always invasive offer this in support of their concept. Penetration to the submucosa with lateral extension leads to the formation of the typical flask-shaped crateriform ulcers (Fig. 3-9) with shaggy, yellowish-brown

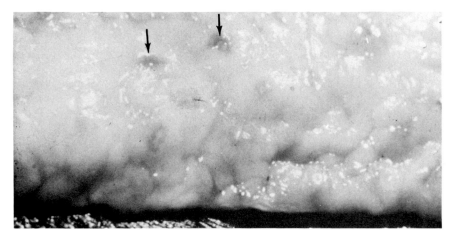

Fig. 3-8. Section of large intestine from patient with amebic dysentery. Arrows indicate "button-hole" lesions with normal mucosa between points of invasion. (Courtesy Dr. Rodolfo Céspedes, Department of Pathology, Hospital San Juan de Dios, San José, Costa Rica.)

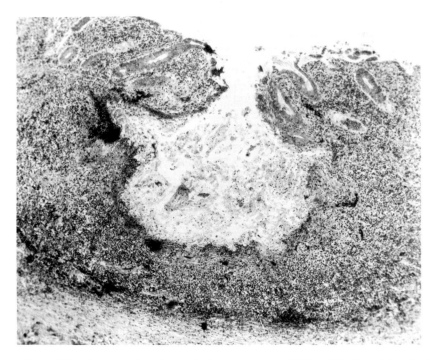

Fig. 3-9. Typical flask-shaped amebic ulcer in the large intestine. (AFIP N-44718. From Schmidt, G. D., and Roberts, L. S.: Foundations of parasitology, St. Louis, 1977, The C. V. Mosby Co.)

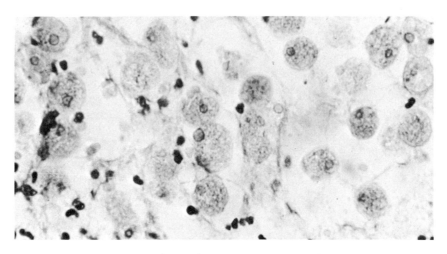

Fig. 3-10. Photomicrograph of *Entamoeba histolytica* trophozoites in rectal mucosa. (Courtesy Dr. James S. Magidson, Brookhaven Memorial Hospital, Patchogue, N.Y.)

edges and a floor formed by submucosa and muscular coats. Viewed from the surface such ulcers show normal mucosa between lesions although coalescing of the ulcers may cause an undermining and eventual sloughing of large areas of tissue and resultant sequelae. Initially there is very little inflammatory infiltration, but bacterial invasion from the intestine usually follows, resulting in leukocytic infiltration and further tissue destruction. Some studies suggest that living bacteria transfer an episomal virulence factor to the amebas after their ingestion. Granulation tissue eventually appears at the base of the ulcers. Invasion of the serosa may result in a fibrinous serositis. Further penetration in severe infections, although not common, may lead to perforation of the muscularis and serosa with peritonitis or the formation of adhesions in the area. Although lesions occur most commonly in the cecum, flexures of the colon, and rectosigmoid area, partly because of reduced peristalsis, any area of the large bowel may be involved. As indicated, early lesions show almost no cellular response, the process being mainly one of cell lysis. Regeneration rather than inflammation takes place and hyperemia and edema are usually

absent. Granulomatous lesions called amebomas may occur anywhere in the colon, simulating appendicitis when found in the cecum. Clinically they may suggest a carcinoma. When seen by sigmoidoscopy in the rectosigmoid area the lesions, which are relatively firm, nodular, and with a fibrous outer wall under the edematous mucosa, will reveal in the granulating zone eosinophils, lymphocytes, a few fibroblasts, and internal abscesses containing active trophozoites (Fig. 3-10). Infections of the skin and genitalia are being increasingly seen in reports from Uganda and Papua, New Guinea. Amebic infections of hemorrhoidectomy wounds may produce lesions resembling rectal carcinomas.

Through the use of hemagglutination and gel diffusion techniques, autoantibodies in the human colon have been demonstrated in the sera of numerous patients with fatal amebic colitis.

Diagnosis. The diagnosis of intestinal amebiasis depends on the demonstration of the etiologic agent *E. histolytica*. Trophozoites and cysts may be recovered and identified from the stool. The presence of Charcot-Leyden crystals in the stool, though not

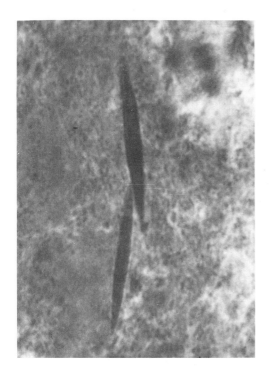

Fig. 3-11. Charcot-Leyden crystals in stool. Trichrome stain. (From a nonprofit cooperative endeavor by numerous colleagues under the editorship of Dr. Herman Zaiman, Valley City, N.D.)

pathognomonic, may be suggestive of infection (Fig. 3-11).

When trophozoites are observed and there is doubt about species, the use of a supravital stain, such as Quensel's or buffered methylene blue, may be very helpful. The nucleus is stained dark blue to black in 15 to 20 minutes in a wet mount and, in appearance, resembles the nuclei of an iron-hemotoxylin preparation, while the cytoplasm takes on a blue coloration. MIF (Merthiolate-iodine-formaldehyde) stain may also be employed. Fixation of the trophozoites and cysts by formalin occurs with staining by eosin and iodine. The nucleus of the trophozoite and cyst appears much as a nucleus with iodine alone, and the delicacy of the chromatin granules and the karyosome is readily discernible. The cytoplasm and background are stained pinkish with eosin.

Although trophozoites occur most commonly in soft, mushy, or watery stools, normal well-formed ones may, in passing down the rectum, scrape off trophic organisms from lesions in the mucosal wall. In such cases, trophozoites found in the bloody mucus patches on the stool surface may be the only evidence of an amebic infection.

Specimens left standing at room temperature will cause deterioration of the trophozoites. Microscopic examination should be made within the hour after passage. If a delay is inevitable, refrigeration (4° C) will hold the organisms for several hours; otherwise, part of the specimen may be placed in 5% formalin and part in polyvinyl alcohol (see Appendix A) for future examination. The prior treatment of the patient with such agents as barium, bismuth, kaolin compound, magnesium hydroxide, various oils, antibiotics, antiprotozoan drugs and hypertonic salt, and soap enemas interferes with the routine stool examination.

In amebic dysentery many trophozoites may show explosive pseudopod formation with marked differentiation between ectoplasm and endoplasm, sluglike forms with directional movement (galloping amebas), and ingested red blood cells. Diagnosis can be readily made from fresh specimens. Many stools show trophozoites not presenting these characteristics to a degree sufficient for positive identification. Trophozoites recovered by sigmoidoscopy may present the same problem of identification, enhanced by the fact that various motile tissue cells that can be mistaken for amebas, such as macrophages, may be present. When dysentery is present, the nature of the stool might be suggestive of the disease, since few pus cells, pyknotic bodies caused by cytolysis of cells, clumped red blood cells, and, sometimes, Charcot-Leyden crystals may be present. However, since bacterial invasion usually accompanies amebic invasion, this picture is rarely as clear as described. Cysts are more reliable for identification purposes, and with careful search they can usually be found. Since young cysts frequently contain a diffuse glycogen mass and unorganized chromatoidal material, obscuring of the nucleus or confusion with dividing nuclei may occur. Such cysts in saline solution present little of diagnostic value. The presence of refractile masses, however, might lead one to be suspicious of *E. histolytica*. When stained with iodine, young cysts may be easily identified.

As the cysts mature, nuclear division continues, until quadrinucleated cysts are produced. The glycogen becomes less pronounced and the chromatoidal material becomes organized into bars with rounded or squared ends. Over 50% of the cysts will show this diagnostic feature. In saline these bars appear as light refractile masses and aid materially in identification. Care must be taken to avoid confusing bars standing on end with nuclei. When stained with iodine, these bars are less visible as refractile masses in the stained cytoplasm. The mature, quadrinucleated cysts without bars can be differentiated from similar quadrinucleated cysts of *E. coli* by the delicacy of the chromatin granules and karyosome in the nuclei, as well as the tendency of the cyst to be smaller in size. When stained with MIF, nuclear and chromatoidal structures appear much as with iodine alone, and identification follows much the same pattern. When permanent records are desired or trouble is experienced in identification with the various wet-mount stains, iron-hematoxylin-, trichrome-, or chlorazol back E-stained slides should be made. One can then clearly distinguish *E. histolytica* from inflammatory cells, macrophages, and other amebas.

It is difficult to say how many stool examinations should be made before a patient is declared free of the disease. Much depends on the circumstances surrounding the case, such as history, laboratory facilities available, and, not the least consideration, the financial status of the patient. It should be remembered that the cysts fluctuate in numbers and are more abundant at one time than another. This fluctuation is cyclic and usually occurs every 1 or 2 weeks. Patients who are not seemingly ill cannot be retained in the hospital solely for stool examinations. When treated as outpatients, they may lose interest in returning repeatedly for the same purpose over long periods of time. Good judgment must be exercised by the physician in attendance in determining how many and how frequently stool examinations should be made. In most cases, examination of three normally passed stools on alternate days, followed by examination of a purged specimen, if still negative, will yield the diagnosis. However, no limit can be set on the number of stools to be examined—the more the better. If these techniques fail and there is a high index of suspicion of intestinal amebiasis, sigmoidoscopic specimens, rectal biopsy, or both are very helpful.

The sensitivity of the various serologic tests varies with the type of infection. Sera from patients with acute amebic dysentery show higher sensitivity than do sera from asymptomatic carriers. When the indirect hemagglutination (IHA) test is used, reports show 85% to 98% positive indications of acute amebic dysentery. The diagnosis of the asymptomatic carrier is quite variable and appears to be dependent on the geographic area from which the sample is taken. According to Kagan and Norman, the IHA test was positive in 2% to 6% of noninfected controls and in hospitalized patients with bacillary dysentery and other diseases, while other areas showed reactors up to 44%. The indirect fluorescent antibody (IFA) test appears to be almost as sensitive as the IHA test, but specificity varies. Gel diffusion and IHA seem to agree fairly well. IHA titers of 1:128 (see Tables 15-1 and 15-2) are considered significant by the Center for Disease Control diagnostic laboratory.

Treatment. The treatment of intestinal amebiasis is dependent on the general health of the patient. Asymptomatic carriers are treated differently than patients with a mild to moderate disease, while severe intestinal amebiasis may require even more intense therapy. The drugs of choice and alternatives, the adult and pediatric dosages, and the adverse effects of these drugs are given in Table 3-2. As indicated in Table 3-2, the toxic effects on the heart necessitate electrocardiographic monitoring and bed rest for patients receiving emetine. Tachycardia, arrhythmia, marked weakness, dyspnea on exertion, diarrhea, and vomiting are signs of emetine toxicity. Emetine has a cumulative action, with asthenia, emaciation, mental depression, and cardiac irregularity occurring. Desquamation of the skin and an atropic brittle condition of the nails frequently follow.

E. histolytica and enteropathogenic bacteria are frequently regarded as the chief cause of diarrhea or dysentery among travelers in the tropics, no doubt partly because of the highly publicized prevalence in these areas. This has led to some degree in the promulgation of the use of chemotherapeutic drugs among travelers often without medical supervision. One such drug, iodochlorhydroxyquin (clioquinal), marketed under the name Entero-Vioform or in a combination product called Mexaform, has shown indications of inducing a syndrome of a subacute myelo-optic neuropathy (SMON), characterized by sensory and motor disturbances of the extremities and visual disturbances including optic atrophy. The Australian Drug Evaluation Committee has recommended that clioquinal and related halogenated hydroxyquinolines should, at least for the time being, be available only by prescription by a physician.

Caution in the use of such drugs prophylactically is further indicated by the report that many diarrheas of travelers are frequently associated with changes in drinking water and resultant changes in osmotic pressures in the gut as well as bacterial infections.

Cure can be ascertained only by repetitive stool examinations for at least 6 months after treatment. Patients who have had successfully treated amebiasis may have recurrent diarrhea, presumably attributable to residual colon damage, and should not be needlessly subjected to repeated therapy for amebiasis unless the stool examination demonstrates the presence of E. histolytica. In endemic areas reinfection makes evaluation of therapy difficult.

Extraintestinal amebiasis

Symptomatology. Invasion of the bloodstream and lymphatics following erosion of the intestinal mucosa results in the transportation of the trophozoites via the portal system to the liver. Extraintestinal amebiasis may occur in the absence of any past history of symptomatic intestinal infection. Cutaneous amebiasis, resulting from an extension of infection from the colon or hepatic tissues to the genital, abdominal, and perianal regions, has been reported. A rare incidence of cutaneous amebiasis of the eyelid with extension into the orbit caused by E. histolytica is recorded. Morphologically the amebas could not be mistaken for the free-living limax Acanthamoeba polyphaga, which has also been reported from the eye. Abscess formation has been reported in the brain, kidneys, lungs, and other parts of the body. Infection by metastasis may develop anywhere in the body. Pericardial infection, a life-threatening complication, is rare, but when present is usually associated with an abscess of the left lobe of the liver. Though the trophozoites may establish foci of infections in various organs of the body, most commonly they remain in the liver where they become established in the lobules with necrosis of capillaries and parenchymal tissue. Initially the patient remains asymptomatic, the blood count remains normal, and liver function tests remain negative; later symptoms of pain, fever, chills, and sweating develop. The liver usually becomes enlarged and tender. A moderate leukocytosis

Table 3-2. Treatment for amebiasis caused by *Entamoeba histolytica*

Infection	Drug	Adult dose*	Pediatric dose*
Asymptomatic			
Drug of choice	Diiodohydroxyquin[1]	650 mg tid × 20d	30-40 mg/kg/d in 3 doses × 20d (max. 2 gm/d)
Alternatives	Diloxanide furoate[2]	500 mg tid × 10d	20 mg/kg/d in 3 doses × 10d
	OR		
	Paromomycin	25-30 mg/kg/d in 3 doses × 5-10d	25-30 mg/kg/d in 3 doses × 5-10d
Mild to moderate intestinal disease			
Drug of choice	Metronidazole[3] *plus*	750 mg tid × 5-10d	35-50 mg/kg/d in 3 doses × 10d
	diiodohydroxyquin[1]	650 mg tid × 20d	30-40 mg/kg/d in 3 doses × 20d (max. 2 gm/d)
Alternative	Paromomycin	25-30 mg/kg/d in 3 doses × 5-10d	25-30 mg/kg/d in 3 doses × 5-10d
Severe intestinal disease			
Drug of choice	Metronidazole[3,4] *plus*	750 mg tid × 5-10d	35-50 mg/kg/d in 3 doses × 10d
	diiodohydroxyquin[1]	650 mg tid × 20d	30-40 mg/kg/d in 3 doses × 20d (max. 2 gm/d)
Alternatives	Dehydroemetine[2,5] *plus*	1 to 1.5 mg/kg/d (max. 90 mg/d) for up to 5d	1 to 1.5 mg/kg/d (max. 90 mg/d) in 2 doses for up to 5 d
	diiodohydroxyquin[1]	650 mg tid × 20d	30-40 mg/kg/d in 3 doses × 20d (max. 2 gm/d)
	OR		
	Emetine[5] *plus*	1 mg/kg/d (max. 60 mg/d) for up to 5d	1 mg/kg/d in 2 doses (max. 60 mg/d) for up to 5d
	diiodohydroxyquin[1]	650 mg tid × 20d	30-40 mg/kg/d in 3 doses × 20d (max. 2 gm/d)
Hepatic abscess			
Drug of choice	Metronidazole[3,4] *plus*	750 mg tid × 5-10d	35-50 mg/kg/d in 3 doses × 10d
	diiodohydroxyquin[1]	650 mg tid × 20d	30-40 mg/kg/d in 3 doses × 20d (max. 2 gm/d)
Alternatives	Dehydroemetine[2,5]	1 to 1.5 mg/kg/d (max. 90 mg/d) for up to 5d	1 to 1.5 mg/kg/d (max. 90 mg/d) in 2 doses for up to 5d
	followed by chloroquine phosphate	1 gm (600 mg base) daily × 2d then 500 mg (300 mg base) daily × 2-3 wk	10 mg base/kg/d × 21d (max. 300 mg base/d)
	plus diiodohydroxyquin[1]	650 mg tid × 20d	30-40 mg/kg/d in 3 doses × 20d (max. 2 gm/d)
	OR		
	Emetine[5]	1 mg/kg/d (max. 60 mg/d) for up to 5d	1 mg/kg/d in 2 doses (max. 60 mg/d) for up to 5d
	followed by chloroquine phosphate	1 gm (600 mg base) daily × 2d then 500 mg (300 mg base) daily × 2-3 wk	10 mg base/kg/d × 21d (max. 300 mg base/d)
	plus diiodohydroxyquin[1]	650 mg tid × 20d	30-40 mg/kg/d in 3 doses × 20d (max. 2 gm/d)

*See opposite page.

Table 3-2. Treatment for amebiasis caused by *Entamoeba histolytica* —cont'd

Adverse effects of antiparasitic drugs

Diiodohydroxyquin USP
  Occasional: rash; acne; slight enlargement of the thyroid gland; nausea; diarrhea; cramps; anal pruritus
  Rare: optic atrophy and loss of vision in children after prolonged use in high dosage for months
Diloxanide furoate (Furamide)
  Frequent: flatulence
  Occasional: nausea; vomiting; diarrhea; urticaria; pruritus
Metronidazole (Flagyl)
  Frequent: nausea; headache; metallic taste
  Occasional: vomiting; diarrhea; insomnia; weakness; stomatitis; vertigo; paresthesia; rash; dark urine; dry mouth
  Rare: ataxia; depression; irritability; confusion; mild Antabuse-like reaction with alcohol
Paromomycin (Humatin)
  Frequent: GI disturbance
  Rare: eighth-nerve damage (mainly auditory); renal damage
Dehydroemetine—Similar to emetine, but possibly less severe
Emetine HCl USP
  Frequent: cardiac arrhythmias; precordial pain; muscle weakness; cellulitis at site of injection
  Occasional: diarrhea; vomiting; peripheral neuropathy; heart failure
Chloroquine HCl and Chloroquine phosphate USP (Aralen; and others)
  Occasional: pruritus; vomiting; headache; confusion; depigmentation of hair; skin eruptions; hemolysis especially
    with G6PD deficiency; corneal opacity; irreversible retinal injury (especially when total dosage exceeds 100
    grams); weight loss; partial alopecia; extraocular muscle palsies; exacerbation of psoriasis, eczema and other ex-
    foliative dermatitis
  Rare: discoloration of nails and mucous membranes of mouth; nerve-type deafness; blood dyscrasias; photophobia

From The Medical Letter, Inc., 56 Harrison Street, New Rochelle, N.Y.
*The letter d indicates day.
1. Dosage and duration of administration should not be exceeded because of possibility of causing optic neuritis. Available from Panray Division, Ormont Drug and Chemical, 520 South Dean Street, Englewood, New Jersey 07631
   and from Glenwood Laboratories, Inc., 83 North Summit Street, Tenafly, New Jersey 07670. Alternatives to
   diiodohydroxyquin in amebiasis are paromomycin or diloxanide furoate in the same dosage recommended for asymptomatic amebiasis.
2. In the U.S.A., this drug is available from the Parasitic Diseases Division, Center for Disease Control, Atlanta,
   Georgia 30333; telephone 404-329-3311.
3. Metronidazole is carcinogenic in rodents and mutagenic in bacteria; it should generally not be used in pregnant
   women, particularly in the first trimester.
4. An occasional treatment failure has been reported when metronidazole has been used alone for the treatment
   of liver abscess or intestinal infection.
5. Because of the toxic effects on the heart, patients receiving emetine should have electrocardiographic monitoring
   and should remain sedentary during therapy. Dehydroemetine is probably as effective and probably less toxic
   than emetine.

may occur. Chills and fever may raise a suspicion of malaria. Abscess formation frequently follows, most commonly in the right
lobe. In most instances, a large, single abscess is formed, though after amebic dysentery, multiple abscesses seem more common. Pain is often referable to the upper
right quadrant. Direct extension through the
diaphragm may occur, followed by amebic
pneumonitis, with symptoms similar to those

seen in liver infections, plus a cough. If a
pulmonary abscess ruptures through a bronchus, the sputum may contain an anchovy-
sauce-like exudate containing trophozoites.
Other foci of infections, though rare, may
occur in almost any organ of the body, producing symptoms referable to the area in
question.

Pathology. Some patients with a present
and past history of intestinal amebiasis have

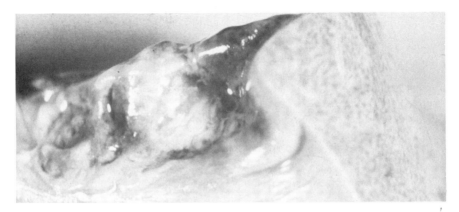

Fig. 3-12. Partial section of right upper quadrant of liver showing an amebic abscess. (Courtesy Dr. Rodolfo Céspedes, Department of Pathology, Hospital San Juna de Dios, San José, Costa Rica.)

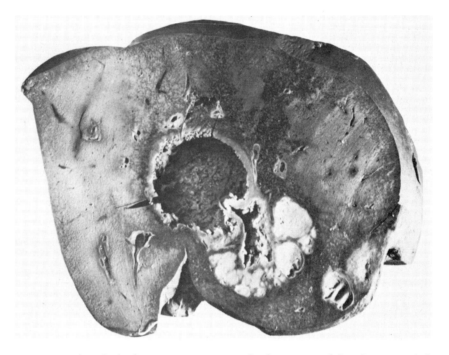

Fig. 3-13. Liver with multiple abscesses. Necrotic tissue has been removed from large central abscess. (AFIP 58-4839-2.)

an enlarged tender liver, abnormal liver function tests, and an increased sedimentation rate. Studies for abscess may be negative, liver biopsy does not reveal amebas, and treatment for intestinal but not hepatic amebiasis results in resolution of hepatic findings; therefore the diagnosis of "amebic hepatitis" is believed by most workers to be the result of toxic products from the intestinal tract rather than actual amebic invasion. It is interesting that there is little pathologic evidence for a clinical stage of liver disease

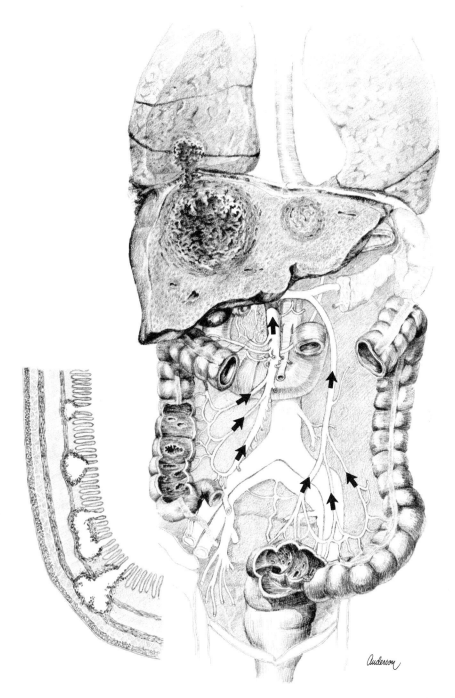

Fig. 3-14. Major pathology of amebiasis. Invasion of the intestinal mucosa occurs most commonly in the cecum and next most commonly in the rectosigmoid area. Passage of trophozoites via the portal circulation may result in liver abscess formation. Metastasis through the diaphragm may result in secondary abscess formation in the lungs. Trophozoites carried in the bloodstream may cause foci of infection anywhere in the body.

prior to abscess formation. Abscess formation is associated primarily with active intestinal invasion and comes about because of destruction of parenchymal tissue by cytolysis. Thrombi in the interlobular veins produced by the amebas lead to lysis and necrosis with passage of the parasites to the periportal sinusoids and thence to the parenchymal tissues of the liver. Possibly, multiple foci with no inflammatory reaction appear first, later coalescing to form the true abscess accompanied by infiltration of leukocytes and fibroblasts. In chronic lesions a fibrous wall rarely develops. Because of the minimal cellular response around an amebic abscess, healing after therapy is usually complete and no pathologic evidence of an old abscess is seen (Fig. 3-12).

Invasion of the liver results in eventual destruction of parenchymal tissue by cytolysis. (Fig. 3-13). The trophozoites live in the border of the forming abscess, destroy the living tissue, and leave a necrotic mass of lysed liver cells. This viscid material or "pus," often described as resembling anchovy sauce, is chocolate brown to red-orange in color and contains relatively few amebas (Fig. 3-14). The detection of autoantibodies against normal human liver in the sera of patients with high titers to *E. histolytica*, as shown by the indirect hemagglutination (IHA) test, and with clinically proven amebic abscess suggests that, in addition to damage from the parasite itself, immunologic damage could result from the attachment of circulating antigen to the cell surface of host tissues such as the liver.

Diagnosis. Although the diagnosis of extraintestinal amebiasis depends heavily on the clinical evidence, the sensitivity of the serological tests (Tables 15-1 and 15-2) is very high. The indirect fluorescent antibody (IFA) test and the IHA test appear almost equally sensitive, but reports vary on the specificity of the IFA. IHA titers of 1:128 are considered significant by the Center for Disease Control diagnostic laboratory More than

90% of proved cases are positive while more than 75% of intestinal infections are positive with the IHA test.

Abscesses of the liver may be aspirated and the exudate examined for trophozoites. Since the organisms have a predilection for living tissue, they are seldom found in the necrotic process, unless the most peripheral part of the aspirate (last obtained) is examined. If feasible, scrapings of the abscess wall should be made and examined for the amebas. The technique for recovery of organisms from the exudate is given in Chapter 15. A bacteriologically sterile liver abscess in a patient who has not received antibiotics is very suggestive of amebiasis.

Doming and fixation of the diaphragm on the right side, as seen by x-ray film, are highly suggestive of a liver abscess. Pleural effusion may be observed and is said to be more common than in pyogenic abscesses of the liver. A liver scan might help in determining the location of the abscess, although a normal picture does not rule out its presence (Fig. 3-15).

The accidental discovery of a hepatic amebic abscess through the use of a nephrotomogram and an intravenous infusion of sodium diatrizoate (Hypaque) on a patient with a suspected abnormal right kidney affords another procedure for diagnosis. Ultrasound reveals liver abscesses with a hollow cavity, often with scattered internal echoes. Arteriography, a more intensive procedure, usually shows an avascular mass with distortion of the normal vascular architecture.

The finding of the organisms in the stool at this time, or the confirmation of a previous intestinal infection, may add further support to the signs and symptoms mentioned, along with the radiologic evidence present, but at least half of the patients with extraintestinal amebiasis have no concurrent intestinal infection.

The ultimate diagnosis rests on a critical evaluation of all signs and symptoms present, along with the laboratory data available.

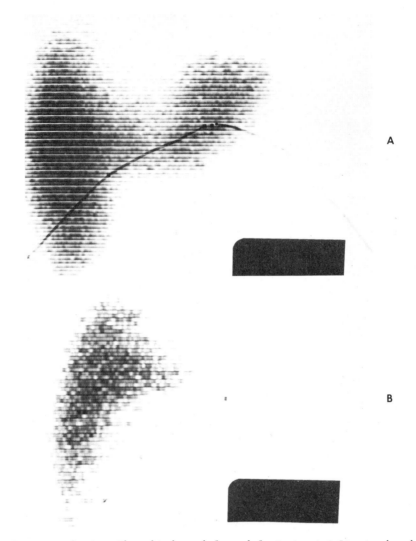

Fig. 3-15. Liver scans of patient with amebic abscess before and after treatment. **A,** Liver is enlarged, extending toward the left and inferiorly below the rib cage outlined by a black line. Note the large filling defect in the superior middle portion of the liver. **B,** Several months after treatment liver has returned to normal size with filling defect no longer visible. (Courtesy Department of Nuclear Medicine, University of Miami, School of Medicine.)

Proof of an infection with *E. histolytica* requires either aspiration of the liver abscess, a technique neither as dangerous nor as formidable as expounded in the American literature on this subject, discussed later, or serologic tests.

Treatment. Metronidazole (Flagyl) plus diiodohydroxyquin are the drugs of choice for extraintestinal amebiasis as indicated in Table 3-2 under hepatic abscess. Alternative drugs and adverse effects of antiamebic drugs are also listed.

Because a percentage of amebic liver abscesses are secondarily infected, some physicians recommend antibiotics also. It is important to note that the use of metronidazole has in no way altered the indications for aspiration of a liver abscess and that failure to

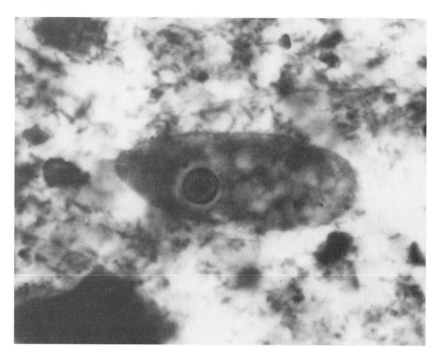

Fig. 3-16. *Entamoeba coli* trophozoite. Note the large eccentric karyosome. (From a nonprofit cooperative endeavor of numerous colleagues under the editorship of Dr. Herman Zaiman, Valley City, N.D.)

aspirate some abscesses may result in relapses no matter what drugs are used. Reports indicate that the best results with metronidazole have been obtained in those institutions where therapeutic aspiration is frequently practiced. The cardiac toxicity of emetine or dehydroemetine, as indicated, requires ECG monitoring and bed rest for the patient during therapy. Dehydroemetine is available in the United States from the Parasitic Disease Drug Service of the Center for Disease Control, Atlanta, Georgia.

Most patients with extraintestinal amebiasis improve within 7 days of treatment. Failure to respond usually reflects the necessity for drainage. Evacuation of pus from a liver abscess usually results in a dramatic decrease in fever, pain, and leukocytosis. Under local anesthesia a large-bore needle is inserted over the area of fluctuance, maximum tenderness, or defect demonstrated on liver scan, or, lacking any of these, in the anterior axillary line in the eighth or ninth

interspace. Pus should be aspirated into serial containers and the last one examined for trophozoites, which are most likely to be detected at the edges of the abscess. A single dose of emetine or metronidazole prior to aspiration is said to reduce the danger of any leakage of the abscess material. Recurrence of symptoms after aspiration and while the patient is on therapy may indicate a need for reaspiration. Abscesses of the left lobe and those that do not respond to appropriate drugs and cannot be reached by closed aspiration should be drained surgically.

Entamoeba coli

Like *E. histolytica*, *Entamoeba coli* also has two stages in its life cycle, the trophozoite and the cyst. It is similar in almost all other respects, except morphology and the fact that it does not invade tissue and thus is nonpathogenic. Trophozoites (Fig. 3-16) vary from 12 to 30 μm in diameter and are usually larger than the vegetating forms of *E.*

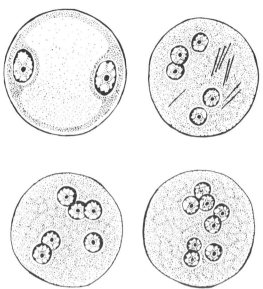

Fig. 3-18. *Entamoeba coli* cysts. Note the glycogen mass, splintered sticklike chromatoidal bars, and typical nuclei, up to eight in number.

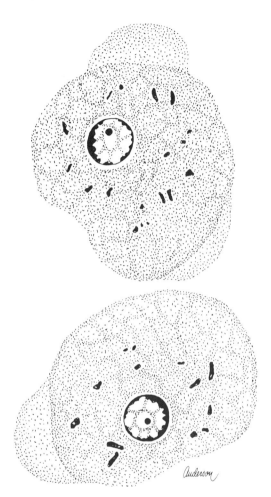

Fig. 3-17. *Entamoeba coli* trophozoites, Note the broad, blunt pseudopodia, typical nucleus, and ingested bacteria.

histolytica, although, as indicated, there is a marked overlapping in size. In fresh stools they move by short, blunt, broad pseudopodia, seldom show progressive, directional movement, and are very sluggish in their activity. They do not normally ingest red blood cells, and differentiation between the ectoplasm and endoplasm can be made only with difficulty. It is important to remember, however, that the more aggressive organisms may sometimes be mistaken for *E. histolytica* and that the latter organism, particularly when left standing in a stool for some time

before examination, can seldom be differentiated from any of the amebas. The cytoplasm of *E. coli* usually presents a "dirty" appearance, caused by the abundance of ingested bacteria, fungi, and other food particles (Fig. 3-17). The nucleus may be visible in saline solution and appears as a grayish to black ring. When stained with Quensel's, buffered methylene blue, MIF, iron-hematoxylin, or trichrome, the thick, coarse, nuclear membrane with dense, coarse, irregular-sized, coalescing chromatin granules on the inner surface can be seen. The karyosome appears coarse, thick, and usually eccentrically located.

Cysts, such as those of *E. histolytica*, are more reliable for identification and can usually be found in the stool. Young cysts appear first, most commonly as binucleated organisms with a large, well-defined glycogen mass centrally located and often displacing the nuclei to each side. The nuclei, except for being smaller, are similar in morphology to those seen in the trophozoite stage. They

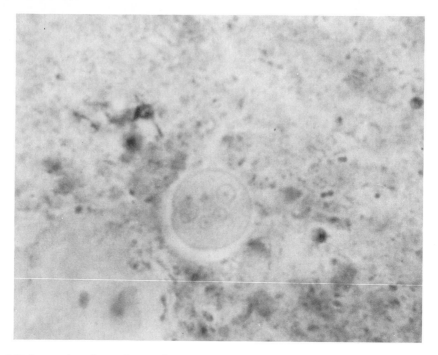

Fig. 3-19. *Entamoeba coli* cyst showing five nuclei in the plane of focus. (From a nonprofit cooperative endeavor of numerous colleagues under the editorship of Dr. Herman Zaiman, Valley City, N.D.)

divide rapidly and, in maturing cysts, up to eight nuclei can be seen (Fig. 3-18). Chromatoidal material may be present, first unorganized, but later becoming differentiated into bars with splinterlike ends. Though present in less than 10% of the cysts, when they are seen, they are diagnostic of *E. coli*. Like *E. histolytica*, the cysts (Fig. 3-19) are predominately spherical, although aberrant shapes may be seen. In diameter they average 18 μm and display a much thicker cyst wall than do those of *E. histolytica*.

Entamoeba polecki

Entamoeba polecki is a very rare intestinal ameba of humans that, when present, may be confused with *E. histolytica*. About 20 cases in humans have been reported in the literature. It was first reported in pigs and monkeys. Both trophozoites and cysts occur in the life cycle.

Trophozoites range in diameter from 10 to 25 μm. Their motility resembles that of *E.*

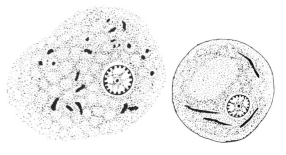

Fig. 3-20. *Entamoeba polecki* trophozoite and cyst. Note the angular tapering chromatoidal bars and inclusion mass in cyst.

coli in normal stools, but with diarrhea they may show more activity, thus resembling the activity of *E. histolytica*. The cytoplasm is "dirty" and contains ingested bacteria, yeast, and other food particles. In stained smears the nucleus often resembles that of *E. histolytica*. Vacuolation of the cytoplasm, unlike that of the other amebas in humans, is common (Fig. 3-20).

Cysts, varying from 10 to 18 μm in di-

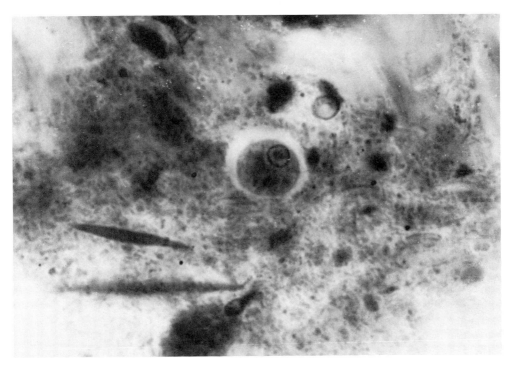

Fig. 3-21. *Entamoeba polecki* cyst showing angular chromatoidal bars. Note presence of Charcot-Leyden crystals in the stool specimen. (Courtesy of G. T. Strickland.)

ameter, remain uninucleated. Glycogen, though occasionally seen as a single mass, usually appears in several smaller masses and is diffuse in appearance when stained with iodine. Chromatoidal bars, unlike those of *E. histolytica*, which are rounded or squared, appear with angular, (Fig. 3-21) tapering to pointed ends. Approximately half the cysts present show an inclusion mass that is oval to round and that stains less distinctly with iron-hematoxylin than does chromatoidal material. Little is known about this ameba, but it is generally believed to be nonpathogenic. However, two symptomatic cases have been recorded. Intermittent bouts of abdominal cramps, nausea, diarrhea, and malaise have been noted with numerous cysts present in the feces. Successful therapy was reported in one case in which a 10-day course of 750 mg of metronidazole was given three times a day, followed by 10 days of 500 mg of diloxamide three times daily.

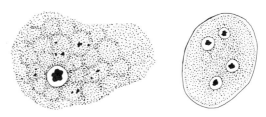

Fig. 3-22. *Endolimax nana* trophozoite and cyst. Note the large karyosome and absence of chromatin granules on nuclear membrane.

Endolimax nana

Endolimax nana, likewise, has a trophozoite and a cyst stage in its life cycle. It is nonpathogenic and in all essential aspects is like the other nonpathogenic amebas. The trophozoites are small, averaging 6 to 12 μm in diameter, and sometimes fall within the size range of small trophozoites of *E. histolytica*. In most respects they are similar to those of *E. coli*. The nucleus usually is invisible in saline solution. When stained, the nuclear membrane, intermediate between that of *E. histolytica* and *E. coli*, shows no chromatin granules present. The karyosome is large and may be centrally or eccentrically located. Sometimes the mass may be divided into two parts (Fig. 3-22).

Cysts are more reliable for identification and appear in the stool in predominantly oval forms. Nuclei, as described, may be one to four (Fig. 3-23) in number, but quadrinucleated cysts are most common. Glycogen is rarely discernible and no chromatoidal material of diagnostic value can be seen. The nuclei, when stained with iodine, usually appear as distinct dots surrounded by a halo or clear zone. The nuclear membrane, since it contains no chromatin granules, is rarely seen, except when stained with iron-hematoxylin, trichrome, or other permanent stains. After zinc sulfate flotation, cysts may often show a characteristic indentation at one end.

Iodamoeba bütschlii

Iodamoeba bütschlii is a nonpathogen and also has a trophozoite and a cyst stage in its life cycle. Its life history is similar to the other nonpathogenic amebas in humans. Trophozoites, not commonly seen in stools, average 6 to 12 μm in diameter. They resemble those of *E. coli* in many respects. The nucleus, usually invisible in saline, when stained gives an appearance quite similar to the nucleus of *E. nana*. It differs only in that the large karyosome is surrounded by achromatic granules. One or more glycogen masses are usually present and are detectable with iodine (Fig. 3-24).

Cysts, which appear more commonly than trophozoites in the stool, average about 10 μm in diameter. They are typically varied in

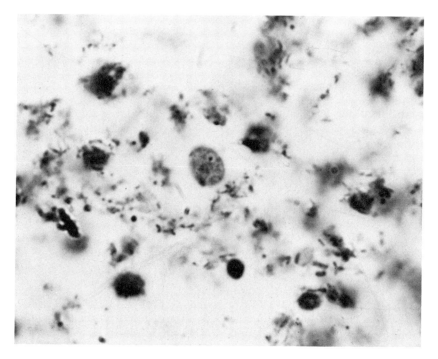

Fig. 3-23. *Endolimax nana* cyst showing typical nuclei. (From a nonprofit cooperative endeavor of numerous colleagues under the editorship of Dr. Herman Zaiman, Valley City, N.D.)

shape—round, oval, elliptical, or rhomboidal. The inconsistency in shape from organism to organism becomes very helpful in identification when they are seen in the microscopic field. The well-defined glycogen mass (Fig. 3-25) persists throughout the life of the cyst and is characteristic of this organism. It is readily discernible with iodine stain, hence the name *Iodamoeba*. Care must be taken, however, to avoid confusion with young cysts of other amebas, particularly those of *E. coli* and possibly *E. histolytica*, both of which may have glycogen masses stainable with iodine. Size, shape, and nuclear differences will aid in the differentiation. The nucleus of *Iodamoeba bütschlii* does not undergo division and differs only from that in the trophozoite stage by a displacement of the karyosome to the periphery with the achromatic granules at one end of

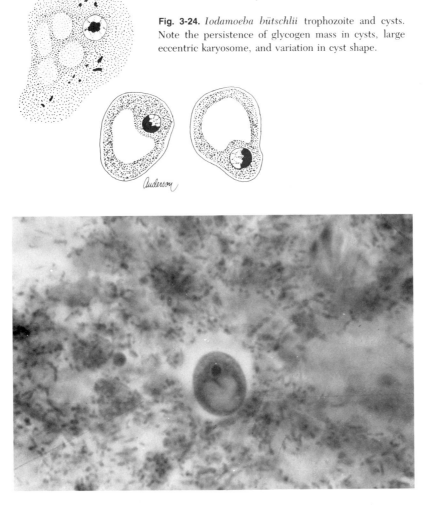

Fig. 3-24. *Iodamoeba bütschlii* trophozoite and cysts. Note the persistence of glycogen mass in cysts, large eccentric karyosome, and variation in cyst shape.

Fig. 3-25. *Iodamoeba bütschlii* cyst. Note the large glycogen mass vacuole. (Photograph by James Jensen. From Schmidt, G. D., and Roberts, L. S.: Foundations of parasitology, St. Louis, 1977, The C. V. Mosby Co.)

the karyosome, like the handle of a basket. No chromatoidal material of diagnostic significance is present.

Other pathogenic amebas

Although *E. histolytica* had been considered to be the only ameba that normally invades tissue and causes infection in humans, exceptions are noted in the literature. A single case of a fatal systemic infection caused by an ameba morphologically resembling *I. bütschlii* was reported in a debilitated Japanese prisoner of World War II. Autopsy revealed dissemination of the trophozoites in extraintestinal lesions, such as in the lungs and brain. In the light of the more recent discoveries of a number of cases of fatal meningoencephalitis caused by the free-living ameba *Naegleria fowleri*, one may raise doubts about the identification of the ameba in this case.

The family Dimastigamoebidae is composed of free-living organisms inhabiting the soil and water. Feeding chiefly on fecal bacteria, they are coprophilic and are found living mainly in stagnant water, sewage systems, and polluted soil. Affiliation with the Mastigophora is reflected in the presence of a flagellate stage as well as the ameboid forms. The free-living organisms are commonly referred to as "limax" (Latin meaning slug or snail) amebas because of their sluglike form and movement. Some workers classify two families on the basis of the type of nuclear division, Vahlkampfiidae and Hartmanellidae. Adaptation of some species to vertebrates, including man, has occurred. The first human infection was observed in Australia in 1961, followed 18 months later by a case in Florida. The first publication appeared in 1965. Butt (1966), in describing the Floridian case, coined the term "primary amebic meningoencephalitis," the name by which the disease is generally known. The consensus of opinion is that the organism involved is *N. fowleri* (Vahlkampfiidae) and

that previous reports in the literature of other species are in error or highly questionable. Reports of the Hartmanellid organisms (*Hartmanella* and *Acanthamoeba*) as caustive agents of primary amebic meningoencephalitis in man have, for the most part, been discredited, but there is one report of a brain granuloma in which amebas were identified as *Acanthamoeba*. No mention, however, was made of finding cyst forms in the tissues, a diagnostic feature of *Acanthamoeba* and the accuracy of identification is questionable to some.

The Hartmanellid amebas, however, should not be dismissed lightly since they do cause severe disease in animals, can be grown in vitro on human tissue, and have often been isolated from the nasopharynx of persons with upper respiratory tract infections. Cases of *Acanthamoeba* ulceration of the cornea of the eye leading to blindness have been reported, substantiated by the demonstration of cyst forms in histologic sections. Several differences between *Naegleria* and *Acanthamoeba* can be noted. *N. fowleri* does not form cysts in tissues, does not respond to sulfadiazine therapy, and does not produce thornlike projections (acanthopodia), all features characteristic of *Acanthomoeba*.

Immunodiagnosis of *Acanthamoeba* is difficult. However, immunofluorescence and immunoenzymatic tests have confirmed the *Hartmanella* and *Acanthamoeba* species in brain tissue from a typical case. Positive tissue staining has been reported by some using the indirect fluorescent antibody (IFA) test. A two-and-a-half-year-old boy from El Paso, Texas, with no history of swimming or wading in ponds, puddles, or lakes, or of traveling outside the United States, succumbed to amebic meningoencephalitis. Brain biopsy revealed trophozoites suggestive of *Acanthamoeba*, but negative to immunodiagnosis, and unsuccessful in being cultured. No cyst forms were noted.

Primary amebic meningoencephalitis

N. fowleri is a free-living limax ameba, ubiquitous in nature, and found in fresh-water lakes and ponds. It occurs also in brackish waters. The elongated flagellate has two long flagella and does not form pseudo-podia, while the ameboid form (trophozoite) develops blunt pseudopodia. Only trophozoites are found in human infections, the cyst stage with its single nucleus appearing only in nature. Human infections occur primarily in the warmer climates of the world, mainly during the summer months of the year. Clinical manifestations usually appear about a week after the patient has been swimming in a warm, fresh, or brackish body of water. More than 80 cases from around the world have been reported in the literature, 35 of which have occurred in the United States. None of those in the United States have been associated with man-made swimming pools. The widespread practice of swimming in ponds and lakes attests to the rarity of this disease. Seven confirmed cases and one suspected case (all fatal) were reported to the Center for Disease Control from four states and Puerto Rico in August 1980.

It is believed that entry occurs through the nasal mucosa (Fig. 3-26) overlying the cribriform plate. The usual presentation of symptoms has been the sudden appearance of headache and mild fever, sometimes associated with a sore throat and nasal infection. Symptoms increase rapidly during the following three days, with vomiting and neck rigidity. Before the end of the week the patient becomes disoriented or even comatose, and a presumptive diagnosis of acute pyogenic meningitis can be made. Lumbar puncture usually will reveal a purulent spinal fluid under increased pressure. Cardiorespiratory failure usually follows quickly, and then death. A feature of significant importance is the failure to find pathogenic bacteria (assuming no antibiotic therapy has yet been initiated) as would be expected in a purulent spinal fluid. The simple procedure of microscopically examining a wet mount of the well-mixed spinal fluid (avoid centrifugation or refrigeration) will usually reveal the trophozoites. The organisms will grow on plain agar seeded with *Escherichia coli* at temperatures between 21° C and 37° C. Maximum proliferation occurs at 37° C. The typical limax movement and shape can be readily detected. The absence of thorn-like pseudopodia so characteristic of *Acanthamoeba* will be obvious. Stained smear may be made as for any ameba trophozoite (see Appendix A) and nuclear detail can be studied.

The pathology of the disease has been well described by Carter in his study of nine Australian cases and substantiated by others. The

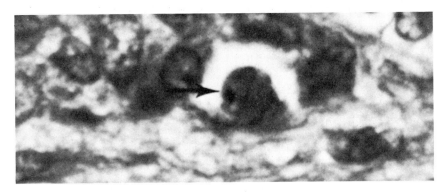

Fig. 3-26. *Naegleria (arrow)* within the nonmyelinated nerve fibers of the olfactory submucosa. (AFIP 75-7092-4.)

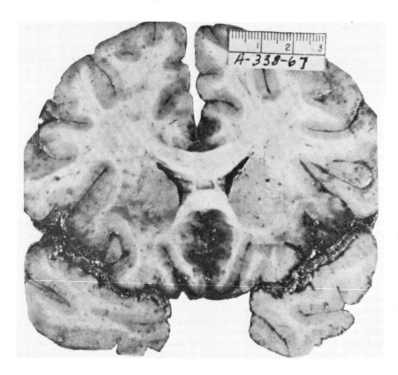

Fig. 3-27. Coronal section of brain showing hemorrhagic necrosis from *Naegleria* rhinomeningoencephalitis. (AFIP 75-7092.)

brain shows moderate swelling with the meninges diffusely hyperemic. Except over the sulci and in the basal subarachnoid cisterns there is no evidence of a purulent exudate. Slight focal hemorrhages occur in the superficial cortex. Inflammation is minimal. The olfactory bulbs, however, are hemorrhagic and necrotic, or at least noticeably reddened. Throughout the brain and spinal cord a fibrinopurulent meningeal reaction containing many polyps and mononuclear cells is observed microscopically. Except in the sylvian fissures, subarachnoid cisterns, and basal parts of the brain, where it is often very prominent, this reaction is not usually seen in bacterial meningitis. Trophozoites can be found on the exudate, although they are usually sparse, degenerate, and engulfed by macrophages. In the Virchow-Robin spaces, however, the amebas are well preserved, often clustered around blood vessels in large numbers, and produce little or no inflammation (Fig. 3-27).

Some encephalitis is usually present, rang-

ing from a slight to massive invasion by the amebas. Very little extension of the purulent exudate into the white matter occurs. Severe ulceration and inflammation of the olfactory mucosa is present, sometimes revealing the presence of amebas. Numerous trophozoites, however, are found in the olfactory nerve filaments, which are inflamed and sometimes necrotic. The pathologic changes become more noticeable as the nerves penetrate the cribriform plate, the ventral portions of the olfactory bulb, more so than the dorsal, becoming completely disorganized by massive amebic invasion with severe hemorrhage and inflammatory exudate. Thus, the pathology suggests that invasion occurs primarily by way of the olfactory nerves, destruction of the olfactory bulbs, and dissemination by way of the subarachnoid space. The higher levels of phospholipase produced by the pathogenic strains of free-living ameba, as opposed to the lower levels produced by the nonpathogens, has been suggested as the partial explanation for their invasiveness and virulence that serves as an initial step in preparing host tissue for endocytosis. Both phagocytosis and pinocytosis of host tissue by *N. fowleri* have been observed. IgA, found normally in highest concentration in external secretions at the mucous membrane level forming a first-line defense against invasion, may possibly play an important role in primary amebic meningoencephalitis infection. Studies in this area are indicated by the finding of low serum IgA in one fatal case of a patient with a history of upper respiratory complaints that suggests a lowered resistance to infection.

Therapy has been far from satisfactory. The usual antibacterial, antiamebic, or antiparasitic drugs have not been effective. Amphotericin B shows some clinical effectiveness in the dosage of 1 mg/kg of body weight intravenously daily. Prompt diagnosis, early treatment with micanzole, amphotericin B, and rifampin, along with careful management, were attributed to for the survival of a patient in California. Intrathecal therapy seems crucial since amphotericin B and micanzole do not reach therapeutic levels in the cerebral spinal fluid otherwise.

Coprozoic amebas and artifacts

At times, free-living amebas may be found in the stool, their presence resulting either from the ingestion of cysts and their passage unharmed through the body, or, more commonly, from carelessness in leaving a stool specimen uncovered, or the use of a dirty container, resulting in contamination by flies and air currents. These cysts may excyst and the trophozoites may develop under proper conditions of moisture and temperature. However, they may be readily differentiated from parasitic trophozoites by the presence of one or more contactile vacuoles. The cyst itself has a very thick wall, and the nuclei within have thick membranes with very dense karyosomes.

Numerous artifacts in the feces may be mistakenly identified as amebas and other protozoa. Their number and kind are dependent on the diet of the host and the host tissue cells, which may pass into the feces.

REVIEW QUESTIONS

1. Name the amebas found in humans. Give the chief habits of each. Which are considered to be pathogenic?
2. Differentiate the cyst stage of *E. histolytica* from *E. coli*, *Endolimax nana*, and *I. bütschlii*. The trophozoite stage. Why is this differentiation important to the medical parasitologist?
3. Discuss the epidemiology of amebiasis.
4. Discuss the diagnosis and treatment of intestinal amebiasis. Of extraintestinal amebiasis.
5. Discuss how the nature of the stool should aid in differentiating amebic from bacillary dysentery.
6. What is primary amebic meningoencephalitis?
7. What is the significance of the *Hartmanellidae* amebas?
8. How can one differentiate *N. fowleri* from *Acanthamoeba* sp?
9. What is the treatment for primary amebic meningoencephalitis?
10. What is a "limax" ameba?

REFERENCES

Ahmad, H., and G. B. Ball. 1963. Increase in size of *Entamoeba hartmanni* trophozoites cultured on an enriched medium. Am. J. Trop. Med. Hyg. **12:**709-718.

Archivos de Investigación Médica 4 sup. 1. 1973. Quinto seminario sobre amibiasis. Inst. Mex. de Seguro Social, Publicada.

Australian Drug Evaluation Committee. 1971. Subacute myelo-optic neuropathy and the halogenated hydroxyquinolines. Med. J. Aust. **2:**1090.

Beaver, P. C., A. Lopez Villegas, C. Cuello, and A. D'Alessandra. 1978. Cutaneous amebiasis of the eyelid with extension into the orbit. Am. J. Trop. Med. Hyg. **27:**1133-1136.

Bos, H. J., and A. A. Van den Eijk. 1976. Enzyme linked immunosorbent assay (ELISA) in the serodiagnosis of amebiasis. Pages 721-727. In Sepúlveda, B., and L. S. Diamond, Editors. Proc. Int. Congr. on Amebiasis. Centrole estudios sobre ambiasis, Mexico.

Bunnag, D., and T. Harinasuta. 1974. Clinical trial of tinidazole in amoebic liver abscess using low doses. Proc. 3rd Int. Congr. Parasitol. **3:**1276.

Butt, C. G. 1966. Primary amebic meningoencephalitis N. Engl. J. Med. **274:**473-476.

Cahill, K. M., and others. 1971. Symposium on amoebiasis, Bull. N.Y. Acad. Sci. **47:**435-507.

Carter, R. F. 1972. Primary amoebic meningoencephalitis: an appraisal of present knowledge. Trans. R. Soc. Trop. Med. Hyg. 66:193-208.

Center for Disease Control. 1974. Blindness after Diiodoquin (diiodohydroxyquin). Morbidity and Mortality Weekly Report 23:254.

Center for Disease Control. 1978. Primary amebic meningoencephalitis: California, Florida, New York. Morbidity and Mortality Weekly Report 27:343-344.

Center for Disease Control. 1979. Amebic meningoencephalitis: Texas. Morbidity and Mortality Weekly Report 29:117-119.

Cerva, L. 1971. Studies of *Limax* amoeba in a swimming pool. Hydrobiologica 38:141-161.

Chang, S., W. Holdenbrandt, and S. E. Silvis, 1974. The accidental discovery that sodium diatrizoate (Hypaque) infusion will visualize amebic abscesses on hepatic tomograms. Am. J. Trop. Med. Hyg. 23:31-34.

Chang, S. H. 1974. Etiological, pathological, epidemiological and diagnostical consideration of primary amoebic meningoencephalitis. CRC Crit. Rev. Microbiol. 3:135-139.

Cursons, R. T. M., and others. 1979. IgA and primary amoebic meningoencephalitis. Lancet 1:223-224.

Cursons, R. T. M., T. J. Brown, and E. A. Keyes. 1978. Virulence of pathogenic free-living amebae. J. Parasitol. 64:744-745.

Faubert, G. M., E. Meerovitch, and J. McLaughlin. 1978. The presence of liver auto-antibodies induced by *Entamoeba histolytica* in the sera from both naturally infected humans and immunized rabbits. Am. J. Trop. Med. Hyg. 27:892-896.

Ganguly, N. K., and others. 1978. Immunoglobulin and complement levels in cases of invasive amoebiasis. Indian J. Med. 67:221-226.

García, Tiguera, J., and others. 1978. Meningoencephalitis amebiana primaria: estudio de in caso sospechoso y revision de la literatura medica. Rev. Cub. Med. Trop. 30:161-168.

Geller, M., and others. 1978. Serum IgE levels in amoebiasis. Clin. Allergy 8:565-567.

Goldman, M. 1969. *E. histolytica*-like ameba occurring in man. Bull. WHO 40:355-364.

Hitchcock, D. J. 1950. Parasitological study on Eskimos in the Bethal area of Alaska. J. Parasitol. 36:232-234.

Juniper, K., and others. 1972. Serodiagnosis of amebiasis. Am. J. Trop. Med. Hyg. 21:157-168.

Kagan, I. G., and L. Norman. 1970. Serodiagnosis of parasitic diseases. Manual Clin. Microbiol., pp. 454-486.

Knight, R., and S. G. Wright. 1978. Progress report: intestinal protozoa. Gut 19:940-953.

Krogstad, D. J., H. C. Spencer, and G. R. Healy. 1978.

Current concepts in parasitology: amebiasis. N. Engl. J. Med. 298:262-265.

Krupp, I. M. 1977. Definition of the antigenic pattern of *Entamoeba histolytica* and immunoelectrophoretic analysis of the variation of patient response to amoebic disease. Am. J. Trop. Med. Hyg. 26:387-392.

Lawless, D. K., and V. Knight. 1966. Human infection with *Entamoeba polecki*; report of 4 cases. Am. J. Trop. Med. Hyg. 15:701-704.

LeMaistre, C. A., and others. 1956. Studies of a waterborne outbreak of amebiasis, South Bend, Indiana: epidemiological aspects. Am. J. Hyg. 64:30-45.

Levin, R. L., and D. E. Armstrong. 1970. Human infections with *Entamoeba polecki*. Am. J. Clin. Path. 54:611-614.

Meerovitch, E. 1965. Some biological studies on the Laredo strain of *Entamoeba histolytica*. In Progress in protozoology, abstracts. Papers Read at the Second International Congress of Protozoology, Excerpta Medica International Congress Series. no. 91., p. 194.

Mithal, S., H. K. Panigrahi, L. N. Mohapatra, and S. Sunder. 1978. Indirect fluorescent antibody test in amoebiasis using axenic *Entamoeba histolytica*. Indian J. Med. Res. 67:367-373.

Nagington, J., and others. 1974. Amoebic infection of the eye. Lancet. 2:1537-1540.

Neal, R. A. 1971. The pathogenesis of amebiasis. Gut 12:483-486.

Phillips, B. P. 1974. *Naegleria*: another pathogenic ameba. Studies in germ free guinea pigs. Am. J. Trop. Med. Hyg. 23:850-855.

Powell, S. J. 1971. Therapy of amebiasis. Bull. N.Y. Acad. Med. 45:469-477.

Powell, S. J., E. J. Stewart, and R. Elsdon-Dew. 1973. Metronidazole combined with diloxamide furoate in amoebic liver abscesses. Ann. Trop. Med. Parasitol. 67:367-368.

Powell, S. J., A. J. Wilmot, and R. Elsdon-Dew. 1969. Single and low dosage regimens of metronidazole in amoebic dysentery and amoebic abscesses. Ann. Trop. Med. Parasitol. 63:139-142.

Report of WHO Expert Committee. 1969. Amoebiasis. WHO Technical Report Series, no. 421. Geneva, Switzerland.

Salaki, J. S., J. L. Shirley, and G. T. Strickland. 1979. Successful treatment of symptomatic *Entamoeba polecki* infection. Am. J. Trop. Med. Hyg. 28:190-193.

Schmidt, G. D., and L. S. Roberts. 1977. Foundations of parasitology. The C. V. Mosby Co., St. Louis.

Schultz, M. G. 1972. Entero-Vioform for preventing travelers' diarrhea. J.A.M.A. 220:273.

Sharma, P., B. N. Krishna Prasad, and G. P. Dutta. 1978. Coproantibodies in intestinal amoebiasis using axenic *Entamoeba histolytica* antigen. Indian J. Med. Res. 68:423-427.

Sharma, R. 1959. Effect of cholesterol on the growth and virulence of *Entamoeba histolytica*. Trans. R. Soc. Trop. Med. Hyg. **53**:278-281.

Spencer, H. 1973. Amoebiasis. Pages 271-297. In Spencer, H., Editor. Tropical pathology. Springer Verlag, Heidelberg.

Stillman, A. E., V. Alvarez, and D. Grube. 1974. Hepatic amebic abscess: unresponsiveness to combination of metronidazole and surgical drainage. J.A.M.A. **229**:71-77.

Tschl-hyon, J. 1974. Use of tinidazole (Fasigyn) in treatment of intestinal and hepatic amebiasis. Proc. 3rd Int. Congr. Parasitol. **3**:1279.

Visvesvara, G. S., and G. R. Healy. 1975. Comparative antigenic analysis of pathogenic and free-living *Naegleria* species by the gel diffusion and immunoelectrophoresis techniques. Infect. Immun. **11**:95-108.

Visvesvara, G. S., D. B. Jones, and N. M. Robinson. 1975. Isolation, identification, and biological characteristization of *Acanthamoeba polyphaga* from a human eye. Am. J. Trop. Med. Hyg. **24**:784-790.

Warhurst, D. C., W. P. Stamm, and E. A. Phillips. 1976. *Acanthamoeba* form a new case of corneal ulcer. Trans. R. Soc. Trop. Med. Hyg. **70**:279.

Wolfe, M. 1973. Nondysenteric intestinal amebiasis: treatment with diloxamide furoate. J.A.M.A. **224**:1601-1604.

CHAPTER 4

The flagellates (Mastigophora)

The following flagellates are parasitic in humans:

Intestinal
  Giardia lamblia
  Dientamoeba fragilis
  Chilomastix mesnili
  Enteromonas hominis
  Retortamonas (Embadomonas) intestinalis
  Trichomonas hominis
Atrial
  Trichomonas tenax
  Trichomonas vaginalis
Blood and tissue (hemoflagellates)
  Leishmania tropica
  Leishmania braziliensis
  Leishmania donovani
  Trypanosoma cruzi
  Trypanosoma b. gambiense
  Trypanosoma b. rhodesiense
  Trypanosoma rangeli

The class Mastigophora is by far the largest of all the protozoa. The flagellates differ perceptibly from the amebas in that the cytoplasm is surrounded by a well-defined pellicle that imparts shape to the organism. Organelles such as flagella and undulating membranes protrude from the organism and aid in locomotion and in obtaining food. Though more complex in appearance than the amebas, the flagellates actually are more primitive from an evolutionary standpoint. Like the amebas, most intestinal flagellates have a trophozoite and a cyst stage. The cyst stage, when present, is the infective or transmissible stage to humans. Otherwise, the trophozoite assumes this role. Most species absorb their nutriment directly through the body wall, whereas some have a definite mouth, or cytostome, for food ingestion. No digestive tract, however, is present. Reproduction takes place by longitudinal division in the trophozoite or vegetative stage. Flagella arise from basal granules in the cytoplasm and may be single or multiple. One or more nuclei may be present and, for the most part, are not as useful in diagnosis as are nuclei in the amebas. When encystation occurs, the process is similar to that of the amebas. Organelles are lost, but internal structures that become useful in identification remain.

The intestinal flagellates, unlike the amebas, are found in the small intestine as well as in the cecum and colon and, in some instances, like *Giardia lamblia*, chiefly in the duodenum. As with the intestinal amebas, transmission occurs primarily through contaminated food or drink and by hand-to-mouth contact. Likewise, not all are pathogenic, but all must be studied and identified to differentiate one from another and, at times, from the amebas (Table 4-1).

The geographic distribution of the intestinal and atrial forms is cosmopolitan. The blood and tissue forms, more commonly referred to as hemoflagellates, have a restricted distribution dependent on the ecology of their respective arthropod vectors. In contrast with the intestinal forms, they require both vertebrate and invertebrate hosts to complete their life cycle. Since adult, sexual, or larval forms cannot be differentiated in dealing with these parasites, the terms "definitive host" and "intermedi-

Table 4-1. Differential characteristics of trophozoites and cysts

	Trichomonas hominis	Chilomastix mesnili	Giardia lamblia	Dientamoeba fragilis
Trophozoites				
Size	Average 10 μm	Average 12 μm	Average 14 μm	Average 10 μm (6-20 μm)
Shape	Ovoid or piriform	Cone shaped	Pear shaped with concave disk ventrally in anterior portion	Ameboid
Motility	Rapidly repeated quick jerks	Rolling, rhythmic motion on longitudinal axis	Falling leaf motion, no direction	Sluggish, rarely progressive; similar to *Entamoeba coli*
Characteristic structures	Undulating membrane, lashing flagella	Spiral groove, cleft-like cytostome	Bilateral symmetry showing two nuclei, flagella, fibrils	Thin, veillike, leaflike pseudopodia with edges or sharp corners
Cysts				
Size	No cyst stage present	Average 8 μm	Average 12 μm	No cyst stage present
Shape		Lemon shaped with nipple	Football shape	
Characteristic structures		Clear zone near nipple; fibrils of cytostome faintly present; sometimes nucleus visible	Fibrils; nuclei (2 to 4); parabasal bodies; cytoplasm retracted from cyst wall	

ate host" cannot aptly be applied. The terms "vertebrate host" and "arthropod host (or vector)" are more commonly used. All hemoflagellates except *Trypanosoma rangeli* are pathogenic.

INTESTINAL FLAGELLATES
Giardia lamblia

Life cycle and morphology. *Giardia lamblia*, an intestinal pathogen, has both a trophozoite and a cyst stage in its life cycle. Trophozoites, rarely seen in the stool except when marked diarrhea is present, are unique among the protozoa in humans in that they are the only organisms that are bilaterally symmetrical. In size, they average around 15 μm (9 to 21 μm) along the longitudinal axis, and show greater girth in the anterior portion (5 to 15 μm), tapering to a conical posterior end. In thickness they vary from 2 to 4 μm. When it is viewed dorsally, the organism, with its two nuclei and adjacent fibrils, presents the appearance of a wizened old professor with pince-nez glasses. Between the two nuclei, each of which has a large central endosome with no chromatin granules on the nuclear membrane, are two slender rodlike structures, often referred to as axostyles, but which actually are formed by the fusion of the axonemes of the ventral flagella and associated groups of microtubules. Four pairs of flagella are arranged as shown in Fig. 4-1. They are described as anterior, posterior, ventral, and caudal. Each one arises from a corresponding axoneme which in turn has its origin in a basal granule or kinetosome. Posterior to the adhesive disk are two curved median bodies which stain deeply and are often mistaken as chromatid bodies or parabasal bodies. Their function is uncertain but some suggest that they may give support to the posterior portion of the organism. Others suggest that they may be involved in energy and metabo-

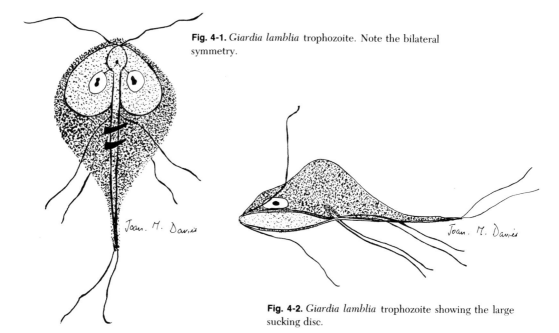

Fig. 4-1. *Giardia lamblia* trophozoite. Note the bilateral symmetry.

Fig. 4-2. *Giardia lamblia* trophozoite showing the large sucking disc.

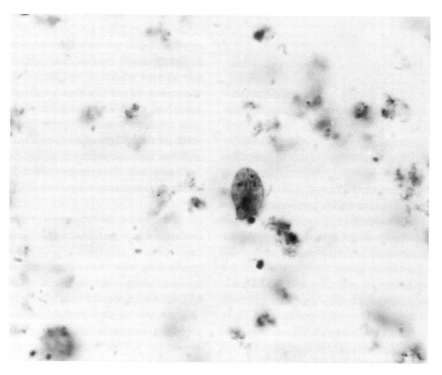

Fig. 4-3. *Giardia lamblia* cyst. Note the presence of three nuclei and the fibrils in the cytoplasm. (Photograph by Charles M. Bailey.)

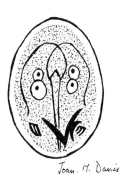

Fig. 4-4. *Giardia lamblia* cyst. Note the retraction of the cytoplasm from the cyst wall.

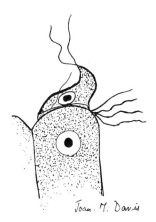

Fig. 4-5. *Giardia lamblia* trophozite perched on top of an epithelial cell.

lism. Of interest is the report that no mitochondria, smooth endoplasmic reticulum, Gogli apparatus, or lysosomes are present in this organism. Dorsally, the trophozoite is convex (Fig. 4-2), while ventrally it is flat, giving the appearance of a uterus cut in sagittal section, the adhesive disk corresponding to the uterine cavity and the tapering end corresponding to the cervical portion. Division occurs longitudinally following duplication of all organelles. Billions of trophozoites may occur in heavy infections. Encystation (Fig. 4-3) takes place as the trophozoites move into the large bowel where dehydration of the fecal mass makes an environment

unsuitable for survival. Flagella are lost and a cyst wall develops around the contracting cytoplasm. Following the duplication of nuclei in young cysts, as maturation takes place all organelles are duplicated. Cysts may survive in water up to three months, but they are highly vulnerable to desiccation and temperatures of 50° C. They may survive up to a week in a watery, urine or fecal sample. Like *Entamoeba histolytica*, *G. lamblia* cysts will survive the normal chlorination of a city water supply. Cysts are typically football shaped, averaging 8 to $12\,\mu$m in length by 7 to 10 μm in width. In saline solution, refractile fibrils can usually be seen, along with the retraction of the cytoplasm from some part of the cyst wall (Fig. 4-4). Identification can often be made without staining. At times, the cysts may be viewed standing on end. Gentle tapping of the coverslip will roll them over and a longitudinal side view will be obtained. With iodine the nuclei and fibrils are more pronounced. Starch-containing cysts, when stained with iodine, appear blue and are referred to as "blue giardia." Young cysts may show diffuse glycogen that may obscure the structures within.

Habitat. An ingested cyst undergoes excystation in the duodenum, and the trophozoite attaches its large sucking disk to the epithelial cells (Fig. 4-5). Crypts of the duodenum and upper jejunum (Fig. 4-6), where the pH of 6 to 7.0 is favorable for growth, are heavily invaded, with the numbers decreasing as the cecum is approached. In heavy infections the floor of the small intestine may be literally carpeted with giardias, their flagella waving freely in the lumen (Fig. 4-7). Trophozoites may also occasionally invade the bile ducts and gallbladder. The adhesive quality of the sucking disk, which is due chiefly to the striated rim of cytoplasm which is flexible and contractile surrounding the rigid bilobed disk itself, prevents trophozoites from appearing in the stool except in severe diarrhea. When seen, their erratic,

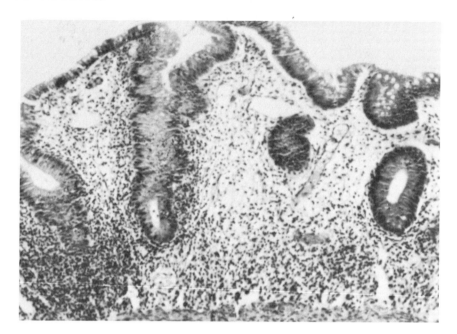

Fig. 4-6. Jejunal biopsy from patient with diarrhea, malabsorption, low IgG, and absence of IgA and IgM. Note the absence of villi and crypts. (AFIP 75-2969-9.)

swaying motion has been aptly described as like that of a falling leaf.

Epidemiology. *G. lamblia* is cosmopolitan in distribution. Waterborne epidemics occur sporadically among world travelers, tourists, and residents in established communities. Tourists returning from Russia, Portugal, and elsewhere in the world have suffered the ill effects of this ubiquitous parasite. In Camas, Washington (population 6,000), in the spring of 1966, 128 laboratory-confirmed cases were reported. And, in 1978, in a study of 100 patients in Cuba in whom clinical manifestations were compatible with an ulcerous syndrome, 56% had *G. lamblia*. In both instances raw surface water supplying the water treatment plants was found positive for *G. lamblia* cysts. Failures in the treatment system or inadequate procedures accounted for the outbreaks in both cases. An outbreak in Vail, Colorado, in 1978, likewise was associated with the contaminated water resulting from a sewer-line obstruction and leakage into the creek supplying the water to the city. An

outbreak in the ski resort of Aspen, Colorado, was traced to contaminated well water. It has been shown that, while routine chlorination is inadequate to destroy cysts (same for *E. histolytica*), properly functioning sedimentation, flocculation, and filtration procedures will remove any particles the size of *G. lamblia* cysts, thus rendering surface water safe for drinking as far as *G. lamblia* and other organisms of the same or larger size are concerned.

Symptomatology. The role played by this parasite in pathogenesis is not fully known. A wide variety of symptoms, none of which is pathognomonic of the disease, is attributed to this organism. Acute manifestations of giardiasis are nausea, anorexia, explosive watery stools, steatorrhea, malabsorption, severe flatulence with abdominal distension, and midepigastric cramps. Acute amebic or bacillary dysentery, at times, might be a prime suspect, but the foul-smelling stool, flatus, and marked abdominal distension, along with the absence of pus and blood,

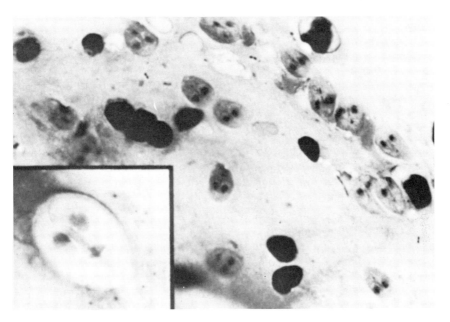

Fig. 4-7. *Giardia lamblia* trophozoites in smear made from jejunal biopsy. Insert shows single trophozoite. (AFIP 75-2969-1.)

are more suggestive of giardiasis. Subacute symptoms with periodic episodes of mushy, foul-smelling stools, at times with evidence of steatorrhea, may last for months. The most common chronic complaints are periodic bouts of soft, mushy, foul-smelling stools, flatulence, and abdominal distension. Remission may occur in some untreated patients. Biliary disease is often simulated, particularly in adults, whereas children show predominantly a diarrheal syndrome, often steatorrheal in nature. Infection is most common in children, particularly in orphanages, camps, and similar institutions. Many patients with a heavy parasitic infection have no symptoms at all.

Pathology. Reports vary concerning the pathogenicity of *G. lamblia*. Mucosal suction biopsies from the duodenum and adjacent jejunum have shown invasion of the mucosa but no signs of host cell injury according to some investigators. Electron microscope studies, however, suggest that the organism may be attacking the fuzzy coat of the micro-villi. Trophozoites have been demonstrated inside host cells by others. Autopsy findings, in some instances, have shown extensive ulceration and sloughing of mucosa in the presence of heavy infections. Passage of parasites up the bile duct to the gallbladder, although rare, sometimes occurs with signs and symptoms of biliary tract disease. Secondary vitamin A deficiency has been suggested by the lower carotene levels in children infected with *Giardia*.

Host susceptibility varies in individuals—some with heavy infections showing few or no symptoms at all, while others with only a few parasites displaying severe disease manifestations. Two predisposing factors to symptomatology appear to be achlorhydria and hypogammaglobulinemia. Giardiasis appears also to cause a general disaccharidase deficiency, resulting in a lactose intolerance, which is usually, but not always, restored after chemotherapy. Immunoglobulin deficiency has suggested to some workers that the lack of secretory IgA in patients may lead to colonization of bacteria in the jejunum and increased susceptibility to *Giardia*. By deconjugating bile acids the bacteria may cause steatorrhea, but opportunistic *Giardia* greatly aggravate the condition.

Diagnosis. The diagnosis of giardiasis depends on the recovery and identification of the parasite. Cyst formation and passage down the intestinal tract, influenced by rate of peristalsis, may be sporadic, so that numerous cysts are present at one time and few, if any, at another; therefore repeated stool examinations at scattered intervals may be necessary. Purgation is not dependable. In saline mounts typical cyst morphology can usually be readily recognized. Retraction of the cytoplasm from the cyst wall, in part or complete, nuclei within, and refractile fibrils render verification relatively easy. Iodine-stained preparations assure identification. Permanent stained mounts for reference purposes may be made, but are not necessary for routine diagnosis. Because this parasite lives in the duodenum, trophozoites are not uncommonly found in duodenal drainage. On occasion, parasites are not found in the stool and can only be detected in duodenal aspirate. An ingenious method of sampling the duodenum with a recoverable nylon yarn swallowed in a weighted capsule has been used successfully.

Treatment. The drug of choice in the treatment of giardiasis is quinacrine hydrochloride (Atabrine) in the dosage of 100 mg three times daily for 5 to 7 days. The pediatric dose is 6 mg/kg/day in three doses after eating for 5 days with a maximum of 300 mg/day. Dizziness, headache, and vomiting are frequent, and occasionally this drug causes toxic psychosis, blood dyscrasia, urticaria, severe exfoliative dermatitis, yellow staining of skin and sclera, blue and black nail pigmentation, and ocular effects similar to those caused by chloroquine. Acute hepatic necrosis is rare. Metronidazole (Flagyl) at the level of 250 mg three times daily for 10 days as an alternative drug is considered

as an investigational drug by the U.S. Food and Drug Administration for *Giardia* infections. The pediatric dose is 15 mg/kg/day in three doses for 5 days. Nitrimidazine (Naxogin) and tinidazole, which are 5-nitroimidazole derivates, and furazolidone (Furoxone) are considered effective in giardiasis but do not supercede metronidazole. Most symptomatic patients respond to treatment. The physician must decide whether treatment is indicated in the asymptomatic patient.

Dientamoeba fragilis

Dientamoeba fragilis, although long recognized as being different from the amebas, has for some time been classified with that group. The presence of two nuclei, connected to one another by a filament (a division spindle) and representing an arrested telophase, is present in over half the trophozoites. The organism is also characterized by the absence of a cyst stage, although one of the amebas, *Entamoeba gingivalis*, also shares this feature. On the basis of immunologic evidence and ultrastructure, this organism has been placed among the trichomonads, even though movement is by pseudopodia and not flagella.

Trophozoites (Fig. 4-8) range from 6 to 20 μm in diameter, the size range of *Iodamoeba bütschlii*. Mobility is sluggish, rarely directional, with thin, veillike or leaflike pseudopodia showing edges or sharp corners. In many respects the organisms resemble *Entamoeba coli*, containing food vacuoles with bacteria, yeasts, starch granules, and cellular elements. The nuclei are usually invisible in saline. When stained, the nuclear membrane, like that of *Endolimax nana*, shows the absence of chromatin granules. The karyosome or endosome is divided into four to six distinct chromatin granules, usually eccentric but variable in position. These trophozoites differ from amebic trophozoites in that although they swell and rupture like the amebas, when mounted in water prep-

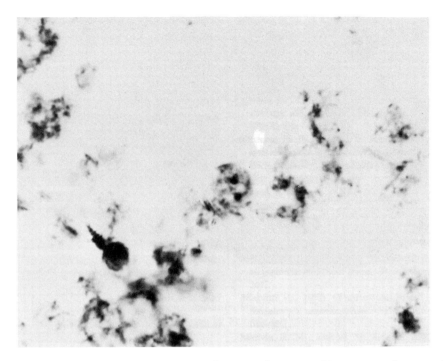

Fig. 4-8. *Dientamoeba fragilis* trophozoite. Note the two nuclei present. (From a nonprofit cooperative endeavor of numerous colleagues under the editorship of Dr. Herman Zaiman, Valley City, N.D.)

arations they return to a semblance of normal size with numerous granules present in brownian movement. This is called the "Hakansson phenomenon" and is a diagnostic feature of *D. fragilis*.

Along with the amebas, *D. fragilis* lives chiefly in the cecum but is found throughout the large intestine. It is found in the mucosal crypts living chiefly on lumen debris. It is considered by many as a commensal, but episodes of diarrhea, vomiting, nausea, flatulence, and other gastrointestinal disorders have been noted. Under such circumstances, antiamebic therapy, as used for *E. histolytica*, may be indicated. Diiodohydroxyquin (Diodoquin) is most commonly used. Tetracycline in the adult dosage of 500 mg four times daily for 10 days has been recommended by some, with a pediatric dosage of 10 mg/kg four times daily for 10 days with a maximum of 2 gm/day. This is considered an investigational drug for this infection by the U.S. Food and Drug Administration.

Chilomastix mesnili

The flagellate *Chilomastix mesnili* is a nonpathogen with a trophozoite and a cyst stage in its life cycle. Like the amebas, trophozoites are more common in soft, loose stools, whereas cysts occur chiefly in firm, well-formed ones. The parasite lives mainly in the cecum and colon (but some believe it lives also in the small intestine). Its importance lies only in its differentiation from other parasites.

The trophozoite averages 12 μm (6 to 24 μm) along its longitudinal axis, being broader in girth anteriorly (3 to 10 μm) and tapering conelike posteriorly. A typical spiral groove running longitudinally is readily discernible as the organism is seen in saline solution, spinning on its longitudinal axis as it moves along. A cleft-shaped cytostome, or mouth,

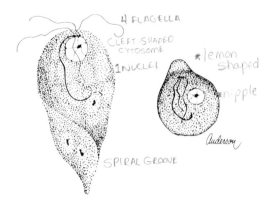

Fig. 4-9. *Chilomastix mesnili* trophozoite and cyst. Note the spiral groove, flagella, and cytostome in trophozoite. Note the nipple and cytostome in cyst.

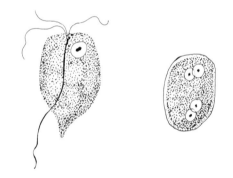

Fig. 4-10. *Enteromonas hominis* trophozoite and cyst.

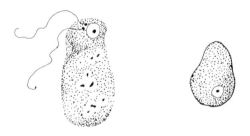

Fig. 4-11. *Retortamonas (Embadomonas) intestinalis* trophozoite and cyst.

is present and can likewise be seen in saline. Along either side of the cytosome is a fibril which probably gives support to the lips. Four anterior flagella (one larger than the others) are present. One of the short and delicate flagella curves backward into the

cytosome and undulates, which probably aids in obtaining food. A single vesicular-type nucleus is anterior in position, and contains a distinct endosome with no chromatin granules on the nuclear border. The typical movement and the features mentioned usually suffice for identification. The anterior flagella, at times, may be discernible (Fig. 4-9).

The cyst stage is quite small, averaging 6 μm in diameter. It is lemon shaped with a characteristic nipple present. The apparently clear area between the cytoplasm and the nipple end, along with the characteristic shape and size, often suffice for diagnosis in saline mounts. When stained with iodine, the nucleus and fibrils forming the cytostome can be seen. Sometimes the coverslip must be gently tapped to roll the cysts over into correct position in order to see the characteristic nipple. Aberrant forms sometimes occur, resulting in frequent confusion with yeast cells.

Enteromonas hominis

The flagellate *Enteromonas hominis*, a nonpathogen, has a trophozoite and a cyst stage in its life cycle. It is rare in humans and, when present, persists for only a few days or weeks. Trophozoites are oval with changeable shape and average 4 to 10 μm × 3 to 6 μm. There are three anterior flagella and a posterior flagellum present. The latter follows along the flattened side of the organism before becoming free (Fig. 4-10).

Cysts are oval, average 7 μm × 4 μm, and contain from one to four nuclei. Binucleated cysts are most common, and the nuclei are usually at opposite ends of the cyst. Confusion with cysts of *E. nana* can occur.

Retortamonas (Embadomonas) intestinalis

The flagellate *Retortamonas* (or *Embadomonas*) *intestinalis*, a nonpathogen and having both the trophozoite and the cyst stages in its life cycle, is also rare in humans. Members of this species are found in a variety of insects, particularly aquatic forms, as well as in frogs and turtles. This fact suggests that the infections in humans may be acquired from these hosts. It is doubtful that it is a normal human parasite. The trophozoite averages 6 μm $\times$ 3 μm. Two flagella are present (Fig. 4-11).

Cysts are pear shaped and average about the same size as the trophozoites. When stained, a single nucleus and a cytostome can be seen. *Embadomonas sinensis* from China is believed by some to be identical to *E. intestinalis.*

Pentatrichomonas hominis

Three species of the trichomonads are found in humans. All three are quite similar in morphology, and confusion in identification is possible when they are seen together. The restriction of species to specific habitats in humans considerably simplifies diagnosis. The trichomonads are unique in that only a trophozoite is found in the life cycle. This stage then becomes the transmissible stage to humans.

Members of this family are oval and taper to a point posteriorly. They have three to five anterior flagella and an undulating membrane extending along the longitudinal axis, the length depending on the species in question. A stiff rod or axostyle running the length of the organism within gives rigidity to the parasite and protrudes posteriorly as a caudal spine. The trichomonads move by a quick, jerky motion, and the undulating membrane coming in and out of the plane of focus gives a cogwheel appearance. A nucleus and a cytostome are present but not readily discernible in a fresh mount. Reproduction occurs by longitudinal fission.

The diagnosis of these organisms depends on the identification of the features mentioned in a fresh saline mount. Species diagnosis for practical purposes depends on the habitat in the human host. Trichomonads

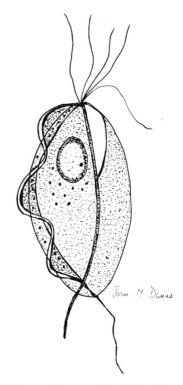

Fig. 4-12. *Pentatrichomonas hominis* trophozoite. Note the five anterior flagella.

characteristically lose their organelles upon standing outside the body, round up, and even send out protoplasmic projections resembling pseudopodia. They may easily be mistaken for amebas. This is particularly true for the intestinal species.

P. hominis is found only in the intestinal tract, presumably the small as well as the large intestine, and is considered by most workers to be a nonpathogen. The absence of a cyst stage and the inability of the trophozoite to survive the gastric juices leaves the method of transmission unresolved. Survival of the trophozoites in the eggs of parasitic nematodes has been suggested as in its close relative *Histomonas.* Ameboidlike organisms resembling *D. fragilis* have been found in the eggs of *Enterobius vermicularis,* the common pinworm, and epidemiologic evidence has been offered to support this concept.

P. hominis has been known as *Trichomonas hominis* for some time, but most trophozoites have five anterior flagella and accordingly it has been assigned to the genus *Pentatrichomonas*. It is found in other primates and domestic animals, as well as in humans. Some clinicians have attributed diarrhea and gastrointestinal upsets to this parasite, but no evidence substantiates this claim (Fig. 4-12).

Diagnosis is made by identification of a typical trichomonad in a fresh stool. The organism averages 10 μm in length (8 to 20 μm) and has an undulating membrane extending the full length of the body, continuing posteriorly as a free-trailing flagellum. A conical cytosome at the anterior end lies ventrally, opposite to the undulating membrane. A vesicular-type nucleus is also anterior in position with a small endosome. Since old stools may show atypical or degenerating trophozoites that resemble amebas, it is helpful to know the time of stool passage or, preferably, to obtain fresh specimens for examination.

ATRIAL FLAGELLATES
Trichomonas tenax

Trichomonas tenax is restricted to the mouth and is nonpathogenic for humans. It lives around the gumline in the same environment as *Entamoeba gingivalis* (Fig. 4-13). Scrapings smeared in saline solution on a slide will reveal the typical organisms when present. Since their habitat is restricted to the mouth, no problem of confusion with intestinal parasites occurs. The organism averages 6 to 8 μm in length with great variation in size and shape, but it is typically ellipsoid or ovoid. It more closely resembles *Trichomonas vaginalis* than *P. hominis*, but it is more slender and smaller. The posterior flagellum on the margin of the undulating membrane (which does not reach the posterior end of the body) likewise terminates at this point. Trophozoites have been recovered

from mouth washings and sputum smears in patients with respiratory tract infections.

Trichomonas vaginalis

Morphology. The flagellate *Trichomonas vaginalis*, the only pathogenic trichomonad in humans, is found in the vagina and male urethra. Diagnosis is relatively simple, depending on the identification of a typical trichomonad moving among the epithelial cells in a fresh vaginal or urethral smear in saline solution. This organism averages 15 μm in length with great variation in size, and is quite robust in appearance. The undulating membrane is short, never extending beyond the middle of the body (Fig. 4-14). Granules along the axostyle are more numerous and constant, a dependable criteria in differentiating *T. vaginalis* from other species in living, as well as properly fixed and stained, specimens.

Symptomatology and pathology. Although most clinicians regard this organism as the

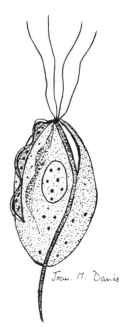

Fig. 4-13. *Trichomonas tenax* trophozoite.

causative agent of a persistent vaginitis, some parasitologists are not yet convinced that it is a primary pathogen. Patients show vaginal inflammation and complain of a burning, itching sensation and discharge. This discharge is frequently frothy, creamy, and yellowish and is full of bacteria, epithelial cells, pus cells, and organisms. The vulva and surrounding areas may be red and inflamed. The urethra as well may be involved.

Incidence in the male is higher than believed formerly. Symptoms are frequently absent, although an irritating urethritis or prostatitis may be present, and infection often remains unnoticed unless aggravated by a secondary bacterial invasion.

Sexual intercourse accounts for much of the incidence in women, with the males serving as a reservoir source of infection. In unsanitary environments and congested

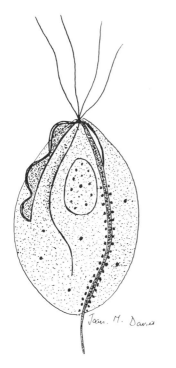

Fig. 4-14. *Trichomonas vaginalis* trophozoite. Note the short undulating membrane and numerous granules along the axostyle.

housing conditions, transmission from female to female possibly may occur through contaminated clothing and unclean toilet facilities. The normal vaginal environment has a pH around 3.8, a flora rich in Döderlein's bacilli, and a healthy epithelium rich in glycogen. The bacilli convert glycogen into lactic acid, which in turn keeps the environment acidic. Such an environment is not conducive to growth of *T. vaginalis*. The organisms flourish best when the pH is elevated, bacilli reduced in number, and a thinning of the epithelium yielding a lower concentration of glycogen occurs. This explains the rationale of many treatments using acid douches and insufflation agents.

Diagnosis. As previously indicated, the diagnosis can readily be made by the recovery and identification of the trophozoites in a saline smear. With a speculum in place, a specimen should be obtained from the cervix, vaginal wall, and urethra and transferred to a saline mount for early microscopic examination. Urethral discharge, prostatic fluid, and centrifuged urine from the male may also reveal the organism. The typical robust trichomonads can be seen in their characteristic jerky motion moving among the epithelial cells, with the undulating membrane giving a cogwheel effect as it comes in and out of focus. Degenerating organisms that have lost their organelles resemble sluggish amebas, hence the importance of prompt examination of the material. Since *T. vaginalis* is the only trichomonad found in the vagina, species identification presents no problem. In cancer diagnostic centers, infections are readily picked up during the screening of Papanicolaou smears.

Treatment. Successful treatment of women entails detection and eradication of infection in the male partner. Metronidazole (Flagyl) is the drug of choice for both females and males. The recommended dosage for women is 250 mg orally three times daily for 7 days, whereas the male is given 250 mg twice daily for 7 days. In addition to the oral treatment for women a 500 mg vaginal suppository is recommended daily for 7 days. The pediatric dose is 15 mg/kg per day in three doses for 7 days. Some evidence suggests that certain strains of *T. vaginalis* are becoming drug resistant. Metronidazole frequently causes nausea, headaches, dry mouth, metallic taste, and an Antabuse-like reaction with alcohol. Carcinogenicity in rats has also been noted. Occasionally, vomiting, diarrhea, insomnia, weakness, stomatitis, vertigo, paresthesia, and rash are observed. Ataxia is rare. Alcohol is contraindicated from 24 hours before to 48 hours after therapy.

Coprozoic flagellates

As in amebas, free-living flagellates may contaminate the stool. Identification may be difficult. Most of these organisms are present because of carelessness in using dirty containers without lids for collecting the speci-men. Such conditions can be avoided easily by a little forethought.

BLOOD AND TISSUE FLAGELLATES (HEMOFLAGELLATES)

All genera of the blood and tissue flagellates belong to the family Trypanosomatidae and probably stem from ancestors parasitic in various arthropod hosts. Six distinct morphologic types, each representing a genus, have been identified in this family. Of these, four are of medical significance. The amastigote is a small, round, or oval body without a flagellum but containing a nucleus and a kinetoplast. The latter structure consists of a parabasal body and a dotlike blepharoplast from which arises a slender fibril or axoneme. The promastigote is elongated and slender with a free flagellum extending from the axoneme. The kinetoplast is near the anterior end of the organism. The epimastigote, somewhat like the promastigote in body form but less slender, is characterized by the shift-

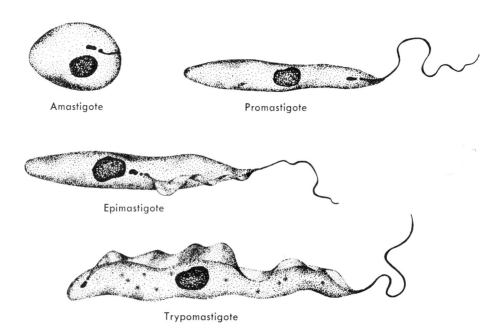

Amastigote

Promastigote

Epimastigote

Trypomastigote

Fig. 4-15. Four morphologic forms of the hemoflagellates.

ing of the kinetoplast to a position anterior to the nucleus and the development of an undulating membrane, which at the extreme anterior becomes the free flagellum. The trypomastigote is characterized by a shift of the kinetoplast to a posterior position with an undulating membrane extending the full length of the body. A free flagellum may or may not be present (Fig. 4-15).

Two genera of medical importance bear names the same as the older nomenclature of the morphologic types. They are *Leishmania* and *Trypanosoma*. The species of medical significance are as follows:

Leishmania tropica
Leishmania braziliensis
Leishmania donovani
Trypanosoma cruzi
Trypanosoma rangeli
Trypanosoma b. gambiense
Trypanosoma b. rhodesiense

In general, adaptation to the vertebrate is an innovation of relatively insufficiently long standing to effect complete severance from the arthropod host. An exception is *Trypanosoma equiperdum* in horses, which is transmitted through coitus.

Leishmaniases

Life cycle and morphology. The differentiation of the species causing the leishmaniases in humans is a clinical rather than a morphologic one, since the organisms, in the opinion of many, are indistinguishable. Life cycles are identical. Small, oval amastigotes are found intracellularly in the reticuloendothelial system of the skin, bone marrow, liver, spleen, and lymph nodes of mammals and reptiles, the vertebrate hosts, and promastigotes are found in the alimentary tract of sandflies of the genera *Phlebotomus* and *Lutzomyia*, the invertebrate hosts. Sandflies, while feeding, regurgitate promastigotes from the blocked foregut into the wound, and thus such flies serve as the arthropod vector. Initial skin lesions are similar in all

infections. The promastigotes, averaging 14 to 20 μm, quickly invade local tissue cells and change to amastigotes, an obligatory intracellular parasite. The latter averages 2 to 4 μm × 1 to 2 μm. Multiplication takes place within the tissue cells by longitudinal division and eventually destroys the host cells. Invasion of more cells occurs, producing initially a small papule that later varies in development according to the strains or species involved. Invasion into endothelial cells of the reticuloendothelial system and into mononuclear macrophages and polymorphonuclear neutrophils of the blood, lymph, and bone marrow follows to an extent dependent on the species involved and the host resistance. The nature and extent of cellular invasion and tissue damage form the chief basis for speciation in the genus *Leishmania*. In the gut of the fly, ingested amastigotes multiply, becoming infective promastigotes in up to 20 days. Migration into the foregut takes place where blockage again occurs.

Not all lesions are as typical for the species as often described in textbooks. Virulence of strains and variations in host susceptibility undoubtedly influence the clinical picture. In the opinion of some workers, all cutaneous leishmaniases are caused by one species, and skin lesions are divided into the following three main types:

Ulcerating
Vegetating or verrucous
Nodular

Others believe that the characteristic geographic distribution of certain types of lesions reflect different species and occasional clinical variations may represent altered host resistance. The genus *Leishmania* is apparently actively speciating. The taxonomy, heretofore based on clinical manifestations, is moving into a phase where intrinsic, physiologic, metabolic, antigenic, and immunogenic characteristics of different strains are being studied as a possible basis for a taxo-

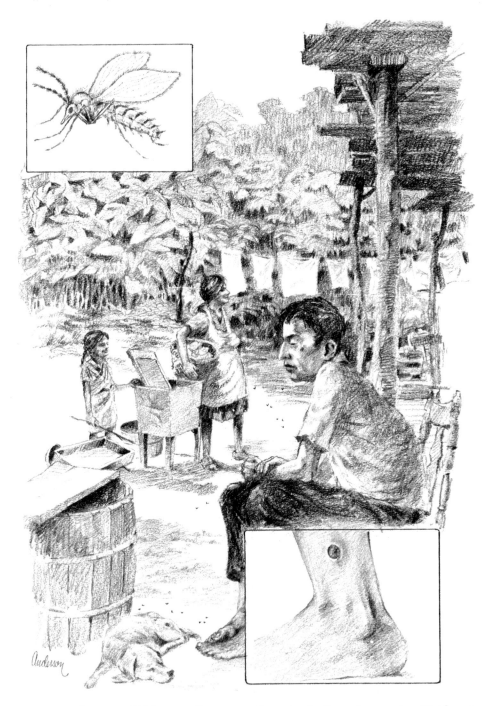

Fig. 4-16. Leishmaniasis. Phlebotomus flies serve as the vector for the various species of *Leishmania*, transmitting promastigotes at the time of biting. Invasion of local tissue cells, with reversion to amastigotes, results in skin lesions of varying kind and degree. Phlebotomus flies, while feeding, ingest amastigotes, which multiply and transform into promastigotes for further transmission.

nomic system based on molecular and immunologic concepts.

The relationship between immunity and infection is complex. Both humoral and cellular factors may be involved in the immunopathologic mechanisms of lesion pathogenesis. Animal model studies indicate that genetically controlled factors regulate the growth of *Leishmania* sp in mice.

Epidemiology. Distribution varies with the species. Natural reservoir hosts are dogs, cats, cattle, horses, sheep, and a variety of wild rodents. A wide variety of laboratory animals can be experimentally infected. The inability to find reservoir hosts among the lower animals in areas where humans have temporarily invaded and become infected represents an unsolved problem. Other arthropods in addition to phlebotomus flies are also being investigated as possible vectors (Fig. 4-16).

In addition to cyclic transmission, mechanical transmission may also occur where skin lesions are present. In some areas, artificial inoculation of the buttocks of children has been used to prevent deforming primary skin lesions from developing on the face. Vaccination against oriental sore has been widely used in the U.S.S.R. Amastigotes in the nasal and intestinal mucosa theoretically enable transmission by respiratory contact or fecal contamination.

Diagnosis. The diagnosis of the leishmaniases depends on the demonstration of the amastigotes in stained smears from skin lesions, blood, and bone marrow and in liver biopsies. Adjuncts such as serology (see Tables 15-1 and 15-2), skin testing, culture, and animal inoculation are often employed. All hemoflagellate infections produce an increase in serum globulin.

The leishmaniases produce both IgG and IgM as detectable by the fluorescent antibody test (FAT) and the indirect hemagglutination test (IHA). Both tests show cross-reactivity with *Trypanosoma cruzi* and *Mycobacterium* sp. Gel diffusion tests are less sensitive but give more detailed and specific information about individual antigenic systems. The leishmanin skin test, which uses an antigen prepared from cultured promastigotes, is analogous to the tuberculin or lepromin tests, the reaction being one of delayed hypersensitivity. The test is genus specific only. In most cutaneous and mucocutaneous infections the test becomes positive (within a few days after infection in some) and may remain positive for years. In visceral and disseminated cutaneous leishmaniases, however, the test remains negative during infection (often for years in the disseminated type), becoming positive after cure. Thus, a positive leishmanin skin test in both kala-azar and disseminated cutaneous leishmaniasis is a good sign indicating that cell-mediated immunity is developing, whereas a positive test in other cutaneous infections indicates infection but does not signify protective immunity.

In uncomplicated, self-curing cutaneous infections, antibody titers are low or negligible. However, when lymphatic involvement occurs serology becomes positive. Amastigotes are preferred to promastigotes as a source of antigen in most tests since the host's defenses are against amastigotes.

The gamma globulins reach high levels in the leishmaniases and their coagulation, flocculation, and precipitation is the basis of the formal gel test, antimony test (see Appendix B), and the older aqueous precipitation test. Although nonspecific, these tests are diagnostic of active kala-azar.

Leishmania tropica

Geographic distribution and epidemiology. Cutaneous leishmaniasis is endemic in the countries surrounding the Mediterranean Sea, in western and southern Asia, and central and northeast Africa. In the western hemisphere it is found in Central America, South America, and probably Mexico. Dogs and rodents serve as the chief reservoir hosts in many areas, although in some areas the

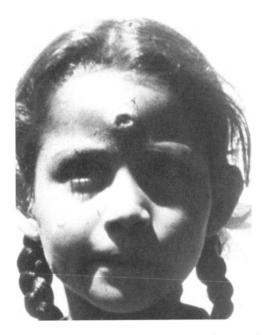

Fig. 4-17. Cutaneous leishmaniasis. Note the typical crateriform ulcer on forehead and also lesions on cheek. (Courtesy Dr. Antonio Peña Chavarría, Hospital, San Juan de Dios, San José, Costa Rica. Photo by J. W. B.)

reservoir hosts are unknown. Three indigenous cases of dermal leishmaniasis have been reported in Texas. Serologic evidence of *Leishmania* infection in another individual and in three dogs in the area suggests that dermal leishmaniasis may be epidemic in parts of south central Texas. *Lutzomyia* sp are the chief vectors in the New World. Since lesions occur in the skin, mechanical transmission by biting flies, such as *Stomoxys calcitrans*, the stable fly, may occur.

Throughout the Orient, infections are known as oriental sore, although other names in specific areas are used, such as Aleppo ulcer, Baghdad boil, Lahore sore, and Delhi boil. Though this disease is coextensive with kala-azar, the two are rarely present in the same area. In India, for example, oriental sore occurs in the dry western half of the Indo-Gangetic plain whereas kala-azar is found in the moist eastern portion. The variations in distribution of their respective vec-

tors are thought to explain this phenomenon. In the western hemisphere it is often difficult to distinguish oriental sore from the more common mucocutaneous forms and many investigators treat them as one entity (Fig. 4-17).

Symptomatology and pathology. The incubation period of cutaneous leishmaniasis is quite variable, ranging from 2 weeks to several years, with an average of 2 to 6 months. The primary lesion may be single or multiple. The initial lesion in all leishmaniases is a focus of proliferating dermal macrophages, some of which contain amastigotes. Multiplication of the parasites eventually destroys the host cell, and other local macrophages ingest the liberated amastigotes. At the site of inoculation a small red papule appears and increases in size, with a dry scaly scab forming on the surface. Satellite foci develop at the margin of the lesion, ulceration occurs, and the foci continue to extend their boundaries peripherally. Sloughing occurs, and a floor of granulation tissue is formed, surrounded by an area of red induration. Secondary bacterial infection is common. Lesions may take various forms. The verrucous, or vegetating, type presents a cauliflowerlike growth, whereas others appear as a keloid or lupoid form. Surrounding lymph nodes may be involved, with parasites present. Subcutaneous nodules that later break down may appear along the lymphatic chain. In the Old World two distinct types, the moist and the dry, have been described, each immunologically distinct from the other. The dry, urban type (*L. tropica* minor) is characterized by unbroken papules lasting for many months, with delayed ulceration, an incubation period of many months, abundant organisms in the lesion, and slight pathogenicity for mice. The moist, rural type (*L. tropica* major) shows weeping lesions that ulcerate rapidly; this type has a short incubation period, a short duration with only a few organisms in the sore, and a marked pathogenicity for

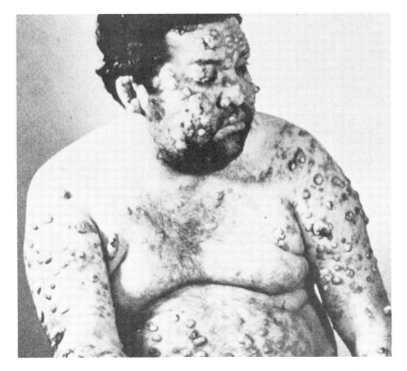

Fig. 4-18. Diffuse anergic cutaneous leishmaniasis. (AFIP 72-2312-13.)

mice. Infection confers lasting immunity only to the type concerned, although infection with the dry form appears to suppress severe development of the wet type when it is contracted.

Both types have also been reported from the western hemisphere. A diffuse cutaneous form, seen mainly in Venezuela, is characterized by a macrophage granuloma that causes thickening of the skin (Fig. 4-18) suggestive of lepromatous leprosy. Some consider this a new species, *Leishmania pifanoi*. The virtual absence of a cell-mediated reaction is suggested by the consistently negative leishmanin skin test and by the absence of lymphocytes in the lesion. Cure, with the aid of chemotherapy, is dependent on developing a cell-mediated immunity. On the other hand, in the ulcerating, satellite-foci-forming lesion, referred to previously, a pathologically hyperfunctioning cell-mediated reaction may be suppressed, for example, with steroids.

A relatively mild cutaneous leishmaniasis in Mexico and South America with reservoir hosts being wild rodents and opossums has been called *Leishmania mexicana*. Some classify Chiclero ulcer, referred to later under *Leishmania braziliense*, as *L. m. mexicana*.

Diagnosis. Diagnosis is made by microscopic examination of Romanowsky-stained scrapings from the indurated edge of the lesion. The amastigotes, normally intracellular, may be expressed from the cells during the trauma of making the dab smear. Culture in suitable blood agar media (an NNN type of medium to which 200 to 500 units of penicillin per ml of overlay are added to control bacteria) yields promastigotes. The Montenegro skin test (leishmanin skin test), a delayed hypersensitive reaction from the intradermal inoculation of dead promastigotes of any species of *Leishmania* or the organism *Trypanosoma cruzi*, although posi-

Table 4-2. Treatment for leishmaniasis and trypanosomiasis

Infection	Drug	Adult dose*	Pediatric dose*
Leishmaniasis			
L. braziliensis (American mucocutaneous leishmaniasis) and			
L. mexicana (American cutaneous leishmaniasis)			
Drug of choice	Stibogluconate sodium[1,2]	Not certain, probably 600 mg IM or IV/d × 6-10d (may be repeated)	10 mg/kg/d IM or IV (max. 600 mg/d) × 6-10d
Alternatives	Amphotericin B	0.25 to 1 mg/kg by slow infusion daily or every 2d for up to 8 wk	0.25 to 1 mg/kg by slow infusion daily or every 2d for up to 8 wk
	Cycloguanil pamoate in oil[3,4]	350 mg base IM	< 1 yr: 140 mg IM; 1-5 yr: 280 mg IM
L. donovani (kala-azar, visceral leishmaniasis)			
Drug of choice	Stibogluconate sodium[1,5,6]	600 mg/d IM or IV × 6-10d (may be repeated)	10 mg/kg/d IM or IV (max. 600 mg/d) × 6-10d
Alternative	Pentamidine[1,5]	2-4 mg/kg/d IM for up to 15 doses	2-4 mg/kg/d IM for up to 15 doses
L. tropica (oriental sore, cutaneous leishmaniasis)			
Drug of choice	Stibogluconate sodium[1]	600 mg/d IM or IV × 6-10d (may be repeated)	10 mg/kg/d IM or IV (max. 600 mg/d) × 6-10d
Alternatives	Topical agents[7]		
Trypanosomiasis			
T. cruzi (South American trypanosomiasis, Chagas' disease)			
Drug of choice	Nifurtimox[1,8]	5 mg/kg/d orally in 4 divided doses, increasing by 2 mg/kg/d every 2 wk until dose reaches 15-17 mg/kg/d	
Alternatives	None		
T. b. gambiense; T. b. rhodesiense (African trypanosomiasis, sleeping sickness)			
Hemolymphatic stage			
Drug of choice	Suramin[1]	100-200 mg (test dose) IV, then 1 gm IV on days 1, 3, 7, 14 and 21	20 mg/kg on days 1, 3, 7, 14 and 21
Alternative	Pentamidine[1]	4 mg/kg/d IM × 10d	4 mg/kg/d IM × 10d
Late disease with CNS involvement			
Drug of choice	Melarsoprol[1,9]	2-3.6 mg/kg/d IV × 3 doses; after 1 wk 3.6 mg/kg/d IV × 3 doses; repeat again after 10-21 days	18-25 mg/kg total over 1 mo. Initial dose of 0.36 mg/kg IV, increasing gradually to max. 3.6 mg/kg at intervals of 1-5 d for total of 9-10 doses
Alternatives	Tryparsamide[4]	One injection of 30 mg/kg every 5d to total of 12 injections; may be repeated after 1 mo.	Unknown
	plus suramin[1]	One injection of 10 mg/kg every 5d to total of 12 injections; may be repeated after 1 mo.	Unknown

*See opposite page.

Table 4-2. Treatment for leishmaniasis and trypanosomiasis—cont'd

Adverse effects of antiparasitic drugs

Stibogluconate sodium (Pentostam) (Antimony sodium gluconate)
  Adverse effects similar to those of antimony potassium tartrate, but less frequent and usually less severe
Amphotericin B USP (Fungizone)
  Frequent: renal damage; hypokalemia; fever; thrombophlebitis; nausea during infusion
  Occasional: hypomagnesemia; normocytic, normochromic anemia
  Rare: hemorrhagic gastroenteritis; blood dyscrasias; rash; blurred vision; peripheral neuropathy; convulsions; anaphylaxis; arrhythmias
Cycloguanil pamoate (Camolar)
  Occasional: tenderness at injection site
  Rare: allergic reactions; blood dyscrasias
Pentamidine isethionate (Lomidine)
  Frequent: hypotension; vomiting; blood dyscrasias; renal damage; pain at injection site
  Occasional: may aggravate diabetes; hypoglycemia; shock; liver damage
  Rare: Herxheimer-type reaction
Nifurtimox (Bayer 2502; Lampit)
  Frequent: anorexia; vomiting; weight loss; loss of memory; sleep disorders; tremor; paresthesias; weakness; polyneuritis
  Rare: convulsions
Antimony potassium tartrate USP
  Frequent: painful local inflammation following leakage during intravenous injection; coughing and vomiting when intravenous administration is rapid; muscle pain and joint stiffness; bradycardia
  Occasional: colic; diarrhea; rash; pruritus; myocardial damage
  Rare: liver damage; hemolytic anemia; renal damage; shock; sudden death
Suramin sodium (Germanin)
  Frequent: vomiting; pruritus; urticaria; paresthesia; hyperesthesia of hands and feet; photophobia; peripheral neuropathy
  Occasional: kidney damage; blood dyscrasias; shock
Melarsoprol (Mel B)
  Frequent: myocardial damage; albuminuria; hypertension; colic; Herxheimer-type reaction; encephalopathy; vomiting; peripheral neuropathy
  Rare: shock
Tryparsamide
  Frequent: nausea; vomiting
  Occasional: impaired vision; optic atrophy; fever; exfoliative dermatitis; allergic reactions; tinnitus

From The Medical Letter, Inc., 56 Harrison Street, New Rochelle, N.Y.
*The letter d indicates day.
1. In the U.S.A., this drug is available from the Parasitic Diseases Division, Center for Disease Control, Atlanta, Georgia 30333; telephone 404-329-3311.
2. Must be used for anergic diffuse leishmaniasis.
3. Alternative for *L. mexicana* only.
4. Not available in the U.S.A.
5. Pentamidine should be used for failures with stibogluconate and sometimes for initial treatment in cases from Sudan (which are often resistant to antimonials). All solutions should be protected from light to avoid production of hepatotoxic compounds.
6. For the African form of visceral leishmaniasis therapy may have to be extended to at least 30 days and may have to be repeated.
7. In patients with few or single lesions that are not cosmetically significant, topical or local treatment may be preferable to the risk of toxicity from systemic antimonial compounds.
8. In infections with *T. cruzi* nifurtimox is useful in destroying extracellular trypanosomes in blood; it may also suppress viable organisms remaining in the chronic phase.
9. In frail patients, begin with as little as 18 mg and increase the dose progressively. Pretreatment with suramin has been advocated for debilitated patients.

tive, is no index of immunity. Response may occur early in infection or many years after cure. The serology is discussed under leishmaniases in general.

Treatment. Those workers who feel that cutaneous leishmaniasis is limited to the skin consider topical applications adequate treatment, along with care to prevent secondary infections with cleanliness and the use of antibiotics. Quinacrine (Atabrine) solution (10%) infiltrated around the lesion, with repeated injections of 2 ml at weekly intervals, is recommended. Some report good results with 2% berberine sulfate. Also employed is solid carbon dioxide (dry ice) applied directly over the lesion. Infrared and radiotherapy are also used. In those areas where self-healing is common, specific treatment is seldom necessary. Where disfiguring, nonhealing lesions of the face or severe, multiple lesions persist for 6 months or longer, antimonial drugs, in spite of their toxicity, are indicated. Secondary bacterial infection is common. Diffuse cutaneous leishmaniasis is difficult to treat. Reports of some success with immersion in hot water twice daily indicate that heat therapy warrants further investigation for skin lesions. Those workers considering cutaneous lesions as capable of metastasizing prefer systemic treatment as well as the use of topical applicants. Sodium stibogluconate (Triostam, Pentostam) is considered the drug of choice in the dosage of 600 mg given intramuscularly or intravenously daily for 6 to 10 days (Table 4-2).

Leishmania braziliensis

Geographic distribution and epidemiology. The species *Leishmania braziliensis* produces a great variety of skin and mucous membrane lesions seen in the western hemisphere (Mexico, Central America, and South America). The greatest disease concentration is in central Brazil, but a high frequency also occurs in the forested areas east of the Andes, namely, Colombia, Venezuela, Para-

guay, Bolivia, Ecuador, and Peru. Some workers prefer to further subdivide *L. braziliensis* into a variety of subspecies, whereas others consider the leishmania as one etiologic agent. Although the term *L. braziliensis* refers to the agent of mucocutaneous leishmaniasis (Fig. 4-19), in many parts of the Americas the disease spares the mucous membranes and is indistinguishable clinically from oriental sore. The name *Leishmania tropica* has been reserved by some for the oriental sore confined solely to the skin in the eastern hemisphere. Some workers believe that the propensity to involve mucous membranes and cartilage is not a characteristic of the organism but varies with host resistance and malnutrition.

Although phlebotomus flies serve as the chief vector, the presence of weeping lesions on the exposed body surface affords an excellent means for mechanical transmission by

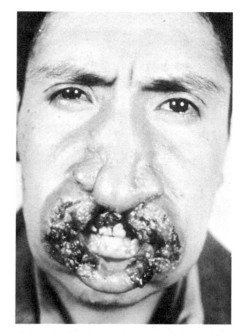

Fig. 4-19. Mucocutaneous leishmaniasis. Note the involvement of the nasolabial structure. (Departmento de Patología, Hospital 2 de Mayo, Lima, Peru. Courtesy of B.H.K.)

biting flies, particularly in crowded areas. In many endemic areas, natural reservoir hosts remain undiscovered. Dogs, though naturally infected, are not as commonly involved as in the Orient. However, in the valleys high in the Andes the sandfly *Lutzomyia* is the vector and the dog is the reservoir host, while in the lowlands forests of Central and South America flies of the *Phlebotomus* genus are the chief vector and forest rodents, such as the agouti and opossum, are the reservoir hosts.

The disease is rural, chiefly of low-lying forest areas where vegetation is dense, rainfall is heavy, and the climate is hot and humid. On the other hand, the disease described from the high mountain areas of the Andes is associated with a dry, cool climate.

Symptomatology and pathology. The primary skin lesions appear 10 days to several months after the infecting sandfly bite. The first lesions, single or multiple, are usually papules that may burn and itch. The papules then become nodules that may or may not ulcerate. Lesions may heal spontaneously at any stage. They have a tendency to metastasize along lymphatic channels. The characteristic type of lesion is to some extent related to the geographic location; this type has been related both to the climate and to the site of fly bites. For example, in some areas of South America, lesions appear as cauliflower masses. In Peru, *Leishmania peruviana* causes a dry skin nodule that resembles a warty growth and is called uta. Neither of these types tends to ulcerate or metastasize. In Mexico, where *L. mexicana* is the organism, and in northern Guatemala the disease is found commonly on the ears of chicle-plantation workers such that extensive erosion of the earlobe cartilage results in marked deformity, but there are few metastatic lesions. In this case, the disease is known as Chiclero ulcer, the badge of the chicle workers. In warmer, moister areas, ulcerating lesions similar to oriental sore predominate.

These may be associated with the simultaneous erosion of nasal, septal, and palatine tissues known as espundia, or the mucocutaneous manifestations may appear decades after apparent healing of the primary skin lesion. Scraping of nasal mucosa may show leishmania long before mucocutaneous disease is recognized. Forest yaws (pian bois) may appear initially as a single, ulcerating lesion or, more frequently, may metastasize by way of the lymphatics and produce multiple cutaneous lesions with no nasopharyngeal metastasis. Panamanian leishmaniasis is characterized by a single or only a few shallow ulcers metastasizing as nodules via the lymphatics with no nasopharyngeal spread.

Epithelial hyperplasia, inflammation, and edema characterize the developing lesions. Ulcers have a granulating base. Developing lesions usually are painful. Involvement of the mucous membranes results not only in mutilating deformity but also paves the way for secondary bacterial invaders. Death may result from sepsis, inanition, or respiratory complications. The high prevalence of granulomatous lesions about the mouth, pharynx, and the cartilaginous parts of the nose has been attributed to the ability of the parasites to grow at sites of lower skin temperatures, the presence of a good capillary filter mechanism, and the lack of a cellular immune response on the part of the cartilaginous tissues.

Diagnosis. The varied appearance of the lesions may result in confusion with some of the dermatomycoses, leprosy, tropical ulcer, and other skin diseases. As with *L. tropica*, organisms can be recovered from the edges of the lesions. Lymph nodes or curettage of nasal mucosa may also reveal the intracellular parasite. Parasites may be very scanty, particularly with chronic disease. In this case, aspirated material may be cultured on a variety of special blood agar media (Appendix B). The Montenegro skin test, using a culture of promastigotes as antigen, will produce an erythematous wheal in 48 hours but is uniformly positive only in late cases. It is considered the method of choice in the diagnosis of mucocutaneous leishmaniasis and is especially useful in those cases where the organisms have disappeared from the lesions.

Treatment. Topical applications may be used as for *L. tropica*, but because of the metastasizing nature of the disease, systemic drugs are recommended. Sodium stibogluconate (Triostam, Pentostam), as indicated for *L. tropica* (600 mg intramuscularly or intravenously daily for 6 to 10 days), is the drug of choice. For details see Table 4-2.

Leishmania donovani

Geographic distribution and epidemiology. Visceral leishmaniasis (kala-azar) has an extensive distribution and a wide variety of clinical forms. In areas around the Mediterranean (North Africa, Greece, Italy, France, and Spain) and eastward through southern Russia to China, it is often coextensive with oriental sore (but distinct in some localities). Common vectors are species of *Phlebotomus*, with dogs, jackals, and foxes as reservoir hosts. Infections occur chiefly in infants. Another variation is found among adults in northeast India and Bangladesh with no known natural reservoir host. In East Africa (Kenya, Uganda, Sudan) a more virulent form uses wild rodents as reservoirs.

Throughout Central and South America dogs and foxes are the chief reservoirs, and a variety referred to by some as *Leishmania chagasi*, which infects infants, is transmitted by *Lutzomyia* sp. Infections have also been reported in Mexico. The disease is primarily one of the home environment in which the flies take up their abode. The finding of organisms in the feces, urine, and nasal discharge of infected patients suggests these as possible sources on occasion. In many areas, dogs are commonly infected and play a major reservoir role. In India, however, where dogs are less commonly involved, it is be-

lieved that the insect vectors maintain a fly-to-human relationship. In Morocco and Iran there is a high incidence of canine infection, but human disease is rare. In the northeastern part of Kenya, where the insect vectors are not domestic, reservoir hosts remain unknown. Experimentally, a wide variety of animals may be infected.

The high incidence of infection in infants in the Mediterranean area at one time gave rise to the creation of a distinct species *Leishmania infantum;* it is now believed to be synonymous with *L. donovani.* In China, infections, when present (rare according to a 1978 survey), occur predominately in young children, whereas in India young adults are most commonly infected. In South America, infants and young children dominate the age groups involved.

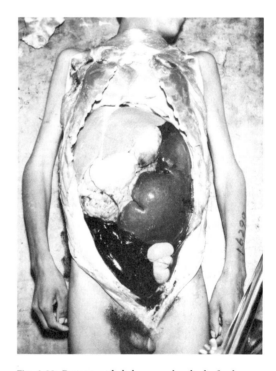

Fig. 4-20. Patient with kala-azar who died of a hemorrhage after spleen biopsy. Note the greatly enlarged spleen. (AFIP A-45364. From Schmidt, G. D., and Roberts, L. S.: Foundations of parasitology, St. Louis, 1977, The C. V. Mosby Co.)

In general, males are more commonly infected than females. Infections throughout endemic areas are associated chiefly with persons living in an environment of poor sanitation, poor housing, and a hot, humid climate.

Symptomatology and pathology. The incubation period of the disease is usually several months but may be as long as 10 years. Skin lesions, when present, are confined to tiny papules that soon disappear. Symptoms are protean in nature and usually begin with undulating fever and chills, lasting for several weeks and frequently confused with malaria. Two fever spikes a day are common with kala-azar and are said to be of differential diagnostic value. Some patients exhibit a characteristic triad of fever, wasting, and protuberant abdomen (secondary to hepatosplenomegaly) but continue to work and feel well despite far-advanced disease. In acute cases, death may occur within several weeks, whereas chronic cases may last 2 to 3 years. Spontaneous cures without treatment are rare.

The disease is primarily one of the reticuloendothelial cells of the liver, spleen, bone marrow, and visceral lymph nodes, and hyperplasia of tissues and organs occurs throughout the body. Invasion of the gastrointestinal tract may produce a dysentery suggestive of invasion by enteric pathogens. Enlargement of the spleen (Fig. 4-20) usually exceeds enlargement of the liver; both result in the typical swollen abdomen. Ascites is noticeably absent. Microscopic examination of internal organs reveals congestion, hyperplasia, numerous parasites, and degeneration. A progressive anemia and leukopenia predispose the patient to secondary bacterial infection, a common sequela. Edema of the skin, emaciation, dys-

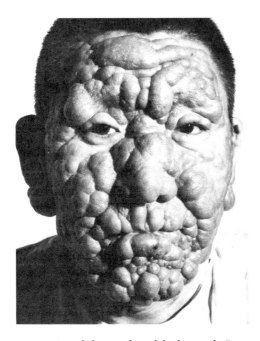

Fig. 4-21. Post–kala-azar dermal leishmanoid. Patient responded very well to treatment. (Photograph by Robert E. Kuntz. From Schmidt, G. D., and Roberts, L. S.: Foundations of parasitology, St. Louis, 1977, The C. V. Mosby Co.)

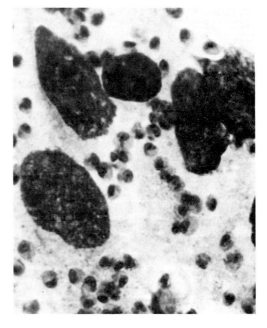

Fig. 4-22. *Leishmania donovani* in macrophages from infected spleen. (Courtesy Department of Epidemiology and Public Health, University of Miami School of Medicine.)

entery, bleeding of the gums and other mucous membranes, cachexia, and eventually death occur in the majority of untreated cases. Immune complexes (IgG, IgM, and C_3) have been found in the glomeruli of patients with kala-azar. The major complications of visceral leishmaniasis are pulmonary- or intestinal-superimposed infections which usually prove fatal in the absence of treatment.

Survivors usually have lasting immunity. The appearance of the pigmented areas in the skin followed by nodule formation in which parasites can be detected may occur, usually a year or so after apparently successful treatment. This condition is known as post–kala-azar dermal leishmanoid (Fig. 4-21).

Diagnosis. In endemic areas clinical manifestations may lead to a presumptive diagnosis, but differentiation from malaria, dysentery, undulant fever, and a variety of other diseases must be made. Confirmation depends on demonstration of the parasites in direct smears or culture of material from the liver, spleen, bone marrow, blood, and lymph nodes (Fig. 4-22). Although splenic aspiration or biopsy produces the greatest diagnostic yield, the safer bone marrow study is usually the preferred technique. Peripheral blood smears may sometimes be positive. Animal inoculation is helpful but requires a month or longer for confirmation. A striking increasing in gamma globulin is suggestive of the diagnosis (Appendix B). The complement fixation test is of value, particularly in early infections before the albumin-globulin (A/G) ratio has been altered. The Montenegro skin test is nonspecific but helpful as supportive evidence, being negative during active disease but positive after successful treatment.

Treatment. Chemotherapy consists chiefly of the use of the pentavalent antimony compounds. Toxicity is much lower than for the trivalent compounds, although the latter are used in some areas of the Orient because of their lower cost. For details see Table 4-2. Because of the severity of the disease, supportive care in the form of a diet rich in proteins, vitamins, and iron is essential.

Trypanosomiases

The trypanosomes, as recommended by Hoare, have been divided into two groups on the basis of characteristics in both the vertebrate and invertebrate hosts. One group, formerly known as the *lewisi* group, is now identified in the section Stercoraria and contains the subgenus Schizotrypanum in which *Trypanosoma cruzi* and *Trypanosoma rangeli* are present. The other group, now section Salivaria, contains the subgenus Trypanozoon in which are found the former *brucei-evansi* group. *Trypanosoma brucei gambiense* and *Trypanosoma brucei rhodesiense* are in this subgenus.

Trypanosoma cruzi

Geographic distribution. The hemoflagellate *Trypanosoma cruzi* causes American trypanosomiasis, or Chagas' disease. It is confined to the western hemisphere, found chiefly in Mexico, Central America, and South America. Various species of triatomid bugs (Reduviidae), or kissing bugs, are the vectors, or arthropod hosts. Infected bugs

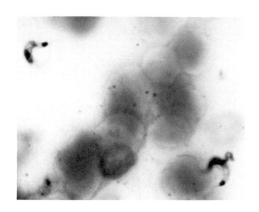

Fig. 4-23. *Trypanosoma cruzi* in blood. Note the short C-shaped trypomastigotes with large kinetoplast. (Courtesy Department of Epidemiology and Public Health, University of Miami School of Medicine.)

and reservoir hosts have been reported in the United States, and authentic human infections have been contracted in the southern states. Dogs, cats, opossums, raccoons, armadillos, monkeys, and other animals may serve as reservoir hosts. The organism has been reported in Maryland, Florida, Georgia, Texas, Arizona, New Mexico, California, Alabama, and Louisiana. Over 14 species of mammals in the United States have been found infected by *T. cruzi*. The presence of naturally occurring infections in animals in the United States, along with the authentic reports of infections in humans, emphasizes the importance of the awareness of physicians in this country to this disease.

Morphology and life cycle. The trypomastigote is quite typical of this species. It is about 20 μm in length, much shorter and stubbier than the other trypomastigotes of humans. The nucleus is centrally located and stains a deep violet to black color. The ki-netoplast, located at the posterior end of the organism, stains similarly. It is quite large, is oval to round, and consists of a blepharoplast and parabasal body appearing as one, because of the fusing of the stain. This kinetoplast is very characteristic of *T. cruzi* because it is much larger than in other *Trypanosoma* species. The organisms are predominately C-shaped in blood smears, another distinguishing feature of this species. The undulating membrane arising from the kinetoplast and extending anteriorly emerges from the border as a free flagellum. It is not as well developed as in *T. b. gambiense* and *T. b. rhodesiense* (Fig. 4-23).

Triatomid bugs defecate at the time of feeding. The metacyclic or infective trypomastigotes are deposited with the feces on the skin or mucous membranes. These parasites may penetrate intact skin and mucous membranes, or enter hair follicles. Trypomastigotes do not multiply in the vertebrate

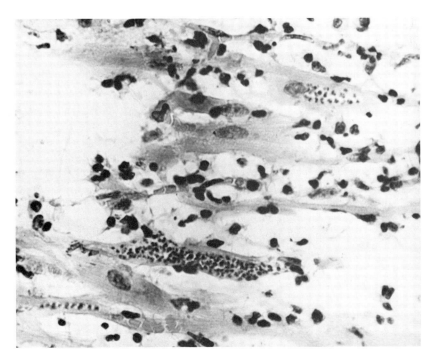

Fig. 4-24. Nests of amastigotes of *Trypanosoma cruzi*, the cause of acute myositis in Chagas' disease. (Photograph by Robert E. Kuntz.)

host. Invading organisms enter tissue cells and revert to amastigotes; in the cells localized multiplication (Fig. 4-24) takes place similar to the species of the *Leishmania*. Other trypomastigotes are carried in the bloodstream and invade leukocytes, monocytes, and lymphocytes with reversion again to amastigotes. Freely circulating trypomastigotes, as well as intracellular amastigotes liberated from destroyed host cells, spread throughout the body, invading any organ system, particularly the reticuloendothelial system and heart muscle. Transitory epimastigotes and promastigotes can be seen in the interstitial spaces.

In the gut of the insect the ingested trypomastigotes become epimastigotes and multiply by longitudinal division. Movement to the hindgut follows, with reversion to the metacyclic trypomastigotes that pass in the feces to initiate infection in humans and other vertebrates.

Epidemiology. The transmission and incidence of this disease are intimately associated with the environment and habitats of both humans and insects. The disease is most common in the tropics where living conditions are primitive, but recently increased incidence of the disease in urban areas of South America has also been reported. Natives, living in adobe mud huts, may bring bugs into the home with firewood; the bugs then take up residence in the cracks and crevices of the mud walls. At night the bugs leave their lairs in the walls and look for warm-blooded hosts. Though quite large, these bugs are able to feed undisturbed, frequently on the conjunctiva of the eye. Animals living in close association with the family become reservoir hosts (Fig. 4-25). *T. cruzi* can cross the placental barrier to the fetus, and infants at birth with advanced Chagas' disease (megaesophagus) have been reported in Chile. The hazards of blood transfusion are apparent.

The prevalence of the disease in sylvatic form in the United States, but very rare in humans, attests to the importance of improved living conditions. Smooth plastered walls and strong sources of light serve as deterrents to the intrusion of the triatomid bug into human abode.

Symptomatology. American trypanosomiasis may be seen as an acute or chronic disease. The acute form, commonest and most severe in children less than 5 years of age, is characterized by an initial chagoma reaction at the site of the infective bite. This hard, red, hot, tender plaque usually appears within a few hours after the bite and may last for months. Although the chagoma may appear on any part of the body, the characteristic location is on the face; on the upper eyelid it causes Romaña's sign (Fig. 4-26). There may be localized adenopathy. The chagoma may or may not be present at the time of the initial febrile response. In the acute form the initial febrile response appears within 2 to 3 weeks of the infective bite and is associated with chills, bone and muscle pain, malaise, hepatosplenomegaly, and varying degrees of cardiac failure; at this stage, trypomastigotes can be demonstrated in the blood. Patients with severe cases may die in a few days; in others, the disease may become chronic, with intermittent attacks of fever and heart failure occurring.

In the chronic type, usually seen in adults, there is frequently no history of an acute illness, and the patient has a low-grade fever and cardiac arrhythmias or failure of varying degree. Particularly in Brazil, this form of the disease is believed to be the cause of sudden death in apparently well young adults. The heart frequently becomes enlarged and flabby, with loss of muscle tone resulting from destroyed nerve ganglia. Electrocardiographic changes most commonly seen are alterations in the primary T waves, an increase of the P-R interval, and an injured ischemic pattern. Surveys in Brazil indicate that 30% of adult deaths result from this organism. In these cases, parasites may not be detected in the blood by either direct

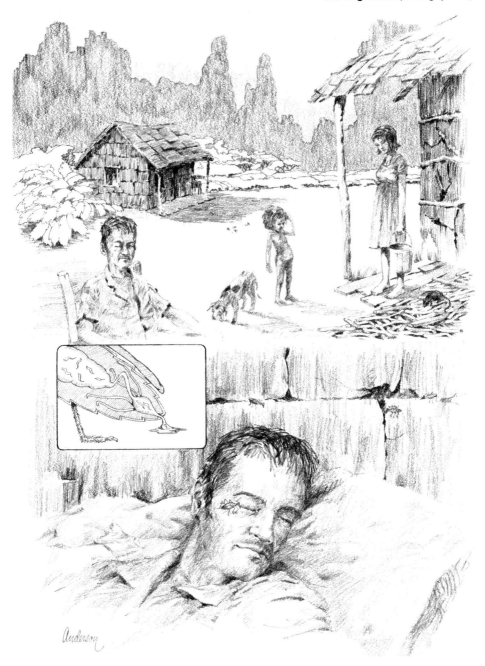

Fig. 4-25. Chagas' disease. Triatomid bugs living in cracks and crevices of adobe mud huts forage at night, searching for warm-blooded hosts. Biting occurs commonly on the conjunctiva, followed by defecation. Metacyclic trypomastigotes in the feces penetrate the wound or possibly the intact mucosa. Reversion to amastigotes occurs after penetration of local tissue cells. Multiplication results in a chagoma. Circulating trypomastigotes may invade cardiac muscle and other tissues of the body. Bugs, feeding on an infected host, ingest trypomastigotes, which multiply in gut, become metacyclic trypomastigotes, and continue the life cycle.

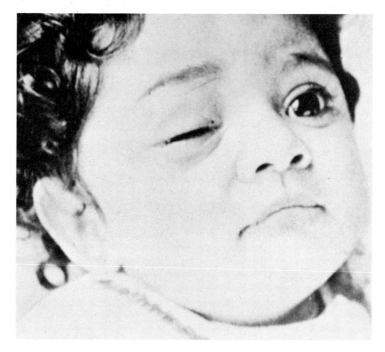

Fig. 4-26. Romaña's sign. Note the unilateral palpebral and periorbital edema. (AFIP 62-3934-6.)

smear or xenodiagnosis, and the diagnosis rests upon the Machado test, a complement-fixation reaction. Although the complement-fixation titers remain high, the absence of parasites suggests some other mechanism for the continuing disease. Also seen are meningoencephalitis, primarily in the acute form in young children, and gastrointestinal symptoms, primarily of the subacute or chronic type.

Pathology. The amastigotes of *T. cruzi* multiply in the cells of many tissues; the heart is most affected. Myocardial fibrosis may result. Studies suggest that a major effect may be the result of destruction of cardiac ganglia, with resultant dilatation and hypertrophy, cardiac arrhythmias, and right bundle branch block (Fig. 4-24).

Reports indicate that T-lymphocytes from patients with Chagas' disease become activated by a cross-reactive heart cell antigen, suggesting that an autoimmune mechanism

can be established in some acute cases and perpetuated in chronic cases by continuous antigenic stimulation. This autoimmune destruction of heart cells is believed to be produced by delayed hypersensitivity and mediated by *T. cruzi*–sensitized T-lymphocytes. There is also evidence of damage to nerves and ganglia in the muscular walls of the viscera, resulting in dilatation and atony (megaesophagus and megacolon) of any part of the alimentary tract. Nodular foci in the brain or meningoencephalitis may ensue. Parasites can be found in the sediment of the spinal fluid or in the neuroglial cells of the brain nodules. Rupturing of packets of amastigotes (pseudocysts) is accompanied by an acute inflammatory response with subsequent sequelae of degeneration and necrosis of nerve cells resulting, it is believed, from the release of toxins. Increases in IgM and IgG during acute infection suggest the inherent danger in the use of immunosuppressive drugs and the presence of debilitating diseases which suppress the immune mechanism.

Diagnosis. Diagnosis is often made clinically in South American countries by Romaña's sign. If lesions are examined early enough, amastigotes may be found in stained scrapings of the chagoma. The scarcity of the trypomastigotes in the circulating blood makes examination of blood smears relatively useless, except during acute exacerbations when examination of the buffy coat may help. Xenodiagnosis, the feeding of clean bugs on the suspected patient and the subsequent examination of the bug's feces for parasites, is very useful. The complement-fixation test (Machado) and the intradermal skin test are also useful aids in diagnosis, as well as animal inoculation and artificial culture of suspected blood and tissue biopsies. For acute infections the complement-fixation test is probably the most useful of all diagnostic procedures. Purified antigen from culture organisms gives a high degree of accuracy. A rising titer in acute Chagas' disease is significant (see Tables 15-1 and 15-2). The anti–sheep cell reactivity shown by the sera of many patients requires absorption with sheep cells prior to being tested for *T. cruzi*. Titers of 1:8 are significant. The indirect hemagglutination antibody (IHA) test, positive in both chronic and acute disease, is also a preferred test with titers of 1:32 as significant. Both tests are recommended for use by the Center for Disease Control diagnostic laboratory.

The presence of a circulating antibody (EVI antibody) in the endocardium, blood vessels, and interstitium of striated muscle of patients with Chagas' disease, and its absence in controls is indicative of heart involvement. The presence of these antigenic determinants in *Trypanosoma b. rhodesiense* also suggests that an EVI antibody may be induced by a cross-reacting antigen in Rhodesian sleeping sickness. Heart in-

volvement has been observed in this disease also.

Since this disease bears a similarity to visceral leishmaniasis in that both are tissue-invading diseases caused by the amastigotes, which are morphologically indistinguishable, one must be careful to differentiate the two by xenodiagnosis and the immunologic and cultural methods available.

Treatment. Treatment for Chagas' disease is generally unsatisfactory. Bayer 2502, a nitrofurfurylidene derivative, has shown some promising results. The dosage schedule is quite complicated but is obtainable from the Parasitic Disease Drug Service of the Center for Disease Control, Atlanta, Georgia. The alternative drug recommended is primaquine phosphate at the level of 26.3 mg (15 mg base) for 7 to 10 days. Dosages in excess of 26.3 mg per day for 14 days may cause hemolytic anemia, particularly in patients with a deficiency of glucose-6-phosphate dehydrogenase (G6PD) in the red cells. This is most common in blacks. The drug, although effective against the trypomastigotes, does not destroy the amastigotes.

Trypanosoma rangeli

Trypanosoma rangeli (*T. ariarii*), a member of the *lewisi* group like *T. cruzi*, is infective for humans but nonpathogenic. It has been reported from monkeys, dogs, and opossums in areas of Central and South America. Unlike *T. cruzi*, trypomastigotes are discharged in the salivary secretion at time of biting and thus initiate the infection in humans. Also, unlike *T. cruzi*, longitudinal division of trypomastigotes takes place in the vertebrate host. No intracellular amastigotes have been observed. The trypomastigotes in humans average 30 μm in length and have a relatively small kinetoplast, more posteriorly located than that in *T. cruzi*. *Rhodnius prolixus*, the triatomid bug, is the chief invertebrate host. Serology, morphology, invasion of the salivary glands by *T. rangeli*, and transmission by bite should be considered in the differentiation between *T. rangeli* and *T. cruzi*.

African trypanosomes

Geographical distribution and epidemiology. The African trypanosomes (section Salivaria) belong to a group of closely related pleomorphic forms. Three subspecies are recognized as distinct, although morphologically indistinguishable. They are *Trypanosoma brucei brucei*, *Trypanosoma brucei gambiense* and *Trypanosoma brucei rhodesiense*. *T. b. brucei* represents the ancestral form in this complex. It is a natural parasite of wild game in Africa, particularly the antelope, the natural reservoir host, and is nonpathogenic and noninfective for humans. *T. b. brucei*, however, is highly pathogenic for domestic livestock (sheep, goats, donkeys, camels, dogs, pigs, horses, and other animals) as well as some native animals, causing the disease "nagana." Trypanosomiasis in domestic animals in Africa has had a far-reaching effect on the retardation in growth and development of that continent. The discovery of fossil remains of tsetses in North America has suggested the ravages of trypanosomiasis as an explanation for the demise of some prehistoric animals.

Normal human serum has been shown in vitro to have a powerful trypanocidal action on a laboratory strain of *T. b. rhodesiense* but none at all on *T. b. gambiense*. *T. b. brucei* cannot infect humans because of this trypanocidal property. However, individuals, either because of other diseases or malnutrition, who have had this trypanocidal property diminished can become infected, and the trypanosomes in such patients become known as *T. b. rhodesiense*. This is an explanation offered for the establishment of trypanosomes in man. The parasite then becomes, it is postulated, serum resistant and capable of being cyclically transmitted to any human. If passaged for any time through animal hosts it then reverts to *T. b.*

brucei. It has been suggested that *T. b. gambiense* arose in a similar manner, but, because of environmental factors, has had a prolonged man-tsetse-man relationship leading to the development of a "fixed" serum resistance not readily lost by passage through nonhuman hosts. This longer human relationship also is supported by the apparent better adaptibility to man than in the case of *T. b. rhodesiense*, which is more virulent.

The trypanosomes in Africa extend from 15°N to 25°S latitude, corresponding with the distribution of their arthropod vectors, the tsetse (*Glossina* sp). The principle vectors for *T. b. gambiense* are *Glossina palpalis* and *Glossina tachinoides* which are found mainly along the banks of rivers and lakes usually close to human habitation. This disease is commonly called West African or Gambian sleeping sickness. The chief vectors for *T. b. rhodesiense* are *Glossina morsitans*, *Glossina pallidipes* and *Glossina swynnertoni*. Infections are more restricted in distribution than for *T. b. gambiense* but overlapping in some areas. They are identified chiefly with the East African coast and the disease called East African or Rhodesian sleeping sickness.

Both sexes of tsetses are involved in the transmission of African sleeping sickness, unlike malaria, in which only female insects are involved. In addition to cyclic transmission, mechanical transmission may occur by means of various species of biting flies that, after having their blood meal interrupted, pass directly to another host with a soiled proboscis. This means becomes significant in congested areas where flies are numerous and the incidence of infection is high.

Tsetses are fairly long lived, have a long flight range, are daytime biters, and congregate in areas called "fly belts." The Gambian disease is more widespread, has a higher endemic rate, and is more commonly associated with epidemics, whereas the Rhodesian form is usually sporadic, more restricted, and of lower endemic intensity. Al-

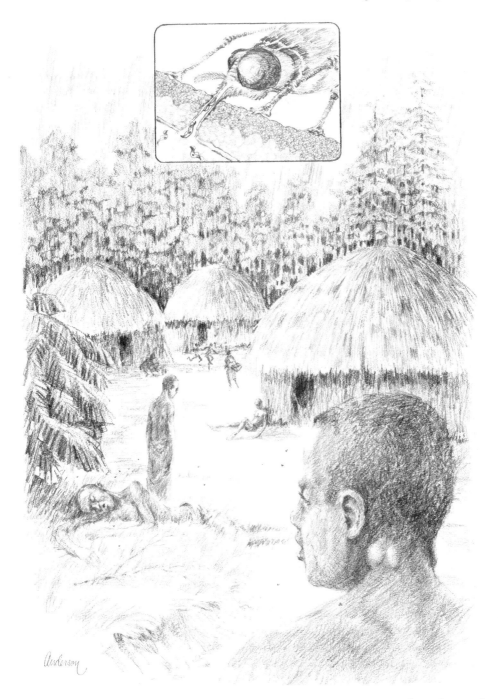

Fig. 4-27. African sleeping sickness. Tsetses of the genus *Glossina* transmit *Trypanosoma b. gambiense* and *T. b. rhodesiense* at time of feeding. Trypomastigotes in the lymphatics produce swelling of the posterior cervical lymph nodes (Winterbottom's sign). Invasion of the central nervous system may result in the sleeping sickness stage. Insects, feeding on an infected host ingest trypomastigotes, which multiply and, as metacyclic trypomastigotes in the salivary glands, reinfect other hosts at the time of biting.

though the general belief is that wild game animals play no role as reservoir hosts for *T. b. gambiense*, it seems apparent that they are the chief source of infections for *T. b. rhodesiense* (Fig. 4-27).

Morphology and life cycle. In the bloodstream and spinal fluid of humans, the trypomastigotes vary as to morphology, measuring 14 to 33 μm in length. The following three types appear: a short, broad form without a flagellum, a medium-sized, broad form with a flagellum, and a long, slender form also with a flagellum. Multiplication takes place by longitudinal division. The kinetoplast is small and oval to spherical in shape, features that help to differentiate the species from *T. cruzi*. C-shaped organisms, in contrast with *T. cruzi*, are rare (Fig. 4-28).

In lower animals the nucleus of the parasite, *T. b. rhodesiense*, shifts to a position posterior to the center, a condition only rarely seen in *T. b. gambiense*. This serves to distinguish the species, which, in humans, are morphologically identical.

Trypomastigotes taken in by tsetses at feeding time multiply by longitudinal division in the midgut. Migration forward into the salivary glands occurs with further multiplication as epimastigotes. Transformation to metacyclic trypomastigotes takes place before transmission to the vertebrate host at the time of biting.

Symptomatology and pathology. Although East African and West African sleeping sickness are generally separated by their place of origin and by course and character of illness (and will be discussed separately), it is well to remember that each clinical type is occasionally seen in the other area, and the clinical differences between the two forms may not always be as clear cut as presented.

In the West African (Gambian) type there is initially an interstitial inflammatory reaction at the site of the bite. This subsides and is followed in about a week by a tender erythematous nodule (chancre) which may or may not ulcerate. Within a few weeks the

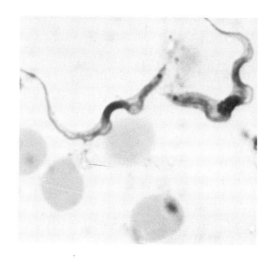

Fig. 4-28. *Trypanosoma b. gambiense* in blood. Note the elongated trypomastigotes with small kinetoplast. (Courtesy Department of Pathology, University of Miami School of Medicine.)

lesion subsides and therefore is rarely seen in natives, whereas it may be brought to the attention of the physician more frequently by infected foreigners. Trypomastigotes appear in the blood within 1 to 2 weeks after exposure. The patient is asymptomatic. Absence of symptoms may continue for weeks or even months. Invasion of the lymphatics and lymph nodes is associated with a painful, febrile period of night sweats, malaise, insomnia, and persistent headache lasting about a week. An afebrile period follows for about a week, and then symptoms appear again. During these repeated attacks trypomastigotes appear in the blood during the febrile period but are scanty or absent during the afebrile episode. In light-skinned races, a circinate, annular, or maculopapular rash, usually on the trunk, may appear at intervals. Each appearance, often elicited by heat, lasts only a few hours. Subcutaneous, peripheral, and facial edema may occur. Generalized lymphadenopathy is present in most cases. The enlarged posterior cervical chain nodes are most striking (Winterbottom's sign, Fig. 4-29). During the early slave-trading days this was used as a screening mechanism for

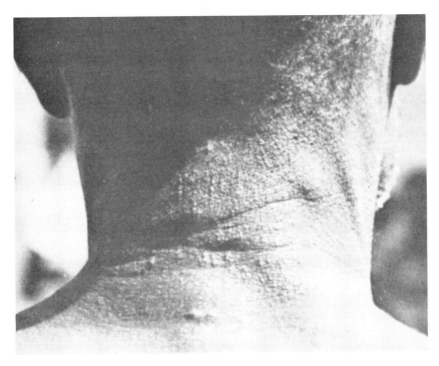

Fig. 4-29. Winterbottom's sign. Note the enlarged posterior cervical lymph nodes. (AFIP 74-8337.)

weeding out unfit slaves for shipment abroad. Aspiration of lymph nodes may reveal parasites. Axillary and inguinal lymph nodes are also often enlarged, accompanied by headache, weakness in the extremities, cramps, and arthritic pain. Dyspnea, interference with vision, anemia, and precordial pains are noted. Spontaneous remission of symptoms occurs, as with *T. b. rhodesiense* infection, from toxemia before the central nervous system becomes involved.

The central nervous system signs and symptoms follow within 6 months to 1 year. These symptoms may be intermittent over a period of months, or at any interval may become progressive and unrelenting. Daytime lethargy, apathy, and character changes appear, often alternating with nocturnal insomnia and irritability. Headache is classically constant. Motor and sensory changes and convulsions appear later. Kerandel's sign, delayed pain after pressure on large nerves such as the ulnar, is suggestive of West Afri-

can sleeping sickness when present. Motor changes include hemiplegia or paraplegia, fine tremors, unsteady gait, and slurred speech. Finally, the patient becomes comatose (Fig. 4-30). At this stage a puffy face may present a distinctive contrast to the marked malnutrition. Death usually results from malnutrition or intercurrent infection.

Because of the long incubation period in this form of trypanosomiasis, symptoms may not appear until the victim has left the endemic area. Craniotomy for brain tumor and shock therapy for psychiatric illness, as well as treatment for tuberculous meningitis, are not infrequent in such misdiagnosed cases.

The African trypanosomes are known to show great variation in antigenicity. Animal models indicate that specific antibodies produced against the parasite are rendered ineffective in controlling the infection because of the continual change and appearance of new antigens. Constant stimulation of the immune mechanism of the host results in

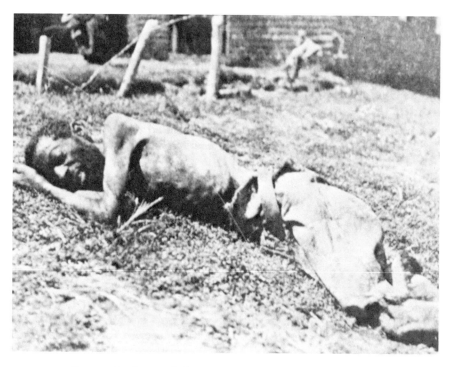

Fig. 4-30. Final stage of African sleeping sickness. (AFIP 219371-45.)

high levels of immunoglobulins, mostly non-specific IgM which appears to have no affinity for the parasites. IgG, likewise, lacks parasite specificity. It has been assumed that the variations in antigenicity have occurred principally in the bloodstream, with fluctuations in parasitemia. However, animal studies show that *T. b. brucei* and *T. b. gambiense* have various tissue forms in the internal organs and that the possibility of an occult visceral phase being present is suggested by the findings of amastigotes in the choroid plexus and other organs of rats infected with *T. b. brucei*. The presence of headaches, associated with increased intracerebral pressure, has been attributed to the swelling of the choroid plexus and the resultant blockage of the flow of cerebrospinal fluid through the foramina. Dilation of the ventricles has been observed at autopsy in patients with Gambian sleeping sickness. Some believe that a basic pattern of pathology underlies all

forms of African trypanosomiasis. Adsorption of some parasite antigens to host cells may lead to specific antigen-antibody complexing in conjunction with complement (C) and the lysis of host cells. Such a mechanism might explain the presence of anemia. It has been hypothesized that some trypanosomes cannot survive in some hosts because of the C-activation, resulting in cytotoxicity. Lysis of mast cells results in the release of kinins, histamine, and other factors resulting in sequelae such as increased vascular permeability in susceptible tissues. Hypertrophy of the reticuloendothelial system accounts for thrombocytopenia, a feature of African trypanosomiasis. Severe damage occurs chiefly in the perivascular connective tissue. Collagen bundles are disrupted. Fibers of voluntary muscle are also damaged, and characteristic of all forms of chronic trypanosomiasis is muscular wasting. There is no hemoglobinuria and no change in the fragility of

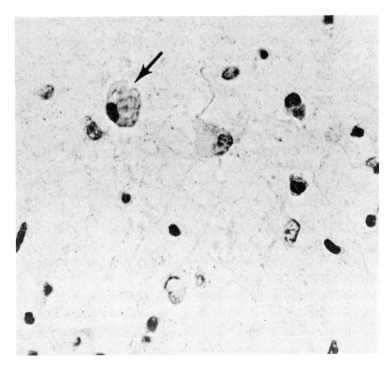

Fig. 4-31. A morula cell *(arrow)* and large astrocytes in the hypothalamus. (AFIP 61-538.)

the erythrocytes. Deposits of hemosiderin appear in the spleen and liver. Injury to the walls of the capillaries by the parasites causes intravascular clotting and perivascular edema. Passage through the injured walls leads to multiplication of the parasites in the edema. Damage occurs whenever the parasites appear, each succeeding lesion seeming worse than the last. Studies in rats suggest that anemia, splenomegaly, and nephritis may be related to the formation of autoantibodies, forming complexes with their antigens in African trypanosomiasis.

Classical East African Rhodesian trypanosomiasis, in contrast, has a shorter incubation period and more rapid progression to central nervous system involvement. The local reaction at the site of the bite is either more severe or more often noted; it is frequently still present when systemic symptoms appear. Fever and chills are said to be more marked and lymphadenopathy less striking,

or absent. Central nervous system involvement appears early, within a month in some cases, but the untreated patient frequently dies of cardiac failure or toxicity before the central nervous symptoms are pronounced.

Diagnosis. Fluid aspirated from the chancre contains actively dividing trypomastigotes. Aspiration of even small lymph nodes is more likely to reveal parasites than blood examination in West African trypanosomiasis. Organisms are more numerous in the blood in East African trypanosomiasis.

Both lymph node aspirate and blood can be examined either in fresh preparations or stained with the usual Ramonowsky stains. Thick blood smears increase the yield of positive cases, as does examination of the leukocyte layer of centrifuged blood. Autoagglutination of red cells, probably caused by altered serum proteins, is common. In the spinal fluid there is usually the picture of aseptic meningitis, with an increase in lymphocytes (30 to 1,000 per mm³) and a normal sugar. Morula cells of Mott (Fig. 4-31) are said to be characteristic. In Africans a spinal fluid protein over 20 mg% is considered abnormal; in non-Africans without malnutrition, a spinal fluid protein as high as 40 mg% can be accepted as normal in the absence of a cellular response. Since high levels of IgM are characteristic of trypanosomiases, their absence rules out infection. The presence of IgM in the spinal fluid is diagnostic of infection.

Treatment. The prognosis is proportional to the duration of the disease and the degree of spinal fluid protein elevation at the onset of therapy. For treatment see Table 4-2.

Drug prophylaxis. Drug prophylaxis offers protection when it is necessary to enter a known endemic area. However, the risk of serious drug toxicity must be weighed against the chance of infection. If only brief visits are anticipated, chemoprophylaxis is not recommended. When indicated, pentamidine is taken as 4 mg/kg intramuscularly every 3 to 6 months. Suramin as an alternative is taken, 0.3 to 0.7 gm intravenously every 2 to 3 months.

REVIEW QUESTIONS

1. As a pediatrician how would you deal with a high incidence of *Giardia lamblia* infection in an orphanage?
2. What is the significance of the various intestinal flagellates to the laboratory technician?
3. Discuss the treatment of *Trichomonas vaginalis* vaginitis.
4. Discuss the clinical relationships of the various leishmaniases.
5. How does Chagas' disease differ pathologically from Gambian sleeping sickness?
6. What is the significance of Chagas' disease to the practicing physician in the United States?
7. How does Rhodesian sleeping sickness differ clinically from the Gambian form?
8. Discuss the status of antigenicity of African trypanosomes.
9. Why are IgM and IgG of little value in controlling African trypanosomiasis?
10. Discuss the relationship of *Dientamoeba fragilis* to the amebas. What is the transmissable stage to man?
11. Is *Dientamoeba fragilis* pathogenic? Discuss.

REFERENCES

Ament, M. E., and C. E. Rubin. 1972. Relation of giardiasis to abnormal intestinal structure and function in gastrointestinal immunodeficiency syndromes. Gastroenterology **62**:216-226.

American Society of Tropical Medicine and Hygiene. 1979. Tropical medicine and hygiene in modern China. Trop. Med. Hyg. News. Suppl. **28**:31-32.

Babb, R. R., D. C. Peck, and F. G. Vescia. 1971. Giardiasis: a cause of traveller's diarrhea. J.A.M.A. **217**:1359-1361.

Barett-Connor, E., R. J. Ugoretz, and A. I. Braude. 1973. Disseminated intravascular coagulation in trypanosomiasis. Arch. Intern. Med. **131**:574-577.

Beal, C. B., and others. 1970. A new technique for sampling duodenal contents. Am. J. Trop. Med. Hyg. **19**:349-352.

Brooks, S. E. H., and others. 1970. Electron microscopy of *Giardia lamblia* in human jejunal biopsies. J. Med. Microbiol. **3**:196-199.

Center for Disease Control. 1977. Waterborne giardiasis outbreaks: Washington, New Hampshire. Morbidity and Mortality Weekly Report. **26**:169-170.

Center for Disease Control. 1978. Giardiasis: Vail, Colorado. Morbidity and Mortality Weekly Report **27**:155.

Cheissin, E. M. 1964. Ultrastructure of *Lamblia duodenalis*. I. Body surface, sucking disc and median bodies. J. Protozool. **11**:91.98.

Convit, J., M. E. Pinardi, and A. J. Rondón. 1972. Diffuse cutaneous leishmaniasis: a disease due to an immunological defect of the host. Trans. R. Soc. Trop. Med. Hyg. **66**:603-610.

Danciger, M., and M. Lopez. 1975. Numbers of *Giardia* in the feces of infected children. Am. J. Trop. Med Hyg. **24**:237-242.

Fabregas Rodríguez, C., P. Velbes Marquéti, M. Artigas Rodríguez, and J. Lasarte Ferrer. 1978. Duodenitis parasitaria. Rev. Cub. Med. Trop. **30**:175-180.

Farrar, Jr., W. E., S. D. Gibbins, and S. T. Whitfield. 1972. Low prevalence of antibody to *Trypanosoma cruzi* in Georgia. Am. J. Trop. Med. Hyg. **21**:404-406.

Geller, M., and others. 1978. Serum IgE levels in Chagas' disease. Clin. Allergy **8**:383-385.

Goldsmith, R. S., and others. 1978. Epidemiologic studies of Chagas' disease in Oaxaca, México. Bull. Pan Am. Health Organ. **12**:236-249.

Goodwin, L. G. 1970. The pathology of African trypanosomiasis. Trans. R. Soc. Trop. Med. Hyg. **64**:797-812.

Hanson, W. L., R. F. Devlin, and E. L. Roberson. 1974. Immunoglobulin levels in a laboratory-acquired case of human Chagas' disease. J. Parasitol. **60**:532-533.

Hoare, C. A. 1962. Reservoir hosts and natural foci of human protozoal infection. Acta Trop. **19**:281-317.

Hoare, C. A. 1967. Evolutionary trends in mammalian trypanosomes. In B. Dawes, Editor. Advances in parasitology. Academic Press, Inc., New York, pp. 47-91.

Honigberg, B. M. 1974. Study of *Dientamoeba fragilis* Jepps and Dobell II: taxonomic position and revision of the genus *Dientamoeba* Jepps and Dobell. J. Protozool. **21**:79-82.

Honigberg, B. M., and V. M. King. 1964. Structure of *Trichomonas vaginalis* Donne. J. Parasitol. **50**:345-364.

Hoskins, L. C., and others. 1967. Clinical giardiasis and intestinal malabsorption. Gastroenterology **53**:265-279.

Hübsch, R. M., A. J. Sulzer, and I. G. Kagan. 1976. Evaluation of an autoimmune type antibody in the sera of patients with Chagas' disease. J. Parasitol. **62**:523-527.

Kagan, I. G., and L. Norman. 1970. Serodiagnosis of parasitic diseases. Manual Clin. Microbiol. pp. 453-486.

Kagan, I. G., L. Norman, and D. Allain. 1966. Studies on *Trypanosoma cruzi* isolated in the United States: a review. Rev. Biol. Trop. **14**:55-73.

Kumar, R., I. K. Kline, and W. H. Abelmann. 1970. Immunosuppression in experimental acute and subacute Chagasic myocarditis. Am. J. Trop. Med. Hyg. **19**:932-939.

Lumsden, W. H. R. 1967. Trends in research on the immunology of trypanosomiasis. Bull. WHO **37**:167-175.

Lumsden, W. H. R., and D. A. Evans. 1976. Biology of the kinetoplastida. Vol. I. Academic Press, New York.

MacKenzie, A. R. 1973. Autoimmunity in African trypanosomiasis. Proceedings of the British Society for Parasitology. Abstracted. Parasitol. **67**:23-24.

Manson-Bahr, P. E. C., and B. A. Southgate. 1964. Recent research on kala-azar in East Africa. J. Trop. Med. Hyg. **67**:79-84.

Marsden, P. D. 1979. Current concepts in parasitology: leishmaniasis. N. Engl. J. Med. **300**:350-352.

Moore, G. T., and others. 1969. Epidemic giardiasis at a ski resort. N. Engl. J. Med. **281**:402-407.

Ormerod, W. E. 1967. Taxonomy of the sleeping sickness trypanosomes. J. Parasitol. **53**:824-830.

Ormerod, W. E., and S. Venkatesan. 1971. An amastigote phase of the sleeping sickness trypanosome. Trans. R. Soc. Trop. Med. Hyg. **65**:736-741.

Ormerod, W. E., and S. Venkatesan. 1971. The occult visceral phase of mammalian trypanosomes with special reference to the lyfe cycle of *Trypanosoma (Trypanozoon) brucei*. Trans. R. Soc. Trop. Med. Hyg. **65**:722-735.

Ormerod, W. E., and S. Venkatesan. 1971. The signifi-cance of the choroid plexus in African trypanosomiasis. Trans. R. Soc. Trop. Med. Hyg. **65**:231-232.

Pampiglione, S., and others. 1975. Studies in Mediterranean leishmaniasis 3: the leishmanin skin test in kala-azar. Trans. R. Soc. Trop. Med. Hyg. **69**:60-68.

Peña Chavarría, A., E. Kotcher, and C. Lizano. 1965. Preliminary evaluation of cycloguanil pamoate in dermal leishmaniasis. J.A.M.A. **194**:1142-1144.

Petena, W. B. 1979. The importance of clinical, psychological and social effects experienced by patients with American trypanosomiasis (Chagas' disease). Bull. Pan Am. Health Organ. **13**:131-133.

Rezai, H. R., S. M. Ardehali, G. Amirhakimi, and A. Kharazmi. 1978. Immunological features of kala-azar. Am. J. Trop. Med. Hyg. **27**:1079-1083.

Robins-Browne, R. M., J. Schneider, and J. Metz. 1975. Thrombocytopenia in trypanosomiasis. Am. J. Trop. Med. Hyg. **24**:226-231.

Schultz, M. G. 1975. Giardiasis. J.A.M.A. **233**:1383-1384.

Seah, S. K. K., P. D. Marsden, A. Voller, and L. E. Pettitt. 1974. Experimental *Trypanosoma cruzi* infection in rhesus monkeys: the acute phase. Trans. R. Soc. Trop. Med. Hyg. **68**:63-69.

Shaw, P. K., and others. 1976. Autochthonous dermal leishmaniasis in Texas. Am. J. Trop. Med. Hyg. **25**:788-796.

Sousa, O. E., and C. M. Johnson. 1971. Frequency and distribution of *Trypanosoma cruzi* and *Trypanosoma rangeli* in the Republic of Panama. Am. Soc. Trop. Med. Hyg. **20**:405-410.

Thornburgh, D. B., C. M. Johnson, and N. W. Elton. 1962. The histopathology of cutaneous leishmaniasis in Panama. Trans. R. Soc. Trop. Med. Hyg. **46**:550-554.

Trussell, R. E. 1947. *Trichomonas vaginalis* and trichomoniasis. Charles C Thomas, Publisher, Springfield, Ill.

Walton, B. C., L. Valverde Chinel, and O. Eguia y Eguia. 1973. Onset of espundia after many years of occult infection with *Leishmania braziliensis*. Am. J. Trop. Med. Hyg. **22**:696-698.

Wolfe, M. S. 1975. Giardiasis. J.A.M.A. **233**:1362-1365.

Woody, N. C., and J. B. Woody. 1961. American trypanosomiasis. I. Clinical and epidemiologic background of Chagas' disease in the United States. J. Pediatr. **58**:568-580.

World Health Organization. 1969. Comparative studies of American and African trypanosomiasis. Report of WHO scientific group. WHO Technical Report Series no. 411. Geneva, Switzerland.

Zuckerman, A. 1975. Parasitological review: current status of the immunology of blood and tissue protozoa. I. *Leishmania*. Exp. Parasitol. **38**:370-400.

CHAPTER 5

The ciliates (Ciliata)

Balantidium coli

Among the ciliates, *Balantidium coli* is of importance as a human parasite. This parasite is rather rare in humans, but very common in hogs throughout the world. It occurs also in monkeys. Infections are most prevalent in the tropics, where malnutrition is widespread and pigs share habitation (Fig. 5-1) with the family. The pig is usually regarded as an important source of human infection. However, once the human infection has been established and adaption to the human host accomplished, person-to-person transfer may occur. This becomes significant in environments where group hygiene is usually poor, as in mental hospitals and other institutions of confinement and in tropical communities where public hygiene needs much improvement. The rarity of human infection in the United States indicates that there is no serious problem in controlling hog infections, but human sources of infection become an important epidemiological problem. Infection rates in New Guinea, where the association between humans and pigs is quite close, reaches 20%. Infections in Moslem countries result from direct transmission or a rodent source. A fully documented epidemic occurred in Micronesia, following a typhoon when surface water became contaminated with pig feces. Person-to-person transmission was also involved.

Morphology and life cycle. Like most of the amebas and intestinal flagellates, *B. coli* has a trophozoite and a cyst stage, the latter being the stage transmissible to humans.

Various authors give a wide range of size for the trophozoite stage. Sargeaunt, in a study of this organism, observed "large" and "small" colonies, with conjugation taking place only between small and large organisms. One colony measured 42 to 60 μm long by 30 to 40 μm wide, while the other measured 90 to 120 μm $\times$ 60 to 80 μm. A pellicle covered with cilia (short hairlike projections) surrounds the cytoplasm of the trophozoite, giving an oval shape to the parasite. The cilia aid in locomotion and the movement of food currents into the cytostome (mouth), which is at the bottom of a large, funnel-shaped peristome. Although no digestive tract is present, opposite the cytostome is an anal pore, or cytopyge. A small, vesicular micronucleus is present, often overshadowed by a large, compact macronucleus (Fig. 5-2). Multiplication occurs by transverse fission. This ciliate is unique among the parasitic protozoa in that two contractile vacuoles are present. Encystation usually occurs in the lumen of the intestine, but may also take place outside the host, although most trophozoites in a stool specimen perish rather quickly. Cysts average 50 μm in diameter and typically show a heavy cyst wall (Fig. 5-3) with discrete cilia often discernible within when newly formed. These are eventually lost.

Symptomatology and pathology. The organism lives chiefly in the cecum but occurs throughout the colon as well. Infection may result in an asymptomatic carrier state, mild colitis, or acute dysentery similar to intes-

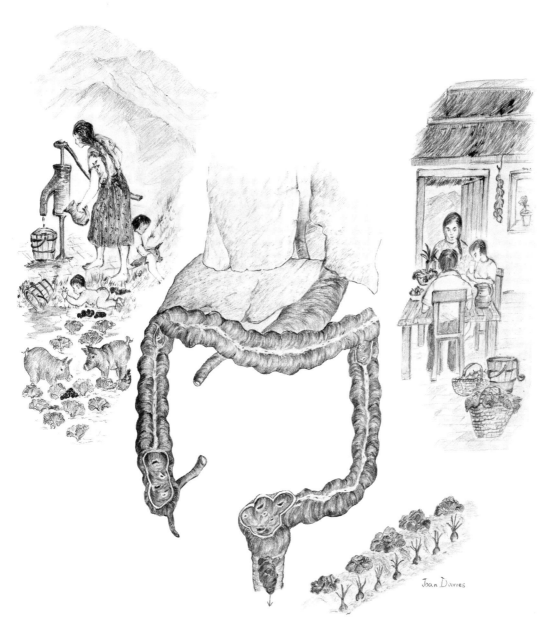

Fig. 5-1. Life cycle of *Balantidium coli.* Food and water contaminated with infective cysts are ingested. Excystation in the ileocecal region results in a colony of trophozoites and cysts becoming established in the cecum and colon. Penetration of the mucosa by trophozoites, with extensive erosion, may occur. Extraintestinal balantidiasis is rare. Cysts passed in the feces contaminate food and water, which, in turn, are ingested by humans. Pigs are a reservoir source of infection.

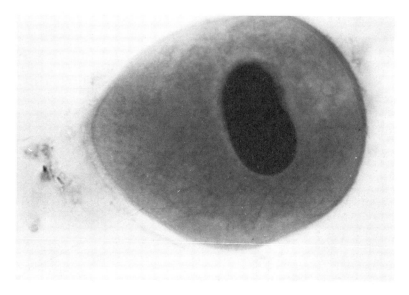

Fig. 5-2. *Balantidium coli* trophozoite. Note the large macronucleus. (Photograph by James Jensen. From Schmidt, G. D., and Roberts, L. S.: Foundations of parasitology, St. Louis, 1977, The C. V. Mosby Co.)

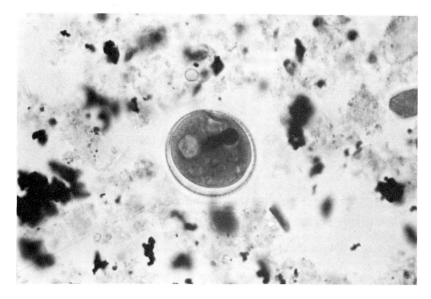

Fig. 5-3. *Balantidium coli* cyst. Note the contractile vacuole present. (Photograph by James Jensen. From Schmidt, G. D., and Roberts, L. S.: Foundations of parasitology, St. Louis, 1977, The C. V. Mosby Co.)

tinal amebiasis. The parasites thrive chiefly on starchy foods and, in such an environment, apparently do not invade the intestinal mucosa. This is evidenced in pigs, wherein the organism is harmless. The scarcity of starchy food in the human intestine may explain the rarity of infection in humans and its propensity for intestinal invasion once infection is established.

Mucosal invasion may cause hyperemia and hemorrhage of bowel surface without ulceration, or flask-shaped ulcers, usually more rounded and with a broader mouth than those of *E. histolytica*, may result. Ulceration, as in *E. histolytica*, at times may extend into the muscularis mucosa, and rare cases of fatal peritonitis following rupture of deep ulcers (Fig. 5-4) have been reported. Clusters of trophozoites may be found in the tissues and, at times, in the capillaries and lymph vessels as well. Concurrent *Trichuris trichiura* infections appear to favor tissue invasion. Unlike amebiasis, extraintestinal disease is rare, but a fatal case of subacute myocarditis apparently caused by this parasite was reported some years ago in a Russian patient. Fatal cases have also been reported from Mexico and Costa Rica. Of the small number of cases reported, fatalities, usually showing extensive ulcerative colitis, have assumed a significant proportion. Infection in the vagina, although quite rare, has also been reported.

Diagnosis. Diagnosis depends on recovery

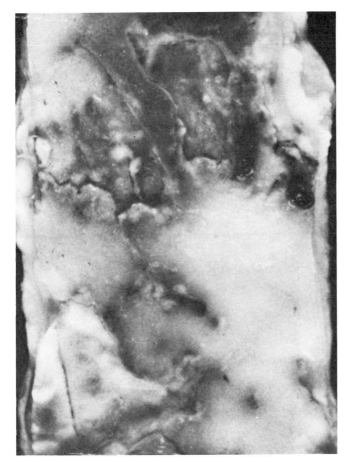

Fig. 5-4. Extensive ulceration of the colon with necrosis by *Balantidium coli* trophozoites. (AFIP 72-17276.)

and identification of the parasites. Trophozoites are more commonly seen in the stool, and since they are the only ciliate parasitic in humans and because of their large size, their identification is easy. Cysts likewise can be readily identified individually by the large size, the heavy cyst wall, cilia discernible within, and the large macronucleus. Because of the density of the cytoplasm, iodine stain should not be employed. To rule out contaminants, repeat specimens should be checked. Techniques employed for the recovery and identification of the amebas and intestinal flagellates are applicable for *B. coli* as well.

Treatment. Oxytetracycline at the level of 500 mg four times a day for 10 days is the drug of choice for the treatment of balantidiasis with diiodohydroxyquin (Diodoquin) at the dosage of 650 mg three times daily for 20 days as the alternative drug. The pediatric dosage of oxytetracycline is 40 mg/kg/day in four doses for 10 days with a maximum of 2 gm/day. For diiodohydroxyquin the dosage is 40 mg/kg/day in three doses for 20 days with a maximum of 2 gm/day. The latter is considered an investigational drug by the U.S. Food and Drug Administration. The therapy should not be continued beyond 20 days because of the danger of inducing optic neuritis.

Coprozoic ciliates

Free-living ciliates may likewise occur in the feces. *Paramecium* sp, for example, closely resemble *B. coli* and can be mistaken for them. Care must be exercised to prevent contamination of the stool container with stagnant water, particularly when washed containers are used. Disposable cardboard cartons with overlapping lids are highly recommended for the collection of stool specimens directly from the patient. No contamination can occur if this method is employed.

REVIEW QUESTIONS

1. Why is balatidiasis of little significance in the United States?
2. What is the chief habitat of *Balantidium coli?*
3. What is probably the common reservoir host for *B. coli?*
4. In what way can the diagnosis be a problem?
5. What is the treatment for balantidiasis?
6. Discuss the symptomatology and pathology of balantidiasis.
7. What is conjugation?

REFERENCES

Alvarez Valverde, R., and R. Garcia Torre. 1967. Estudio de un caso mortal de balantidiasis humana. Rev. Invest. Salud. Publica. **37**:217-224.
Arean, V. M., and E. Koppisch. 1956. Balantidiasis. A review and report of cases. Am. J. Pathol. **32**: 1089-1115.
Botero, D. R. 1972. Effectiveness of nitrimidazine in treatment of *Balantidium coli* infections. Letter. Trans. R. Soc. Trop. Med. Hyg. **67**:145.
Cespedes, R., and others. 1967. Balantidiosis estudio de un caso anatomoclinico masivo con lesions y presencia del parasito en el intestino delgado y pleura. Acta Med. Costaric. **10**:135-151.
Christian, E. C. 1974. Fatal balantidiasis. Ghana Med. J. **13**:86-89.
Delgado y Ganica, R., P. Brito Lugo, and R. Clark y Rodriguez Leal. 1971. Balantidiasis en la Ciudad de México. Rev. de. Salud Pública (Lima) **31**:106-112.
García-Laverde, A., and L. DeBonilla. 1975. Clinical trials with metronidazole in human balantidiasis. Am. J. Trop. Med. Hyg. **24**:781-783.
Hoekenga, M. T. 1953. Terramycin treatment of balantidiasis in Honduras. Am. J. Trop. Med. **2**:271-272.
Isaza Mejia, G. 1955. Balantidiasis vaginal. Antioquia Med. (Colombia) **5**:488-491.
Lumbreras, H. 1964. Balantidiasis humana. Proc. 7th Int. Congr. Trop. Med. and Malaria **2**:375-377.
Radford, H. J. 1973. Balantidiasis in Papua, New Guinea. Med. J. Aus. **1**:238-241.
Sargeaunt, P. G. 1971. The size range of *Balantidium coli*. Trans. R. Soc. Trop. Med. Hyg. **65**:428.
Shookhoff, H. B. 1951. *Balantidium coli* infection with special reference to treatment. Am. J. Trop. Med. **31**:442-457.
Walzer, P. D., and others. 1973. Balantidiasis outbreak in Truk. Am. J. Trop. Med. Hyg. **22**:33-41.
Wenger, F. 1967. Abscesso hepatico producido por el *Balantidium coli*. Kasemera **2**:433-441.
Young, M. D. 1950. Attempt to transmit human *Balantidium coli*. Am. J. Trop. Med. **30**:70-71.
Zaman, V. 1970. Ultrastructure of *Balantidium*. Southeast Asian J. Trop. Med. Public Health **1**:225-230.

CHAPTER 6

The sporozoa (Sporozoa)

The sporozoa parasitic in humans are characterized by the production of spores at some time in their life history. Their life cycles involve an alternation of generations (sexual and asexual) such that usually the intermediate host harbors the asexual forms and the definitive or final host harbors the sexual forms; in some instances, humans may serve as both hosts. A typical sporozoan life cycle is represented by the malarial parasite.

COCCIDIA

The coccidia are a large and diversified subclass of the Sporozoa. The classical coccidia are common parasites of the intestinal tract of birds and mammals and produce in some a devastating diarrhea. Their life cycle takes place in one host (monoxenous), and host specificity is often high. In chickens, for example, coccidiosis is difficult to control (without prophylactic treatment) and, once established, may quickly destroy the younger members of an entire flock. The more advanced coccidia, which form tissue cysts, are two-host parasites (heteroxenous), with part of the life cycle, including the sexual stages, in the intestine of one host (final host) and the main multiplicative stages in various organs of another host species (intermediate host). The intestinal stages usually give rise to little disease, but the multiplicative stages in the liver, lungs, brain, eye, or muscles do give rise to symptoms. Several of these relationships have been known for years in the intermediate host, such as *Toxoplasma* giving rise to pneumonia or encephalitis, and *Sarcocystis* giving rise to myositis. Their coccidian affinities were only recently discovered in carnivores that eat the intermediate host.

Multiplication is by multiple nuclear and cytoplasmic division (schizogony) or division into two daughter cells (endodyogeny). Male (microgamete) and female (macrogamete) sex cells are formed eventually. After fertilization the zygote is called an oocyst. It usually divides into two or four cysts, which sporulate (sporogony) into two or four sporozoites.

Eimeriidae

The family Eimeriidae consists of 14 genera, two of which are of medical interest, *Eimeria* and *Isospora*. The life cycles are believed to be monoxenous, and the oocysts produced usually complete sporogony outside the host. Fortunately, none of the *Eimeria* is parasitic for humans, but many thousands of species exist in a wide variety of hosts, which are ingested by humans because of their dietary habits. The organisms are only itinerant travelers passing through the gastrointestinal tract, but when recovered in the feces they may present a problem in identification (see Diagnosis). The genus *Isospora*, although not as numerous as the *Eimeria* is also found in a wide variety of hosts, including humans. Many species are parasites of dogs, cats, and other carnivores. Once thought to be monoxenous, two species in cats and two in dogs have been found to have stages in the mesenteric lymph nodes of mice, rats, and hamsters. This and other similar findings raises the question as to the authenticity of other monoxenous life cycles among the coccidia.

Isospora

Life cycle and morphology. Two species of
Isospora are parasitic in humans, *I. natalensis* and *I. belli*. *I. belli* is considered a valid
species and has a monoxenous life cycle.
Endogenous stages have been observed in
the epithelium of the small intestine from
the crypts of the mucosal surface, rarely in
the lamina propria and submucosa, and occasionally within epithelial nuclei. Both
sexual and asexual forms of *I. belli* have been
reported in biopsy specimens of the small
intestine. The oocyst is typically oval, somewhat attenuated at one end, and averages
35 μm × 9 μm (Fig. 6-1). *I. natalensis* reported from South Africa is quite rare and is
similar in life cycle and symptomatology to
I. belli. What was formerly identified as *I.
hominis* is now recognized as the sporogonic
stage of *Sarcocystis* species from cattle and
pigs.

Symptomatology and pathology. Infections may persist for a few weeks to several
months or, in some cases, for years. Anorexia, nausea, abdominal pain, and diarrhea
have been observed. A clear deposition of
collagen in the lamina propria, similar to that
found in collagenous sprue, has been noted.
Large numbers of eosinophils, plasma cells,

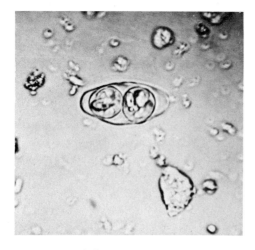

Fig. 6-1. *Isospora belli* oocyst. (Courtesy Department of
Pathology, University of Miami, School of Medicine.)

and lymphocytes have been found in the
lamina propria. The marked dilation of the
vascular spaces and excessive collagen in the
lamina propria suggest that *I. belli* may cause
intestinal malabsorption.

Diagnosis and treatment. The chief difficulty in diagnosis results from confusion between nonpathogenic species of *Isospora*
and *Eimeria* from nonhuman hosts. Immature (unsporulated) oocysts of *Isospora* and
Eimeria cannot be differentiated. After sporulation is completed, however, differentiation is obvious because *Isospora* oocysts
contain two sporocysts, each with four sporozoites (Fig. 6-1), whereas *Eimeria* oocysts
contain four sporocysts, each with two sporozoites. Feces kept in weak $K_2Cr_2O_7$ (2% to
5%) for 72 hours to control bacteria will
reveal this difference. Nonpathogenic species of *Isospora* in humans are only itinerant
travelers and do not persist, as can be observed by repeated stool examination. Therapy is given in Table 6-1. The disease is usually of short duration and self-limiting. *I.
hominis* appears even in fresh stools, only as
sporulated sporocysts; immature oocysts are
usually not present.

Sarcocystis

The taxonomy of *Sarcocystis* is in transi-
tion because much new information on the
life cycle has been discovered in recent
years. The cycle necessarily involves two
hosts. *Sarcocystis* sp form tissue cysts containing numerous bradyzoites in the muscles of intermediate hosts. These are infectious for the final host, a carnivore, in the
gut of which sexual development and sporulation take place. Sporocysts are usually
shed (Fig. 6-2) in the feces. In a review of
the literature, Beaver reports 40 cases in
humans, 35 of which are old and 5 new, in
which seven morphologic types of intramus-
cular cysts have been observed, each possibly representing one to several different
species. All appear to be zoonotic and none
can be designated as *Sarcocystis lindemanni*,

the name previously identifying the species in humans. The rare human infections appear to be caused by species usually found in some animal. This is not surprising with a parasite requiring two hosts, since man is not subject to being eaten often enough to maintain the life cycle of a species specifically adapted to him. Among the four types of cysts found in skeletal muscle, three closely resemble a corresponding species common

Table 6-1. Treatment for coccidiosis and pneumocystosis

Infection	Drug	Adult dose*	Pediatric dose*
Coccidiosis			
Isospora belli			
Drug of choice	Furazolidone[1]	100 mg qid × 10d	6 mg/kg/d in 4 doses × 10d
Alternative	Trimethoprim-sulfamethoxazole	160 mg trimethoprim—800 mg sulfamethoxazole qid × 10d, then bid × 3 wk	
Toxoplasma gondii[2]			
Drug of choice	Pyrimethamine[3] *plus* trisulfapyrimidines	25 mg/d × 3-4 wk 2-6 gm/d × 3-4 wk	1 mg/kg/d × 4 wk after loading dose of 2 mg/kg/d × 3d (max. 25 mg/d) 100-200 mg/kg/d × 3-4 wk
Alternative	Spiramycin[4]	2-4 gm/d × 3-4 wk	50-100 mg/kg/d × 3-4 wk
Pneumocystosis			
Pneumocystis carinii			
Drug of choice	Trimethoprim-sulfamethoxazole	Trimethoprim 20 mg/kg/d—sulfamethoxazole 100 mg/kg/d in 4 doses × 14d	Trimethoprim 20 mg/kg/d—sulfamethoxazole 100 mg/kg/d in 4 doses × 14d
Alternative	Pentamidine[5]	4 mg/kg/d IM × 12-14d	4 mg/kg/d IM × 12-14d

Adverse effects of antiparasitic drugs

Furazolidone (Furoxone)
Occasional: nausea; vomiting; headache; malaise
Rare: Antabuselike reaction to alcohol; hypotension; urticaria; arthralgia; rash; hemolytic anemia; other blood dyscrasias
Pyrimethamine USP (Daraprim)
Occasional: blood dyscrasias; folic acid deficiency
Rare: rash; vomiting; convulsions; shock
Spiramycin (Rovamycin)
Occasional: GI disturbance
Rare: allergic reactions
Pentamidine isethionate (Lomidine)
Frequent: hypotension; vomiting; blood dyscrasias; renal damage; pain at injection site
Occasional: may aggravate diabetes; hypoglycemia; shock; liver damage
Rare: Herxheimer-type reaction

From The Medical Letter, Inc., 56 Harrison street, New Rochelle, N.Y.
*The letter d indicates day.

1. Considered an investigational drug for this condition by the U.S. Food and Drug Administration.
2. In ocular toxoplasmosis corticosteroids should also be employed for anti-inflammatory effect on the eyes.
3. To prevent hematologic toxicity from pyrimethamine, it is advisable to administer folinic acid (leucovorin), about 10 mg/day. Pyrimethamine has been shown to be teratogenic in animals.
4. Not available in the U.S.A.
5. In the U.S.A., this drug is available from the Parasitic Diseases Division, Center for Disease Control, Atlanta, Georgia 30333; telephone 404-329-3311.

in monkeys. Among three types found in human cardiac muscle, one resembles a species seen frequently in the heart of cattle. Most of the infections in humans, reported around the world, have been found at autopsy. Muscle soreness or weakness was noted in seven cases, subcutaneous swelling in five, eosinophilia in two, and periarteritis or polyarteritis in two. The nature of pathogenicity appears to be hypersensitivity.

Tissue cysts are elongated, spindle shaped or cylindrical, and sometimes reach dimensions of 5 cm and are visible to the naked eye. They are often compartmentalized, contain banana-shaped bodies (bradyzoites) within, and average 1 to 2 mm in size; in some instances, however, they reach a diameter of 1 cm. The wall is smooth in some, but others are covered by fibers of varying length and width which radiate out toward the host muscle. The bradyzoites are 5 to

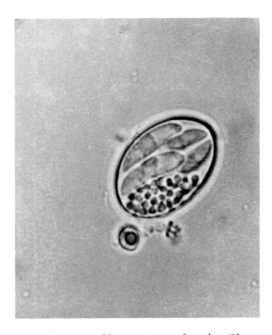

Fig. 6-2. Sporocyst of *Sarcocystis cruzi* from dog. (Photograph by Ronald Fayer. From Schmidt, G. D., and Roberts, L. S.: Foundations of parasitology, St. Louis, 1977, The C. V. Mosby Co.)

12 μm in length, with the anterior end pointed. Differentiation of cysts of *Sarcocystis* from those of *Toxoplasma* is based chiefly on size difference and cyst wall morphology. Although most *Sarcocystis* cysts are larger than those of *Toxoplasma*, some overlapping occurs. Septations and fibers radiating from the wall are not noted in *Toxoplasma* cysts but, as indicated, are not always present in *Sarcocystis* either.

Clean dogs that were fed bovine hearts infected with tissue cysts of *Sarcocystis* have been found to have macrogametes, oocysts, and sporocysts in the intestinal villi. Sporocysts recovered in the feces were morphologically identical to what has been identified as *Isospora bigemina*, suggesting that isosporan oocysts and sporocysts may be the sexual phase of certain *Sarcocystis* species, in this case *S. bovicanis*. As indicated, *S. bovihominis* from cattle and *S. suihominis* from pigs give rise to isosporan sporocysts in humans.

Thus man serves as an aberrant intermediate host for certain *Sarcocystis* normally parasitic in certain animals and as the normal final host for some *Sarcocystis* in cattle and pigs. Since it was not possible to assign the presently recognized forms to previously described names, some new specific names have been coined, composed of the name of the intermediate and the final host. It is of interest to note that cattle are host to at least three *Sarcocystis* species, *S. bovihominis*, *S. bovicanis*, and *S. bovifelis*; pigs are host to at least two, *S. suihominis* and *S. suicanis*; and sheep to at least two, *S. ovifelis* and *S. ovicanis*.

Toxoplasma

Life cycle and morphology. *Toxplasma gondii* was first discovered in a small North African rodent, the gundi (*Ctenodactylus gundi*). Since then the organism has been observed in numerous birds and mammals around the world, including humans. Studies show that *T. gondii* has both a sexual and an asexual phase in its life cycle. Reproduction takes place in the intestinal epithelium of cats by schizogony, leading to gametogony. This has been referred to as the "enteroepithelial" or "enteric" cycle. Oocysts are passed in the feces. The oocysts are ovoid (Fig. 6-3), measuring around 12 μm $\times$ 9 μm and bordered by a thin wall. When mature, each oocyst contains two sporocysts, each with four sporozoites.

Five forms or stages of the organism have been observed in its complete life cycle. The rapidly multiplying forms, characteristic of an acute infection and referred to as tachyzoites or trophozoites (Fig. 6-4), develop within "pseudocysts," now referred to as "groups." Tachyzoites are crescent shaped and average 4 to 8 μm $\times$ 2 to 3 μm. One end, somewhat pointed, contains a truncated, hollow concoid structure. The slowly multiplying forms, characteristic of chronic infections and referred to as "bradyzoites," (Figs. 6-5 and 6-6), develop within cysts. Tachyzoites and bradyzoites appear in the "extraintestinal" or tissue phase (Fig. 6-7) of the cycle, which is the only phase known to exist in humans. The remaining three stages, which have been observed only in the cat, are the "merozoites," produced from schizogony; "gametes," from gametogony; and "oocysts," which mature outside the body by sporogony. This is the phase (three stages) referred to previously as the enteroepithelial or enteric cycle. The cat, like humans and other animals, may also have the extraintestinal or proliferative forms (tachyzoites and bradyzoites) in the body tissues.

Epidemiology. With the ultimate discovery of the cat as the source of oocysts, the importance of this animal in the epidemiology of the disease has assumed significance. Immature oocysts shed by cats are not infective. Sporulation at room temperature (20 to 22° C) requires 1 to 4 days for completion. The mature oocyst with its two sporocysts, each with four sporozoites, will remain infective in the soil for at least a year. Transport hosts, such as cockroaches, filth flies, and

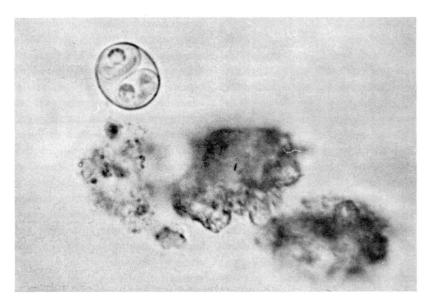

Fig. 6-3. Oocyst of *Toxoplasma gondii* from cat feces. (Photograph by Harley Sheffield. From Schmidt, G. D., and Roberts, L. S.: Foundations of parasitology, St. Louis, 1977, The C. V. Mosby Co.)

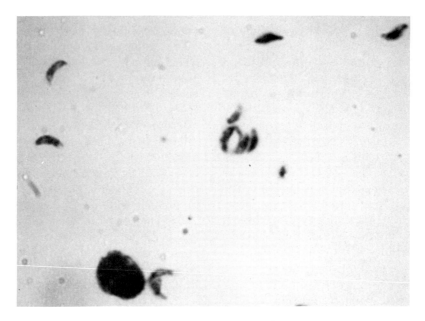

Fig. 6-4. *Toxoplasma gondii* tachyzoites from peritoneal exudate of mouse. (Courtesy Department of Epidemiology and Public Health, University of Miami, School of Medicine.)

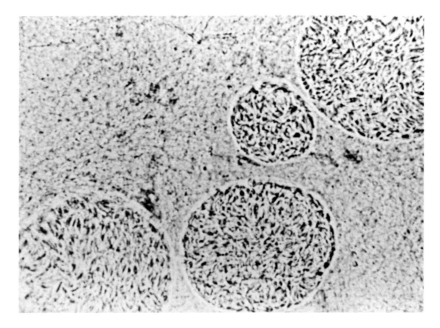

Fig. 6-5. *Toxoplasma gondii* bradyzoites in unstained crush preparation of mouse brain. (Courtesy Dr. B. H. Kean and Dr. Anne C. Kimball, Cornell University, Medical College.)

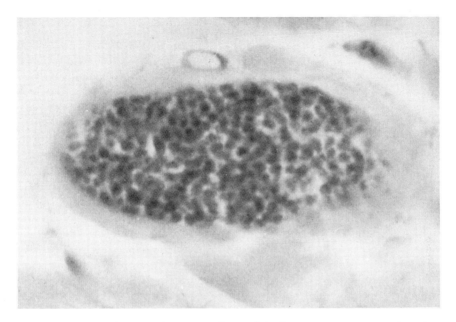

Fig. 6-6. Zoitocyst of *Toxoplasma gondii* in myocardium with bradyzoites. Zoitocyst in muscle is elongated while in brain it is rounded. (AFIP 73-7666.)

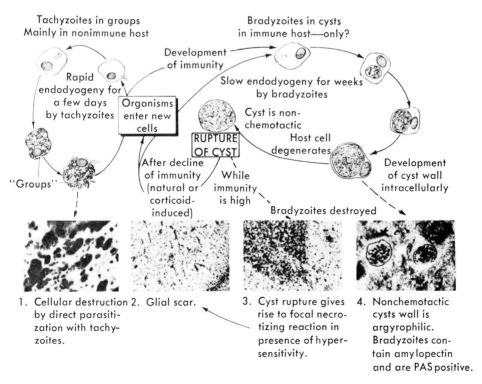

Fig. 6-7. Extraintestinal or tissue phase in humans with histologic response. (AFIP 75-316-2.)

earthworms, may disseminate the oocysts to various environments. The common housefly, *Musca domestica*, for example, has been shown experimentally to acquire and transmit the oocysts of *T. gondii* from infected cat feces to milk over a period of 24 hours. Sandboxes, flower beds, soil around the yard, open fields, and other places where feces are deposited serve as storehouses for oocysts, available for human and animal consumption. An outbreak of toxoplasmosis occurring among the patrons of a riding stable in Atlanta, Georgia, was linked to cats in the stable. Mice trapped near the stable were also found infected. Those attending the stable daily had a higher attack rate than less frequent visitors.

All mammals, including humans, can transmit the infection transplacentally. Thus, pregnant women with pet cats that hunt mice or eat meat scraps must exercise caution in the handling and disposing of cat litter (Fig. 6-8). Wearing of disposable plastic gloves is highly recommended. Besides the fecal contamination of food, water, and hands that come in contact with the mouth, inadequately cooked meat, and raw milk can be important sources of human infection. A group of medical students were infected by eating undercooked hamburgers during a break between classes. During a three-month period at a University in Sao Paulo, Brazil, 110 persons were diagnosed as having toxoplasmosis. Backyard barbecues and the fondness of many for raw beef probably helps to account for the prevalence of antibodies in the United States population. Freezing of meat at $-21°$ C for even a few hours will kill the cysts.

Symptomatology and pathology. Symptomatology varies greatly, depending on the location of the parasites in the body, and may mimic other diseases. Most cases of acquired toxoplasmosis in children and adults result in subclinical or nonspecific illness, although infections resembling mononucleosis, aseptic meningitis, hepatitis, myocarditis, or pneumonitis may ensue. Sponta-

neous recovery usually follows such acute febrile diseases, although the course of illness may be prolonged. The intestine is the first site of invasion in most acute infections. Rapid regeneration of mucosal cells compensates for tachyzoite development. The mesenteric lymph nodes and the parenchyma of the liver are next to be involved. These tissues also show rapid regeneration and usually afford control over the parasites. Swollen lymph glands in the cervical, supraclavicular, and inguinal regions may be painful and accompanied by fever, headaches, anemia, and muscle pain, all very suggestive of influenza. Duration depends on cellular immunity. As indicated, most cases are resolved favorably. However, tachyzoites may spread into the lungs, liver, heart, brain, and eyes, causing serious lesions. Invasion of the central nervous system is more serious than that of other tissues of the body because of its lower immunocompetence. Death may result. In addition, transplacental infection may result in a stillbirth or the birth of an infant severely affected with disseminated disease. About 12% of all such liveborn infants die, and less than 20% of surviving, infected infants are normal by four years of age. Such children have major involvement of the central nervous system, eyes, and viscera. Jaundice, retinochoroiditis, hydrocephalus, or microcephaly may be present at birth, or signs and symptoms may not be apparent until after the neonatal period. Some later manifestations may be related to continuing damage caused by the persistence of infection in the congenitally infected child. In such cases, toxoplasmosis is frequently suspected by finding bilateral retinochoroditis or cerebral calcification in a mentally retarded child. (In adults, retinochoroiditis may be the only evidence of acquired disease, and it is frequently unilateral.)

The parasites can localize and multiply in any organ of the body. They may invade the reticuloendothelial system, parenchymal cells of organs, or the circulatory system.

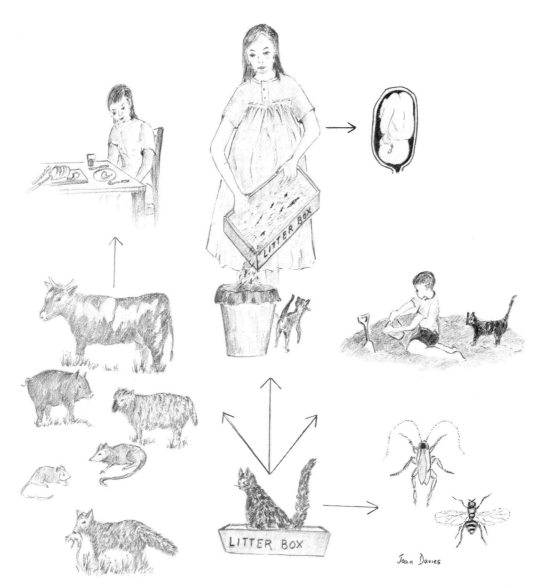

Fig. 6-8. Epidemiology of toxoplasmosis. Domestic cats (and related felines) pass oocysts in the feces which are ingested by humans and various animals. Cockroaches, flies, and other transport hosts disseminate the oocysts in the environment. Soiled hands in the mouth and contaminated food and water lead to infection. Insufficiently cooked meat from domestic animals containing the asexual stages of the parasite results in infection. *Toxoplasma gondii* is transplacentally transmitted to the offspring in infected animals.

They tend to produce serous fluids in body cavities, necrosis of the invaded tissues with minute centers of consolidation, and occasionally granulomatous formation. Only foci of cerebral necrosis calcify in infants. During these periods of quiescence, bradyzoites may be relatively dormant within tissue cysts. An association between toxoplasmosis and polymyositis has been suggested by the fall in IgM antibody titer, clinical improvement, and a decreased need for steroids, with the maintenance of normal muscle enzymes following treatment with pyrimethamine and sulfadiazine.

Diagnosis. Diagnosis most frequently depends on serologic tests (see Tables 15-1 and 15-2). The methylene blue dye (MBD) test, so extensively used previously, has been replaced largely by other methods, particularly the indirect hemagglutination (IHA) test and the indirect fluorescent antibody (IFA) test. Both of these techniques use a killed antigen in contrast to the MBD test, which requires live organisms. These tests are also easier to perform and more economical. The IFA and IHA tests are about equally sensitive and specific, and, in the hands of experts, are comparable in results with the MBD test. Titers of IFA of 1:256 to 1:512 represent chiefly the persistently low antibody titers of the general population but may be indicative of infection in cases of encephalitis under immunosuppressive therapy; lower titers in such patients may be their own or they may have been transfused. Titers as low as 1:2 to 1:16 may be indicative of infection in patients with retinochoroiditis. Titers of 1:1024+ may suggest recent infection in asymptomatic patients, while in the newborn with encephalitis such a titer, if stable or rising, is highly suggestive of toxoplasmosis. In the asymptomatic or jaundiced newborn the same titer rules in the possibility of infection. At least two serologic specimens, preferably taken two weeks apart but a a minimum of one week, are necessary to differentiate low titers, whether they are rising during the early acute phase or are stable and relate to chronic infection. Indicative of chronic infection is a low titer along with a positive skin test. Since antibodies are passively transferred from the mother to the fetus, over 99% of newborns that are asymptomatic or jaundiced are not infected when the antibody titers are 1:32 to 1:128. Such titers decay tenfold over 90 days. Since IHA titers become positive later than IFA, both

are often used simultaneously to facilitate interpretations. However, the ready availability of these tests through kits increases the chance for error from deteriorated reagents, overreading, and unawareness of various pitfalls.

Enzyme-linked immunosorbent assay (ELISA), a relatively new laboratory procedure, offers promise in diagnosis. A quantitative fluorescent antibody test (FIAX), while not readily available to every laboratory because of instrument costs involved, is more accurate than ELISA. An absolute certain diagnosis depends on the demonstration of the organisms in biopsy or necropsy specimens in relation to characteristic lesions compatible with the patient's symptoms. In the diagnosis of acquired adult disease the typical histopathology of a lymph node biopsy specimen is most helpful if verified by finding an antibody titer of 1:1024+. The cerebroventricular fluid in infants shows a high protein level and may contain a *Toxoplasma* antigen demonstrable by a serologic test modified for antigen testing.

Treatment. Treatment for toxoplasmosis is based on the use of pyrimethamine (Daraprim) (25 mg daily for 3 to 4 weeks) plus trisulfapyrimidines (2 to 6 gm daily for 3 to 4 weeks) (Table 6-1). The hematologic toxicity from pyrimethamine can be avoided by giving folinic acid concomitantly in the amount of about 10 mg/kg per day orally. Pyrimethamine will occasionally cause blood dyscrasia and folic acid deficiency. Rash, vomiting, convulsions, and shock are rare. When ocular manifestations occur, corticosteroids should be employed for their anti-inflammatory value on the eyes. Pyrimethamine is considered an investigational drug by the U.S. Food and Drug Administration.

Pneumocystis

Pneumocystis sp have been considered by some workers to be fungi, but the majority believe that they are sporozoan parasites. They are cosmopolitan in distribution in such animals as dogs, guinea pigs, mice, rats, rabbits, foxes, goats, and sheep, as well as in humans. Human infections have been reported from around the world. The organism was named *Pneumocystis carinii* in honor of Carini, who observed these parasites in the lungs of rats infected with *Trypanosoma lewisi*, believing at the time that they were a schizogonic phase of that trypanosome. Frenkel, in a study of *Pneumocystis* in rats and humans, has pointed out that there is no evidence linking human infections to animal sources, while there are many records of human-to-human infection and substantial evidence of humans as carriers. Other workers have reported serologic differences between *Pneumocystis* in rats and humans. On the basis of all evidence, Frenkel has proposed *Pneumocystis jiroveci* as the name to be used for the species in humans in honor of Jiroveci who recognized it as the cause of interstitial plasma cell pneumonia in neonates. Because the name *P. carinii* is well entrenched in the literature, this will be used throughout the discussion.

Morphology and life cycle. The organisms are found in the pulmonary alveoli in a foamy, honeycomblike, extracellular matrix. Impregnation with the methenamine silver staining technique is very useful for screening purposes because the cysts, with their thick walls and nuclei, can be found easily under low-power magnification. However, for verification of the presence of the nuclei and to differentiate from yeast cells, a follow-up stain, such as Gram's, Giemsa, hematoxylin, or trichome, is necessary. The periodic acid-Schiff (PAS) staining technique is the best for revealing the organisms. Numerous forms can be observed in the matrix. The trophozoites, which are ovoid to ameboid and measure 1 to 5 μm in diameter, are enclosed in a double-layered pellicle. Tubular extensions or filopodia project outward from the surface. Their apparent role, analogous to pili on some bacteria, is the attachment of organisms to one another and to the alveolar walls of the lungs. They aid in the attachment to epithelial cells and may inhibit phagocytosis, thereby increasing their virulence. In the cytoplasm are mitochondria, free ribosomes, and endoplasmic reticulum. Precyst forms are also ovoid and measure around 5 μm in diameter. Filopodia are no longer projections from the cytoplasm but may remain adhered to the outer surface. Cysts are 3.5 to 5 μm in diameter with a relatively thick triple-layered wall. Organelles are present in the cytoplasm. Within the cyst are intracystic bodies, usually eight in number and measuring 1 to 2 μm in diameter (Fig. 6-9). Each is enclosed in a double-layered membrane. The cyst is probably the infective stage for man, probably taken into the lungs from the external environment. Intracystic trophozoites, upon release, multiply, probably asexually, and/or develop into trophozoites, precysts, and cysts. Several generations of trophozoites very likely occur before cyst formation. Empty cysts are also seen in the matrix and are frequently crescent shaped because of the collapse of the cyst wall. Cytoplasmic remnants may be seen within.

Epidemiology. *P. carinii* has worldwide distribution in the human race. Studies suggest that babies may acquire an infection between 1 and 2 years of age. Between 3 and 5 years of age, 75% of children show a decline in indirect fluorescent antibody titer, suggesting that immunity has developed. The organism can maintain itself in the immune population, and clinical disease presents itself in those few who are immunosuppressed or immunologically stressed or compromised. Inapparent chronic infections of the carrier state are believed to be uncommon because relatively few immunosuppressed patients develop clinical pneumocystosis. The number is less, for example, than for patients with cytomegalovirus or herpes. Probably rare human carriers are present who infect immunosuppressed patients in hospitals and clinical settings where

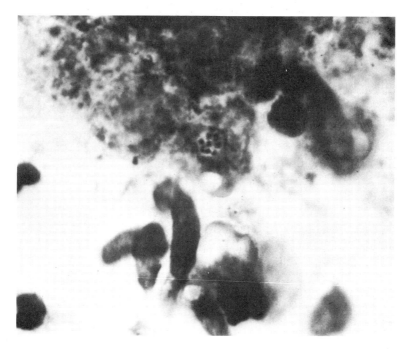

Fig. 6-9. *Pneumocystis carinii* in patient with *Pneumocystis* pneumonia. Note the cystlike structure containing eight parasites. (From a nonprofit cooperative endeavor by numberous colleagues under the editorship of Dr. Herman Zaiman, Valley City, N.D.)

a large population of such patients exists, as in children's hospitals and foundling homes. Patient-to-patient transmission can also occur in such environments.

Studies of confirmed *P. carinii* pneumonias over a three-year period in the United States have revealed that the disease occurs almost exclusively in the immunosuppressed host who has a serious underlying disease. The distribution suggests that physicians will most likely encounter patients in heavily populated states with hospitals or referral centers having large programs in cancer therapy or organ transplantation. The serious underlying disease most commonly encountered is leukemia (acute lymphatic). The highest incidence reported was in children less than 1 year of age, followed by 1- to 9-year-olds and adults 50 to 59 years of age. The predilection of *P. carinii* for certain diseases seems to be largely because of the type and intensity of immunosuppressive agents used in the treatment of those diseases.

Symptomatology and pathology. Dyspnea is the most common symptom observed, followed by fever and nonproductive cough. Physical findings are usually minimal or absent, with cyanosis and rales most frequent. X ray typically reveals bilateral, diffuse or patchy, interstitial infiltrate. Vital signs usually indicate that the average patient has fever, tachycardia, and tachypnea with normal blood pressure. Blood gas determinations usually reveal hypoxia with a mild respiratory alkalosis. Most patients are mildly anemic, with a slight leukocytosis and normal platelet count. Autopsy reveals a heavy infiltrate, consisting of macrophages, lymphocytes, neutrophils, plasma cells, and other cells, in the thickened septa of lung sections. Grossly, the lung appears grayish to tan, firm, but containing a foamy, amorphous

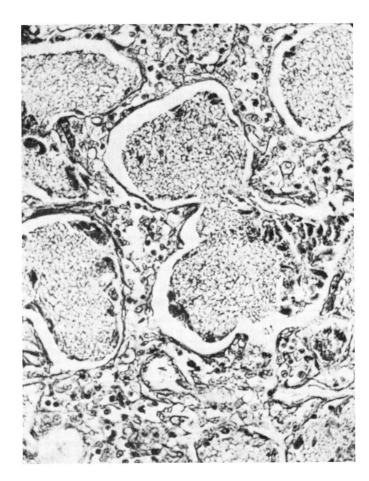

Fig. 6-10. Pneumocystosis. Note the foamy intra-alveolar material and the septal infiltrate. (AFIP 58-5041.)

material (Fig. 6-10). Within this matrix are the various stages of the parasite described. The mortality seems to be relatively high, taking into consideration the prevalence of infection in high-risk patients with an underlying serious disease.

An interesting observation among patients with *P. carinii* infection but with *no* immunodeficiency disease is that serum immunoglobulin levels appear normal except for a lower IgG level. Some workers have pointed out that a deficiency of IgG is the most important link in the establishment of pneumocystosis in malnourished newborns. Plasma cell pneumonia in malnourished newborns, often of premature birth, is considered by many to be a complex immunodeficiency.

IgG, IgM, and IgA are associated with the intra-alveolar masses seen in this disease. A complement deficiency or delayed binding has been suggested by some as the limiting factor. The finding of disease in children with sex-linked agammaglobulinemia emphasizes the importance of antibodies for immunity. It is also interesting to note that children with ataxia-telangiectasia and defects in IgA and cell immunity do *not* develop pneumocystosis. To some this is evidence that IgG and IgM can maintain immunity without help from cell immunity. In summary, *P. carinii* infection appears to be a complex phenomenon dependent on plasma cells, antibodies, T-lymphocytes, macrophages, and probably complement, and it is quite

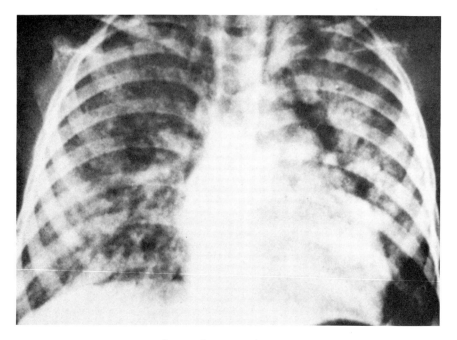

Fig. 6-11. Roentgenogram showing disseminated pneumocytosis. (AFIP 75-12377.)

possible that clinical disease may result from a deficiency in only one of these components.

Diagnosis. Clinical signs and symptoms have been used to make a tentative diagnosis (Fig. 6-11) and serve as the basis for instituting therapy, but demonstration of *P. carinii* in material from lungs is necessary to confirm the diagnosis. Transbronchial lung biopsy via the fiberoptic bronchoscope will provide lung tissue for histologic study without the mortality associated with open or precutaneous lung biopsies, and it is considered by some to be more effective than endobronchial brush biopsy. The complexity of the immune response is reflected also in the various diagnostic serologic tests. At present, serologic diagnosis awaits further study (see Tables 15-1 and 15-2).

Treatment. Therapy for pneumocystosis is given in Table 6-1.

MALARIA

Malaria is a mosquito-borne disease of humans resulting from infection of the paren-chymal cells of the liver and the red blood cells by sporozoa belonging to the genus *Plasmodium*. The following species occur in humans:

Plasmodium vivax—benign tertian (vivax) malaria
Plasmodium ovale—benign tertian (ovale) malaria
Plasmodium malariae—benign quartan (malariae) malaria
Plasmodium falciparum—malignant tertian (subtertian, estivoautumnal, falciparum) malaria

History and geographic distribution. Malaria has been a scourge of mankind through the centuries. It has left its mark on world history, affecting the outcome of wars, movements of populations, and the growth and development of nations. During World War II, five times as many soldiers in the South Pacific area were incapacitated by malaria as by combat. Prior to the Civil War in the United States, it was found as far north as southern Canada. In the early 1920s, it was reported near the Arctic Circle in Russia. It has been reported at altitudes of over 9,000

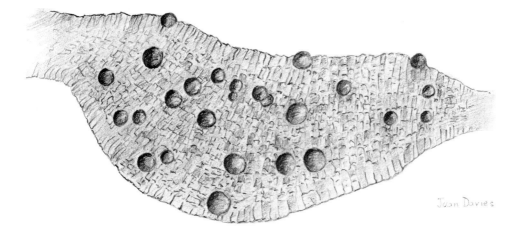

Fig. 6-12. Oocysts on the stomach wall of a mosquito.

feet and at depths of over 1,000 feet below sea level. Over the years there has been a gradual decline in both prevalence and distribution. In the continental United States is ceased to exist as an endemic disease by the early 1950s. Around this time the World Health Organization undertook a worldwide eradication program. The vicissitudes besetting this program are discussed in the section on malaria eradication.

So-called endemic malaria, occurring where the population maintains some degree of constant infection and immunity, is less spectacular as a cause of death but plays a major role in chronic illness, fatigue, malaise, and mental disturbances that result in poor agriculture and malnutrition—a vicious cycle in developing nations.

P. vivax and *P. falciparum* account for over 95% of infections in the world. Some estimates give *P. vivax* as the cause of about 80% of all infections. This species is the most widespread, extending throughout the tropics, subtropics, and into the temperate regions of the world, whereas *P. falciparum* is largely confined to the tropics. *P. malariae*, though coextensive with *P. vivax*, is quite rare and spotty in location. *P. ovale* is confined mainly to central West Africa but also appears in some South Pacific islands, Asia,

and South America. One American serviceman returning from the South Pacific brought back the Donaldson strain of *P. ovale*.

Although *P. malariae* occurs naturally in chimpanzees in central Africa, the major reservoir of this and other species that cause human malaria is man. Several kinds of organisms that cause simian malaria, such as *P. cynomolgi*, *P. knowlesi*, *P. inui*, *P. brasilianum*, *P. shortii*, and others, which are widely used for malaria research, can be transmitted to humans by blood or mosquito inoculation and conceivably can occasionally result in natural infection.

Life cycle. The definitive or final host for the malarial parasite is the female anopheline mosquito. Among the parasites ingested in the blood meal, the only forms that survive in the stomach of the insect are the male and female gametocytes. The zygote formed from the union of the gametes becomes a motile ookinete that penetrates the stomach wall. Embedded on the body cavity side, it rounds up into an oocyst and develops numerous sporozoites within (Fig. 6-12). Rupturing of the oocyst wall results in the displacement of many active sporozoites into the body cavity, some of which migrate forward and enter the salivary glands. The next mosquito bite may result in their discharge into the puncture wound and transport by the blood to the liver, where they penetrate parenchymal cells. Studies in primate malaria suggest that two distinct populations of sporozoites occur, one of which remains dormant (hypnozoites) for varying periods of time to ultimately become reactivated and complete schizogony. The other population immediately undergoes development. Growth in these cells, followed by asexual reproduction, results in progeny called merozoites. This first asexual or schizogonic cycle is called the pre-erythrocytic or primary exoerythrocytic cycle.

In the case of *P. falciparum* and *P. malariae*, all of these merozoites enter red blood cells. In the other species, some but not all merozoites enter the red cells, while the remainder penetrate other parenchymal cells of the liver and initiate a secondary exoerythrocytic cycle or tissue phase. In this manner, a reservoir of parasites (exoerythrocytic [E.E.] stages) is maintained in the liver and may be released at some future time to penetrate red blood cells.

The failure of immunity or therapy to destroy all parasites in the red cells again may result in a buildup with clinical manifestations. This kind of relapse is called a "recrudescence." All species may recrudesce. However, if the erythrocytic phase dies out and a relapse occurs later because of a new invasion of red cells from the liver parasites, this kind is known as a "recurrence." All species may recur except *P. falciparum* and *P. malariae* which have no secondary exoerythrocytic cycles.

Clinical manifestations of malaria are associated with only the erythrocytic cycle. Schizogonic cycles in the red cells continue until either the patient is killed or they are suppressed by immunity or drug therapy. Either of the latter may account for complete cure of the clinical phase (Fig. 6-13). The erythrocytic cycle may also be initiated through blood transfusion, drug addicts sharing a common syringe and needle, malaria fever therapy for treatment of syphilis, and, rarely, congenital infection.

Not all parasites in the erythrocytes are destined to undergo schizogony. Some become differentiated as male and female sex cells or gametocytes. It is these parasites that are destined to continue the life cycle in the stomach of the mosquito.

Epidemiology. Malaria is primarily a rural disease, for it depends on an environment suitable to the anopheline mosquito for its existence and transmission. Only female mosquitoes bite humans. Although most species of *Anopheles* experimentally show some degree of susceptibility to infection, marked variations occur within species. Susceptibility also varies among the species and strains of parasites. The latter is well illustrated by the fact that *Anopheles maculipennis atroparvus* of England can be easily infected with the Italian strain of *P. falciparum*, but not with the strains of the same species from India or Zaire.

The mere presence of suitable vectors in an area does not ensure the establishment of malaria endemically. A definite average number of bites per person per night must be sustained; otherwise a gradual reduction in the disease will occur, until it eventually dies out. This is well exemplified in the United States, where eradication has been achieved primarily by mosquito control. This critical level is conditioned by many factors associated with the ecology of the species in question. Thus, for example, *Anopheles gambiae*, a mosquito fond of human habitation and human blood, may in total numbers be low compared to the other species but, because of its habits, may be a prolific vector for malaria. The introduction of this mosquito into Brazil some years ago resulted in a local epidemic of malaria.

The duration of infection in a given area may also affect the transmission rate as well as the severity of infection. Thus, *P. falciparum*, with no secondary E.E. stages pres-

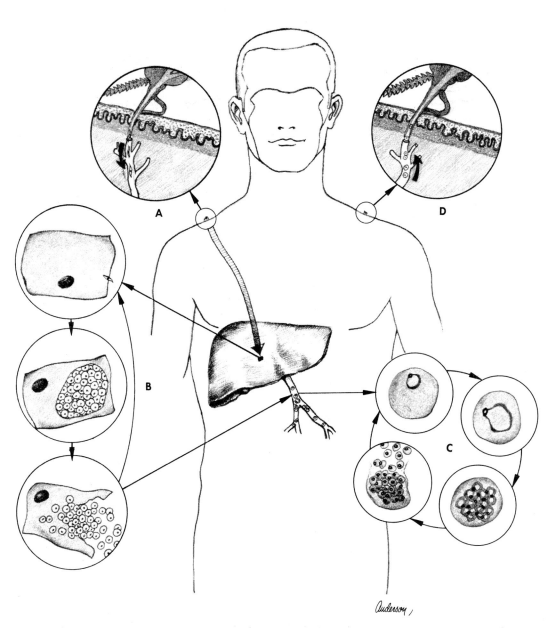

Fig. 6-13. Life cycle of the malarial parasite. **A,** Sporozoites injected by the biting mosquito are carried in the bloodstream to the liver where penetration of the parenchymal cells occurs. **B,** Exoerythrocytic schizogony results in the formation of merozoites, which enter red blood cells. **C,** Erythrocytic schizogony results in the eventual formation of gametocytes, which are ingested by feeding mosquitoes, **D,** in which sporogony takes place, leading to the production of sporozoites.

ent to cause a recurrence, is short lived. Once the blood is free of parasites, the infection is terminated not only clinically but epidemiologically as well. This situation may have some drawbacks, however, because the drop in immunity in a population may predispose to severe epidemics when the infection is reintroduced, whereas in areas where a low level of infection is sustained the "communal immunity" affords protective antibodies against severe attacks.

Although falciparum infections usually last no longer than 10 months, vivax infections for 2½ to 3 years, and malariae infections perhaps for the life of the patient, such infections are of less importance in transmission than are the presence, number, and life span of viable gametocytes in the bloodstream and their exposure to mosquitoes. Mosquito exposure is influenced also by the healthy carrier with asymptomatic parasitemia. The chances for mosquito exposure are enhanced during those periods when the gametocytes are in the bloodstream but the patient is asymptomatic and ambulatory. The patient may also be an important reservoir host during the intervals between paroxysms, when symptoms have abated before the parasitemia, or when parasitemia precedes the primary symptoms.

Morphology and symptomatology. From the time of the mosquito bite until approximately a week or more later no symptoms appear. During this *prepatent period* the parasites develop in the liver. After the merozoites from the preerythrocytic cycle enter the red cells, several broods develop but eventually one dominates (Table 6-2) and suppresses the others. The simultaneous rupture of a large number of red blood cells and liberation of merozoites precipitate the paroxysms of malaria (Fig. 6-14).

Plasmodium vivax. (Fig. 6-14). The young ring forms, which invade only reticulocytes, older red blood cells apparently being resistant to infection, consist of a distinct heavy red chromatin nucleus and a blue margin

Table 6-2. Differential characteristics of plasmodia

	Plasmodium vivax (benign tertian)	Plasmodium malariae (quartan)	Plasmodium falciparum (malignant tertian)	Plasmodium ovale (benign tertian)
Infected red blood cells	Larger than normal, pale, often bizarre in shape; Schüffner's dots often present; multiple infection of RBC not uncommon	Normal or slightly smaller, RBC sometimes darker in early stages; multiple infection of RBC rare	Normal; multiple infection of RBC very common	Somewhat larger than normal, often with fringed or irregular edge, and oval in shape; Schüffner's dots appear even with younger stages; stain more readily and more deeply than in vivax
Small trophozoite (early rings)	Signet-ring form with heavy red chromatin dot and blue cytoplasmic ring	Same as *P. vivax* but blue cytoplasmic circle smaller, thicker, and heavier	Same as *P. vivax* but small threadlike blue cytoplasmic circle with 1 or 2 small red chromatin dots; double chromatin dots common; marginal forms common	Small, darker in color, and more solid generally than those of falciparum; Schüffner's dots regularly present in almost 100% of infected cells
Growing trophozoite	Like small trophozoite as above, with increased cyto-	Chromatin rounded or elongated; cytoplasm	Remains in ring form but grows resembling small tropho-	Resembles closely same stage of *P. malariae* but is consid-

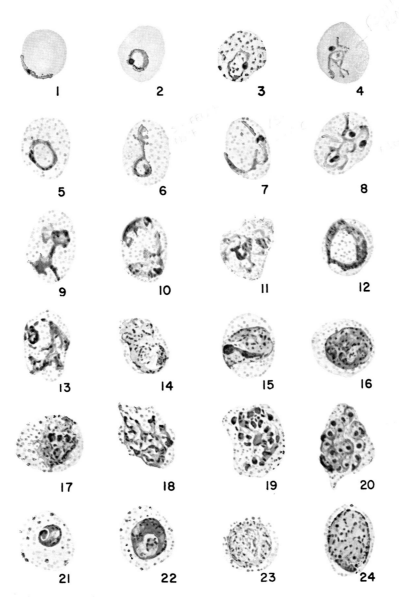

PLATE 1. *Plasmodium vivax*. **1,** Normal-sized red cell with marginal ring form trophozoite. **2,** Young signet ring form trophozoite in macrocyte. **3,** Slightly older ring form trophozoite in red cell showing basophilic stippling. **4,** Polychromatophilic red cell containing young tertian parasite with pseudopodia. **5,** Ring form trophozoite showing pigment in cytoplasm, in enlarged cell containing Schüffner's stippling (dots). (Schüffner's stippling does not appear in all cells containing growing and older forms of *P. vivax*, as would be indicated by these pictures, but it can be found with any stage from fairly young ring form onward.) **6, 7,** Very tenuous medium trophozoite forms. **8,** Three ameboid trophozoites with fused cytoplasm. **9, 11-13,** Older ameboid trophozoites in process of development. **10,** Two ameboid trophozoites in one cell. **14,** Mature trophozoite. **15,** Mature trophozoite with chromatin apparently in process of division. **16-19,** Schizonts showing progressive steps in division (presegmenting schizonts). **20,** Mature schizont. **21, 22,** Developing gametocytes. **23,** Mature microgametocyte. **24,** Mature macrogametocyte. (From Wilcox, A. 1960. Manual for the microscopical diagnosis of malaria in man, Department of Health, Education, and Welfare, Public Health Service, U.S. Government Printing Office, Washington, D.C.)

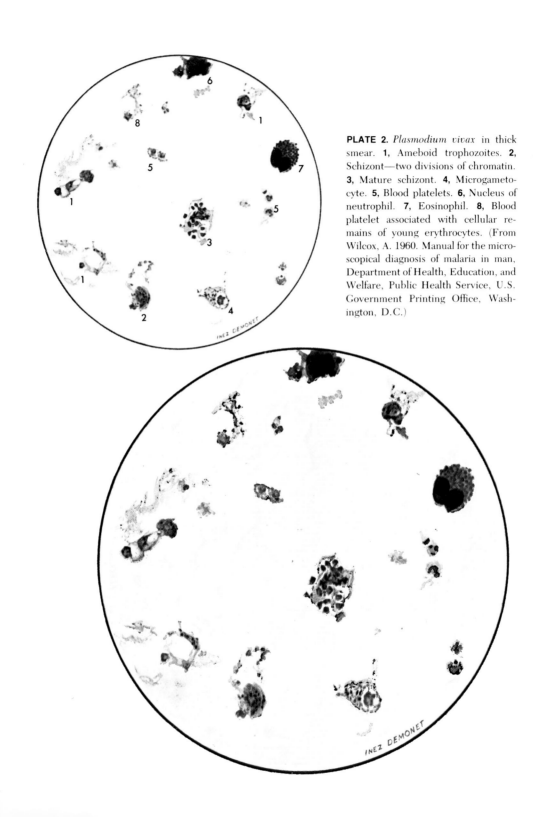

PLATE 2. *Plasmodium vivax* in thick smear. **1,** Ameboid trophozoites. **2,** Schizont—two divisions of chromatin. **3,** Mature schizont. **4,** Microgametocyte. **5,** Blood platelets. **6,** Nucleus of neutrophil. **7,** Eosinophil. **8,** Blood platelet associated with cellular remains of young erythrocytes. (From Wilcox, A. 1960. Manual for the microscopical diagnosis of malaria in man, Department of Health, Education, and Welfare, Public Health Service, U.S. Government Printing Office, Washington, D.C.)

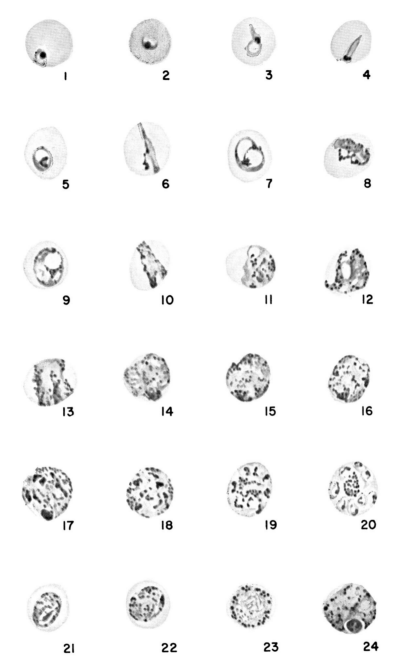

PLATE 3. *Plasmodium malariae.* **1,** Young ring form trophozoite of quartan malaria. **2-4,** Young trophozoite forms of parasite showing gradual increase in chromatin and cytoplasm. **5,** Developing ring form trophozoite showing pigment granule. **6,** Early band form trophozoite—elongated chromatin, some pigment apparent. **7-12,** Some forms that developing trophozoite of quartan may take. **13, 14,** Mature trophozoites—one a band form. **15-19,** Phases in development of schizont ("presegmenting schizonts"). **20,** Mature schizont. **21,** Immature microgametocyte. **22,** Immature macrogametocyte. **23,** Mature microgametocyte. **24,** Mature macrogametocyte. (From Wilcox, A. 1960. Manual for the microscopical diagnosis of malaria in man, Department of Health, Education, and Welfare, Public Health Service, U.S. Government Printing Office, Washington, D.C.)

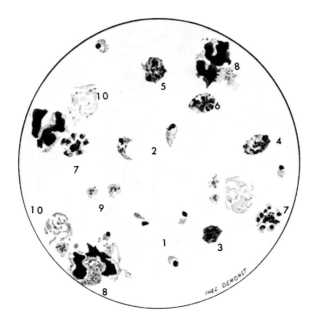

PLATE 4. *Plasmodium malariae* in thick smear. **1,** Small trophozoites. **2,** Growing trophozoites. **3,** Mature trophozoites. **4-6,** Schizonts (presegmenting) with varying numbers of divisions of chromatin. **7,** Mature schizonts. **8,** Nucleus of leukocyte. **9,** Blood platelets. **10,** Cellular remains of young erythrocytes. (From Wilcox, A. 1960. Manual for the microscopical diagnosis of malaria in man, Department of Health, Education, and Welfare, Public Health Service, U.S. Government Printing Office, Washington, D.C.)

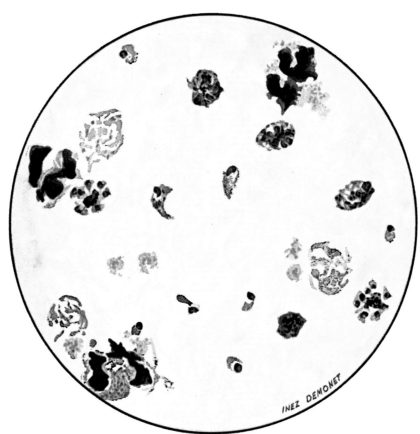

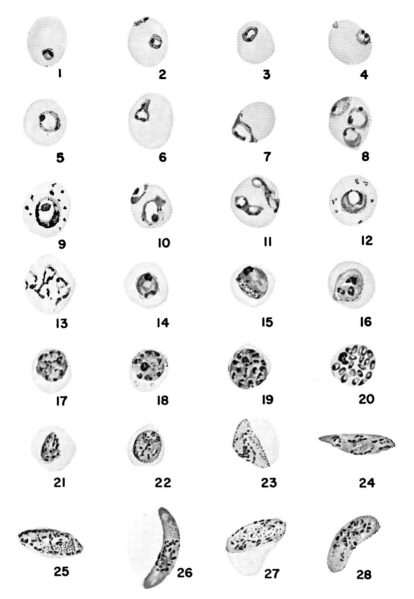

PLATE 5. *Plasmodium falciparum.* **1,** Very young ring form trophozoite. **2,** Double infection of single cell with young trophozoites, one a "marginal form," the other "signet ring" form. **3, 4,** Young trophozoites showing double chromatin dots. **5-7,** Developing trophozoite forms. **8,** Three medium trophozoites in one cell. **9,** Trophozoite showing pigment, in cell containing Maurer's dots. **10, 11,** Two trophozoites in each of two cells, showing variations of forms that parasites may assume. **12,** Almost mature trophozoite showing haze of pigment throughout cytoplasm. Maurer's dots in cell. **13,** Estivoautumnal "slender forms." **14,** Mature trophozoite showing clumped pigment. **15,** Parasite in process of initial chromatin division. **16-19,** Various phases of development of schizont (presegmenting schizonts). **20,** Mature schizont. **21-24,** Successive forms in development of gametocyte—usually not found in peripheral circulation. **25,** Immature macrogametocyte. **26,** Mature macrogametocyte. **27,** Immature microgametocyte. **28,** Mature microgametocyte. (From Wilcox, A. 1960. Manual for the microscopical diagnosis of malaria in man, Department of Health, Education, and Welfare, Public Health Service, U.S. Government Printing Office, Washington, D.C.)

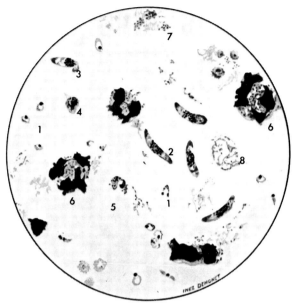

PLATE 6. *Plasmodium falciparum* in thick film. **1,** Small trophozoites. **2,** Gametocytes—normal. **3,** Slightly distorted gametocyte. **4,** "Rounded-up" gametocyte. **5,** Disintegrated gametocyte. **6,** Nucleus of leukocyte. **7,** Blood platelets. **8,** Cellular remains of young erythrocyte. (From Wilcox, A. 1960. Manual for the microscopical diagnosis of malaria in man, Department of Health, Education, and Welfare, Public Health Service, U.S. Government Printing Office, Washington, D.C.)

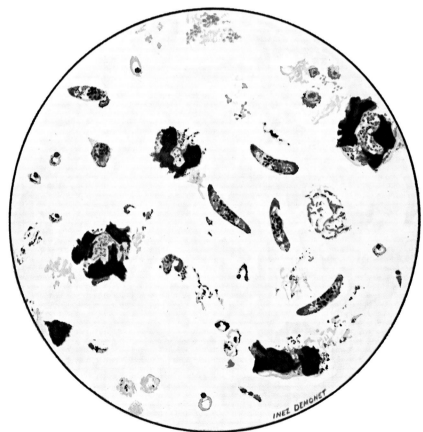

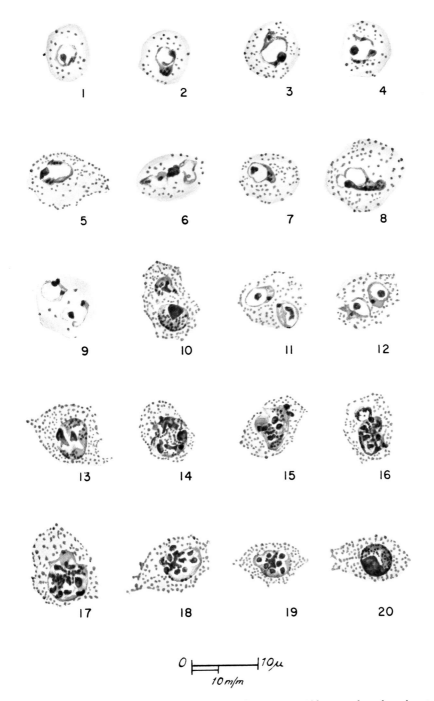

PLATE 7. *Plasmodium ovale.* **1,** Young ring-shaped trophozoite. **2-5,** Older ring-shaped trophozoites. **6-8,** Older ameboid trophozoites. **9, 11, 12,** Doubly infected cells, trophozoites. **10,** Doubly infected cell, young gametocytes. **13,** First stage of the schizont. **14-19,** Schizonts, progressive stages. **20,** Mature gametocyte. (From Wilcox, A. 1960. Manual for the microscopic diagnosis of malaria in man, ed. 2, National Institutes of Health Bulletin No. 180 (Revised), U.S. Government Printing Office, Washington, D.C.)

Know!

Large trophozoite	plasm and ameboid activity; small, yellowish-brown pigment granules in cytoplasm, increasing with age of parasite	compact or in narrow band form across cell; dark brown pigment granules; may have peripheral arrangement	zoite of *P. vivax* in size; usually the oldest asexual stage seen in peripheral blood	erably larger; pigment is lighter in color and less conspicuous
Schizont (presegmenting)	Large mass of chromatin; loose, irregular, or close compact cytoplasm with increasing amount of fine brown pigment; parasite fills cell in 36-40 hr	Chromatin often elongated, indefinite in outline; cytoplasm dense, compact, in rounded oblong or band forms; pigment granules larger, darker than in *P. vivax*; parasite fills cells frequently	Seldom present	Same as above
Schizont (mature)	Chromatin divided; cytoplasm shows varying degrees of separation into strands and particles; pigment collects in parts of the parasite	Same as *P. vivax*, except parasite is smaller, shows less chromatin division, more delayed clumping of pigment	Not present	About 25% of infected cells are definitely oval shaped; usual picture is that of a round parasite in center of an oval cell; many cells with indefinite fringed outline; pigment lighter and less coarse than in *P. malariae*
Gametocyte	12-24 merozoites; pigment in 1-2 clumps; parasite almost fills enlarged cell	6-12 (average 8-10) merozoites in rosette form; parasite almost fills cell	Rarely present; 8-24 merozoites; smaller than other species	Usually 8 merozoites arranged around a central block of pigment
	Microgametocyte: light red to pink chromatin, diffuse central; gives tint to light blue cytoplasm; yellowish brown pigment throughout cystoplasm; usually round about size of normal RBC. *Macrogametocyte:* small, compact, dark red chromatin, eccentric in parasite; cytoplasm dark blue, no vacuoles; abundant dark brown pigment scattered through cytoplasm	Same as *P. vivax* except smaller; fills or almost fills cell	Present in peripheral bloodstream; similar to *P. vivax*; crescent or sausage shape	Distinguished from *P. malariae* by size of infected cells and by Schüffner's dots; less easy to differentiate from *P. vivax*; seldom or never contained in an oval erythrocyte
Stages in peripheral blood	All	All	Ring forms and gametocytes; other stages rare	All
Length of asexual cycle	48 hr	72 hr	48 hr or less	48 hr

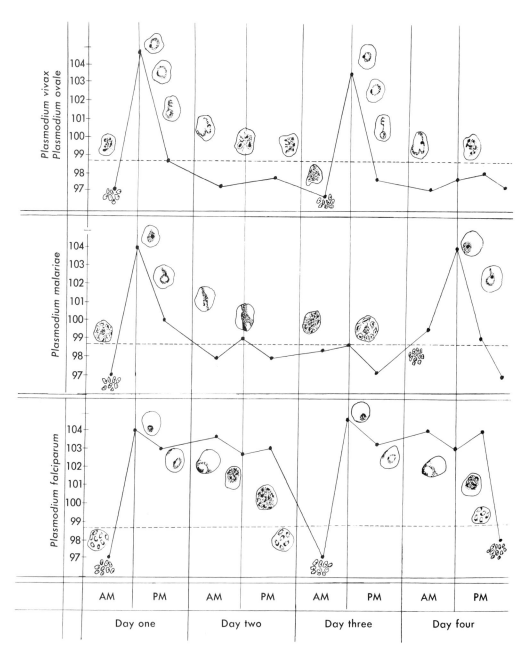

Fig. 6-14. Chart showing the relationship of temperature to erythrocytic schizogony of malarial parasites in the nonimmune host.

of cytoplasm when stained with Giemsa or Wright's. The nucleus is either centrally or peripherally located. Within a few hours after infection the red blood cells become enlarged and Schüffner's stippling appears. All stages thereafter show these characteristics, which are diagnostic of the species *P. vivax.* The growing trophozoites exhibit characteristic ameboid activity, another diagnostic feature (Plates 1 and 2). The early Italian workers, observing this characteristic, dubbed the organism "vivace," meaning vivacious. The organism subsequently became known as vivax. Yellowish brown pigment granules appear in about 5 to 6 hours. After 40 hours the parasite almost fills the enlarged red blood cell, which may be twice its normal size. Ameboid activity ceases, the cytoplasm becomes compact, and the relatively compact nucleus undergoes division to produce 12 to 24 (the average is 16) segments. Cytoplasmic division results in masses collecting around the nuclear fragments to form merozoites. Pigment collects into one or two loose masses. Growth from the small trophozoite through the mature schizont stage takes about 48 hours. Rupturing of the mature schizont releases merozoites which invade other red blood cells to initiate other schizogonic cycles. Gametocytes appear in the peripheral blood early in infection and are believed by some to develop directly from exoerythrocytic stages in the liver. Thick blood films (Plate 2) reveal the highly ameboid trophozoites without red cell morphology, although ghostlike shadows of the red blood cell can sometimes be seen even with stippling. All stages of *P. vivax* may appear in the peripheral blood. In the nonimmune individual the incubation period varies from 8 to 27 days. In some strains a protracted incubation period of 9 to 10 months may occur; in the Netherlands, for example, infections contracted in the fall did not present the primary attack until the following spring.

Broods of parasites with schizogonic cycles out of synchrony with one another first appear in the bloodstream and may produce low-grade symptoms of malaise, general body discomfort, and fever—the latter often quotidian in nature (Plates 1 and 2). Eventually one brood dominates, and the release of merozoites, with the destruction of many red blood cells, results in the first paroxysm of the primary attack. The onset is characterized by a sudden, shaking chill often lasting for several hours. Fever follows, with temperatures reaching 104° to 105° F (Fig. 6-14). Accompanying symptoms persisting for several hours are headache, backache, abdominal discomfort, nausea, and muscle soreness. The fever terminates by crisis with a drenching sweat that may persist for several hours. The entire paroxysm may last 8 to 10 hours or longer. During the paroxysm a moderate leukocytosis appears, followed by a leukopenia, with usually an increase of large, mononuclear cells during the afebrile period. Although exhausted, the patient feels relieved. Coinciding with the release of another brood of merozoites in 48 hours, another paroxysm occurs. A series of such paroxysms of diminishing intensity continues for 2 weeks, more or less, depending on the strain of the organism and the host immune response. This constitutes the primary attack and is followed by a *latent period.* After about 2 weeks a second attack is precipitated, but less intense than the first. A series of such short-term recrudescenses may continue for about 2 months, when a prolonged period of latency follows, indicating that the red blood cell phase has completely died out. About 6 to 9 months after termination of the primary attack, the long-term relapses or recurrences appear. They are often precipitated by such factors as pregnancy, anesthesia, intercurrent infections, or alcoholism. Recurrences may take place up to 2½ to 3 years, and sometimes longer. After this sequence the exoerythrocytic phase is spent, and the infection dies out. Another variation of vivax infection, known as the Western

Pacific pattern, is characterized by the absence of long-term recurrences.

Plasmodium ovale. At one time, *Plasmodium ovale* was considered a variety or strain of *P. vivax.* Craig, in 1900, described it in the Philippines as *Plasmodium vivax minutum.* In 1922 a new species of malaria was observed in East Africa and named *P. ovale* because of the nature of the elongated, infected red blood cells. It proved to be identical to Craig's species. *P. ovale* has been described by some as like a quartan parasite *(P. malariae)* inside a vivax red cell (Plate 7). Like *P. malariae,* multiple infections of the red cell are rare, and cytoplasm of the trophozoites is somewhat compact with a deep blue stain. Schizonts average 8 to 9 merozoites. Thick blood films of *P. ovale* are almost identical in appearance to those of *P. malariae* since Schüffner's stippling is absent. The red blood cell in the thin smear appears oval and irregularly shaped with fimbriated borders.

Clinically, ovale malaria is similar to vivax. The untreated primary course is shorter, and spontaneous recovery without therapy is more common. Fevers are less intense, and parasitemia buildup much slower. Relapses are less frequent than for vivax and usually persist no longer than a year. The disease, on the whole, is usually milder than that caused by *P. vivax.*

Plasmodium malariae. Early ring stages of *P. malariae* are similar to *P. vivax,* but, as development progresses, the cytoplasm becomes more compact with very little ameboid activity. Double chromatin dots are rare. During the growing stage the trophozoites assume broad bands extending across the cell. The chromatin material also stretches across the cytoplasm on one edge. Sometimes it is semicircular, or a rounded mass. Pigment appears early, is usually dark brown, and often is arranged peripherally along the border of the cytoplasm opposite the chromatin on the other side. The parasites infect older red blood cells. The red

cells are never enlarged and sometimes appear shrunken in size. There is no Schüffner's stippling. The mature schizont contains 6 to 12 (the average is 8) merozoites, sometimes arranged around the centrally clumped pigment (rosettes) but more often irregularly arranged in a cluster. Pink staining dots are sometimes seen in the red blood cells, depending on pH and intensity of staining. They are called Ziemann's stippling and are of very little value in diagnosis. *P. malariae* seems to have fewer gametocytes than either *P. vivax* or *P. falciparum* (Plates 3 and 4).

P. malariae in a thick blood film is usually easier to identify than is *P. vivax,* because of the compact cytoplasm and distinct chromatin mass. No ameboid activity is present. Mature schizonts with their 8 merozoites confirm the diagnosis. Rosettes, when seen, are readily identifiable.

The incubation period is longer than that of *P. vivax,* with parasites appearing in the blood from the nineteenth to the thirtieth day. Except for its 72-hour fever cycle, this infection is similar to that of *P. vavix* (Fig. 6-14). Broods of parasites are synchronized and the 72-hour periodicity is regular in the nonimmune host. Paroxysms may be more severe than those in vivax infections. The development of the nephrotic syndrome is a sequel peculiar to *P. malariae* infections (see Pathology). Quartan infections occur in areas where both *P. vivax* and *P. falciparum* are also present, and clinically are dominated by either when mixed infections are present.

Plasmodium falciparum. The incubation period of *P. falciparum* averages 10 to 12 days. The young ring stages (Table 6-2) are usually smaller than those of the other species. The cytoplasm is a delicate threadlike line (Plates 5 and 6) and one or more small chromatin dots are present. Double chromatin dots are much more common in *P. falciparum* than in the other species. Young ring stages appear numerous in the thin blood film, are small, delicate, and highly suggestive of a falciparum infection. Sometimes they appear irregular as streaks, flame-shaped, round, or rectangular. Flattened marginal forms and bridge forms are more common, as are multiple infections of a single cell, than in other species. Falciparum parasites remain as ring forms during most of the early growth phase and are numerous; this makes diagnosis much easier. Older, developing trophozoites, comparable to the ameboid forms of *P. vivax*, are confined chiefly to the capillary beds of internal organs, where development continues, and, only rarely, if ever, appear in the peripheral circulation. Ring forms are found most readily after a chill. If the infection is running a tertian cycle, the parasite density usually will be much higher during the interval between paroxysms than during the paroxysm. Schizogony takes place in the capillary beds of internal organs. In very heavy infections, at times, a schizont may appear in the circulation, dominated, however, by showers of ring forms. The mature schizont has 8 to 24 merozoites and is smaller than those of the other species. The amount of pigment is also less in all stages. Red blood cells are not altered in size by falciparum infection. Sometimes, red-staining dots called Maurer's spots may be seen in the red cell. They are irregular in shape and size and usually much coarser and much less numerous than Schüffner's stippling. Their appearance is dependent on critical staining.

Gametocytes are distinctive in appearance. Often described as banana shaped, sausage shaped, or crescent shaped, they stretch across the red cell revealing a thin film of the cell on the concave side of the parasite (Plate 5). At other times, completely stretching the red cell wall about the parasite, they give the appearance of being free in the blood plasma. In primary infections gametocytes usually do not appear in the peripheral circulation for several days. They are frequently found, however, in older or chronic infections, when ring stages are rare or not seen at all. Unlike those of *P. vivax*,

the gametocytes of *P. falciparum* appear to be produced in showers. In thick blood films, showers of young, delicate ring stages (Plate 6) with numerous double chromatin dots are readily identifiable. Typical gametocyte morphology is obvious, but distortion sometimes occurs in the blood film preparation. Whereas the *P. vivax* complex prefers young red cells and quartan malaria older cells, *P. falciparum* invades old and young red blood cells alike, and massive numbers become readily infected (Plates 5 and 6). Early symptoms of headache, gastrointestinal complaints, malaise, and nausea suggest a cold or flu. The first paroxysm of the primary attack in the nonimmune host may be quite sudden with the chill much less pronounced than in *P. vivax* or hardly detectable. A rise in temperature occurs quickly, with a high sustained fever for many hours. A pseudocrisis appears, but the temperature rises again, and eventually the pseudocrisis is terminated by a true crisis (Fig. 6-14). The sweating period is short and overshadowed by the febrile period. The entire paroxysm may last up to 36 hours. Since the schizogonic cycle may be from 36 to 48 hours, one paroxysm may extend into the next with little or no time between. The patient obtains little or no relief between paroxysms and may remain febrile throughout the entire attack. Following the primary attack, frequent recrudescences occur during the first month. After 3 to 5 months, latent periods are longer between attacks until radical cure occurs in about 10 months. If the patient survives, relapses are diminished in intensity.

Unlike other types of malaria, which are of themselves never fatal, *P. falciparum*, the malignant malaria, can cause death. Pernicious symptoms include temperature elevation to about 105 ° F, up to 108 ° and sometimes 110°. The patient may become delirious or comatose and die within a few hours. Sometimes the patient may lapse into coma without hyperpyrexia.

Cerebral malaria may have a sudden or

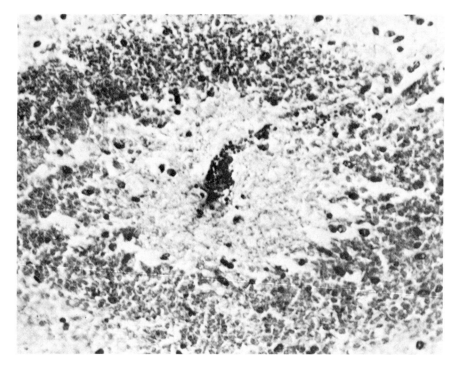

Fig. 6-15. A thrombosed blood vessel in the brain containing parasitized red blood cells and surrounded by a ring hemorrhage. (AFIP 66-6871.)

gradual onset. Manifestations of excitation, depression, behavioral changes with psychotic tendencies, or seizures may appear. The patient may lapse into coma with a noticeable decrease in blood pressure, and cyanosis may develop because of anoxia, cerebral edema, and increased intracranial pressure.

A massive, generalized invasion of the vascular system presents a septicemic form often stimulating a variety of diseases. High fever, headache, delirium, cyanosis, and hemorrhage (Fig. 6-15) in internal organs, resulting from the back pressure built up from clogged capillaries, may occur.

An onset characterized by extreme nausea, severe and continuous vomiting, gastric distress, and pronounced icterus is described as the bilious form. The urine often contains bile pigments, and hemorrhaging in the stomach yields a coffee-ground-like vomitus.

The fever becomes high and remittent rather than continuous. Dehydration and electrolyte imbalance may be present with disturbance of alkali reserve.

A massive, generalized, vascular invasion of the gastrointestinal tract and other abdominal viscera may lead to severe prostration, marked with cold, clammy skin, subnormal temperature, and circulatory collapse. This algid form may be accompanied by severe anemia, and death may ensue without fever.

In the choleraic form, the stools become loose and numerous and somewhat resemble the rice-water stools of patients with cholera. Severe dehydration, followed by anuria and death, may occur. Hemorrhages may occur anywhere in the body.

Researchers in Panama demonstrated the association of malignant tertian malaria with a syndrome of acute hemolysis of the erythrocytes resulting in severe hemoglobinuria. The passage of a dark, mahogany-red urine in falciparum malaria became known as black-water fever. The onset is usually sudden. A severe chill with marked prostration followed by a rapid rise in temperature that may reach 105 ° F with pain over the area of the kidneys characterizes this syndrome. There is severe epigastric distress with nausea and vomiting. The pulse usually is rapid and feeble. Massive hemolysis leads to a rapid and extreme drop in the red blood cell count within 24 hours. There may be recurring hemolytic crises, terminating after the first, or continuing for several days. Because of renal failure, anemia and death may ensue. Mortality rates may reach 50% chiefly as a result of the renal failure. Because blackwater fever is rare in patients who have not had prior experience with malaria or who have not had treatment, particularly with quinine, some have explained the hemolytic crisis as a hypersensitivity reaction to partially treated malaria. According to some, the pathogenesis involves an immuno-allergic mechanism induced by autoantibodies, an etiologic relationship existing between the intake of quinine and the induction of the acute hemolysis. Black-water fever is less common now because of the use of other antimalarial drugs. Those patients with a deficiency of glucose-6-phosphate dehydrogenase in the red cells also are prone to hemolytic crises under treatment with some drugs.

Pathology. Pathologic changes of the parenchymal cells of the liver caused by invasion by exoerythrocytic parasites are minimal. Liver biopsy specimens may show smaller cells containing merozoites. The major pathological findings in all malaria infections are associated with the erythrocytic phase.

Common to all species is red cell destruction and resultant anemia. The antibody-antigen reaction on the red blood cells surface activating complement triggers their destruc-

tion. The spleen becomes enlarged, the pulp tarry, and the malpighian bodies pale gray. Stretching and tearing of the capsule cause perisplenitis in chronic cases. Malaria pigment may be seen in the tissue spaces and within the reticuloendothelial cells. Later, in chronic cases, fibrosis eventually results in a small, shrunken spleen. The liver becomes congested and enlarged, with stretching of the capsule. Lysis of red cells leads to destruction of the bile canaliculi. The Küpffer cells of the reticuloendothelial system become hypertrophied, and blood flow is impaired. The kidneys, in malariae (quartan) as well as in falciparum infections, may show granular casts and fatty degeneration of the parenchyma, suggestive of glomerulonephritis. The bone marrow becomes hypertrophied, congested, and hemorrhagic. Pulmonary capillaries, likewise, show congestion, and mucous membranes show petechiae throughout. Coronary arteries of the heart develop emboli, and resultant ischemia causes anoxia in the heart. Changes also occur throughout the various other organs of the body.

Marked changes occur in the blood-vascular system. In the vivax-ovale group, young red cells are invaded, whereas *P. malariae* prefers older cells. In both instances the total number of red cells destroyed is limited. Likewise, the time between the liberation of merozoites and the invasion of red cells is greatest in these species, thus allowing for phagocytosis to further limit resultant pathology. *P. falciparum*, on the other hand, invades young and old red cells alike. Subterian cycles increase the rapidity with which more cells become infected, whereas phagocytosis between schizogonic cycles is minimal.

During the initial parasitemia, a leukopenia often occurs with a relative monocytosis. A decrease in platelets is commonly associated with a fall in complement but, in falciparum infection, may also reflect disseminated intravascular coagulation. The plasma becomes more viscous during the febrile period, and plasma potassium rises quickly upon rupturing of the red cells, returning to normal about 14 hours later. Bilirubin is also increased during active malaria. Total plasma proteins are reduced with a reversal of the albumin-globulin ratio. The gamma globulin fraction is increased most. IgM, IgA, and IgG show the greatest rise, generally paralleling the rise in parasite density. At the time of the peak, IgM and IgA decline, with IgG remaining sustained for an extended period of time. Persistence of IgG fluorescent antibodies serves as a useful tool in measuring epidemiologically past infections. A high response to IgM and IgG suggests a current infection or one within the past 1 to 3 months. It is a widely accepted view that humoral antibody and cell-mediated reactions collaborate in developing a protective mechansim against malaria, although the extent to which each plays a part is debatable. Antimalarial protection is generally associated with the raised levels of IgG, as attested to in pregnancy when IgG levels fall progressively and exacerbations of malaria increase. Further support to this concept is the protection afforded by passive transfer of antibody.

The quartan malarial nephropathy (QMN) is believed by many to be an immunopathologic phenomenon. Immune complexes of *P. malariae* antigen and antimalarial antibody, by virtue of their binding to the basement membrane of the glomerulus, initiate the nephrotic syndrome involving gross edema with ascites, proteinuria, hypertension, and, eventually, renal failure. It develops in patients with high antimalarial antibody titers and high IgM titers. Granular deposits containing mainly IgM plus complement have been demonstrated in the syndrome. It has been suggested that infection with *P. malariae* may thus cause an immune complex nephritis, which, in turn, is sustained by an autoimmune process.

Malarial parasites take oxygen readily from the oxyhemoglobin in the red cells, the broken-down globin is resynthesized into parasite protein, and the waste product hematin is expelled from the ruptured cells to be phagocytized later by host tissue cells. Glucose-6-phosphate dehydrogenase (G6PD) in the red cells is essential to parasite metabolism; hence patients with this enzyme deficiency are believed to have some natural immunity to infection. The prevalence of the deleterious gene for sickle cell anemia in Africa is also believed to be a result of protection of the gene carrier (patient with sickle cell trait) against fatal falciparum infection.

In falciparum infections the infected red cells become sticky and adhere to the capillary and venule walls in internal organs (Fig. 6-16). The flow of normal red blood cells is impaired (sludge blood), hemostasis occurs, and thrombi develop. However, many feel that circulatory stasis is brought about by the inflammatory response which leads to increased vascular permeability from the release of kinins and subsequent loss of protein and water from the blood to the tissues. Developing pressure within the vascular bed may lead to rupture of weak spots in the walls with petechial hemorrhages. Tissue anoxia and electrolyte imbalance take place in many organs of the body, and death is caused by interference with the normal function of the vascular system, not by toxic products produced by the parasites. The most dramatic changes may be seen in the brain, where low-power microscopy shows all blood vessels clearly defined by the denser-stained parasitized red cells that line the vessel walls. Grossly the brain shows punctiform hemorrhages in the subcortical areas, whereas the gray matter, as a whole, is grayish and there are hemorrhagic spots speckled throughout the white matter. Glial cells, clustered around a central focus of degeneration, present a granuloma-like appearance and are known as "malarial granulomas."

Diagnosis. The diagnosis of malaria is dependent on the recovery and identification of

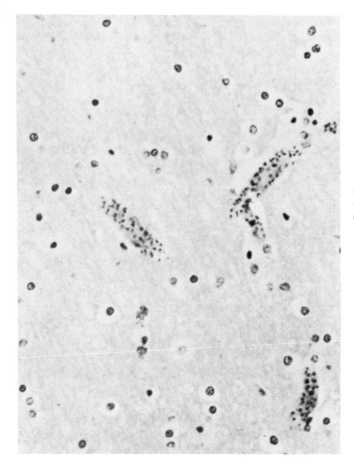

Fig. 6-16. Cerebral capillaries congested with parasitized red blood cells. (AFIP 66-7680.)

the parasites in the circulation. Morphologic characteristics of the four important species are presented in Table 6-2. The question as to the best time to make blood smears may be answered simply by saying as soon and as frequently as possible. If thick blood films, carefully prepared and stained, are examined adequately both morning and afternoon for 3 consecutive days and no parasites are found, one can be reasonably certain that the patient does not have malaria. If doubt persists, more thick films should be made. Bleeding or epinephrine have been recommended in difficult cases to induce release of parasites from the spleen but are too dangerous in an already-ill patient. Techniques for preparing smears are presented in Chapter 15.

The examination of the thick film is the most critical procedure in the diagnosis. After an area where the leukocytes are well stained and numerous cells have been found, the search should begin. A minimum of 100 fields should be thoroughly examined before a patient is declared free of the disease. In mixed infections, the detection of *P. falciparum* parasites among the other species is important so that proper therapy can be instituted at once.

Normally, in vivax, ovale, and malariae infections, parasites in various stages of development are present in the peripheral blood at all times. In malignant tertian malaria, usually only early ring stages and gametocytes appear in the peripheral circulation. In the nonimmune host, ring stages can be detected in the blood about 24 hours before symptoms appear. The typical crescent-shaped gametocytes appear about 8 to 10 days later. Both persist together for several days or weeks before the ring stages clear. The gametocytes may remain a month or longer.

The serodiagnosis of malaria has become available with the significant breakthrough in culturing the three major species of malaria. The indirect hemagglutination (IHA) test and the indirect immunofluorescence (IIF) test, although varying somewhat in sensitivity and specificity, are each useful in their own way. Where previous exposure has occured, as in endemic areas, IHA is nearly twice as reactive, thus indicating more clearly the presence of active transmission. On the other hand, a traveler passing through an endemic area may acquire a primary infection, as indicated by highly reactive IIF (see Tables 15-1 and 15-2). Thus for diagnosing the illness of a single individual, which is the usual case for the average practicing physician, the IIF test is the test of choice. Enzyme-linked immunosorbent assay (ELISA) and fluorescent immunoassay "X" (FIAX) are newer

tests being evaluated. As global travel expands the growing problem of transfusion malaria warrants the screening of blood donors by serodiagnosis.

Attempts to vaccinate humans against malaria, while promising, have had mixed results. Exposure over many weeks to several hundred irradiated, infected mosquitoes gave immunity for 3 months against *P. falciparum* and 3 to 6 months against *P. vivax* in three out of five volunteers. At the present time, it is believed that merozoites of the erythrocytic stage offer the most promising form of vaccine for potential use in human trials. Purified merozoite antigens, in combination with vaccines against the erythrocytic stages or gametes, would help substantially in the interruption of transmission. However, results obtained from animal models cannot necessarily be extrapolated to humans. Basic research is going on in the area of vaccination.

Treatment. Many travelers to malarious areas of the world and their physicians are unaware of the risk of contracting malaria or the need for malaria chemoprophylaxis (Table 6-3). It is essential that the physician

Table 6-3. Indications for malaria chemoprophylaxis

Purpose	Drugs of choice	Alternative drugs
To prevent acquisition of malaria in areas **without** known chloroquine-resistant malaria	Chloroquine phosphate Amodiaquine Hydroxychloroquine Chloroquine sulfate	Pyrimethamine Chlorguanide[1]
To prevent acquisition of malaria in areas **with** known chloroquine-resistant strains of *P. falciparum*	Pyrimethamine-sulfadoxine[1]	Since pyrimethamine-sulfadoxine is not available in the United States and must be obtained overseas (see Table 6-4), travelers should take weekly chloroquine or a comparable drug until pyrimethamine-sulfadoxine can be obtained
To prevent relapses of *P. vivax* and *P. ovale*	Primaquine[2]	

From U.S. Department of Health, Education, and Welfare, Center for Disease Control, Atlanta, Georgia.
[1]Not available in the United States.
[2]Not recommended for all travelers to malarious areas.

Table 6-4. Drugs and doses for malaria chemoprophylaxis

Generic name	Brand names[1]	Manufacturer	Adult dose	Pediatric dose
Amodiaquine	Camoquin Flavoquine Basoquin	Parke-Davis	520 mg (400 mg base) once weekly and continued for 6 wk after last exposure in a malarious area	<1 yr: 65 mg (50 mg base) 1-3 yr: 130 mg (100 mg base) 4-6 yr: 195 mg (150 mg base) 7-10 yr: 260 mg (200 mg base) 11-16 yr: 390 mg (300 mg base)
Chlorguanide	Paludrine Proguanil	Ayerst, ICI Chemicals	100-200 mg daily and continued for 6 wk after last exposure in a malarious area	2 yr & under: 25-50 mg 3-6 yr: 50-75 mg 7-10 yr: 100 mg
Chloroquine phosphate	Aralen Avlocloi Resochin	Winthrop ICI Chemicals FBA Pharmaceuticals	500 mg (300 mg base) weekly and continued for 6 wk after last exposure in a malarious area	<1 yr: 62 mg (37.5 mg base) 1-3 yr: 125 mg (75 mg base) 4-6 yr: 165 mg (100 mg base) 7-10 yr: 250 mg (150 mg base) 11-16 yr: 375 mg (225 mg base) or 5 mg/kg base
Chloroquine sulfate	Nivaquine	May & Baker	500 mg (300 mg base) weekly and continued for 6 wk after last exposure in a malarious area	<1 yr: 62 mg (37.5 mg base) 1-3 yr: 125 mg (75 mg base) 4-6 yr: 165 mg (100 mg base) 7-10 yr: 250 mg (150 mg base) 11-16 yr: 375 mg (225 mg base) or 5 mg/kg base
Hydroxychloroquine	Plaquenil	Winthrop	400 mg (310 mg base) weekly and continued for 6 wk after last exposure in a malarious area	< 1 yr: 50 mg (37.5 mg base) 1-3 yr: 100 mg (75 mg base) 4-6 yr: 130 mg (100 mg base) 7-10 yr: 200 mg (150 mg base) 11-16 yr: 290 mg (225 mg base) or 5 mg/kg base
Primaquine	None	Winthrop	26.3 mg (15 mg base) daily for 14 days or 79 mg (45 mg base) once weekly for 8 wk; start during the last 2 wk of, or following a course of, suppression with chloroquine or a comparable drug	0.3 mg/kg base/day for 14 days or 0.9 mg/kg base/day weekly for 8 wk
Pyrimethamine	Daraprim	Burroughs-Wellcome	25 mg weekly and continued for 6 wk after last exposure in a malarious area	2 yr & under: 6.25 mg 8-10 yr: 12.5 mg Over 10 yr: adult dosage
Pyrimethamine-sulfadoxine[2]	Fansidar Falcidar Antemal Methipox	Hoffmann-La Roche Hoffmann-La Roche	50 mg pyrimethamine and 1,000 mg sulfadoxine every other week and continued for 6 wk after last exposure in a malarious area[3]	In terms of sulfadoxine: 6 to 11 mo: 125 mg 1-3 yr: 250 mg 4-8 yr: 500 mg 9-14 yr: 750 mg

From U.S. Department of Health, Education, and Welfare, Center for Disease Control, Atlanta, Georgia.

[1]Use of trade names is for identification only and does not constitute endorsement by the Public Health Service, U.S. Department of Health, Education, and Welfare.

[2]Countries where pyrimethamine-sulfadoxine can be obtained: Belgium, Brazil, Burma, Cambodia, Germany, Hong Kong, Indonesia, Laos, Malaysia, Philippines, Singapore, Switzerland, Thailand, Venezuela, Viet Nam.

[3]Use of this drug for more than 6 months is discouraged until more information becomes available on its chronic toxicity.

Table 6-5. Treatment for malaria

Infection	Drug	Adult dose*	Pediatric dose*
Malaria *(Plasmodium falciparum, P. ovale, P. vivax,* and *P. malariae)*			
Suppression or chemoprophylaxis of disease while in edemic area (all plasmodia except chloroquine-resistant *P. falciparum)*			
Drug of choice	Chloroquine phosphate[1]	500 mg (300 mg base) once weekly and continued for 6 wk after last exposure in endemic area	*<1 yr:* 37.5 mg base; *1-3 yr:* 75 mg base; *4-6 yr:* 100 mg base; *7-10 yr:* 150 mg base; *11-16 yr:* 225 mg base
Alternative	Amodiaquine hydrochloride[1]	520 mg (400 mg base) once weekly and continued for 6 wk after last exposure in endemic area	*<1 yr:* 50 mg base; *1-3 yr:* 100 mg base; *4-6 yr:* 150 mg base; *7-10 yr:* 200 mg base; *11-16 yr:* 300 mg base
Prevention of attack after departure from areas where *P. vivax* and *P. ovale* are endemic[2]			
Drug of choice	Primaquine phosphate[3]	26.3 mg (15 mg base)/d × 14d (with last 2 wk of chloroquine prophylaxis)	0.3 mg/kg base/d × 14d (with last 2 wk of chloroquine prophylaxis)
Treatment of uncomplicated attack (all plasmodia except chloroquine-resistant *P. falciparum)*			
Drug of choice	Chloroquine phosphate[1,4]	1 gm (600 mg base) then 500 mg (300 mg base) in 6 hr, then 500 mg (300 mg base)/d × 2d	10 mg base/kg (max. 600 mg base); then half this dose once daily beginning 6 hr later × 2d
Alternative	Amodiaquine hydrochloride[1]	780 mg (600 mg base) first day, then 520 mg (400 mg base)/d × 2d	*<1 yr:* 100-150 mg base, then 67-100 mg/d × 2d; *1-3 yr:* 200 mg base, then 134 mg/d × 2d; *4-6 yr:* 300 mg base, then 200 mg/d × 2d; *7-12 yr:* 400 mg base, then 266 mg/d × 2d; *13-18 hr:* 400-600 mg base, then 266-400 mg/d × 2d

From The Medical Letter, Inc., 56 Harrison Street, New Rochelle, N.Y.

*The letter d indicates day.

1. Dosage is oral unless otherwise stated. If chloroquine phosphate is not available hydroxychloroquine sulfate is as effective; 400 mg of hydroxychloroquine sulfate is equivalent to 500 mg of chloroquine phosphate. Recommended prophylactic doses of amodiaquine have been repoted to cause agranulocytosis and pancytopenia.
2. For prevention of attack after departure from areas where *P. vivax* or *P. ovale* are endemic (particularly Africa), many experts prescribe primaquine phosphate daily for 14 days beginning with the day of departure from the endemic area. Some prefer to avoid the toxicity of primaquine and rely on surveillance to detect cases when they occur, particularly when exposure was limited or doubtful.
3. Dosages of primaquine phosphate of 26.3 mg (15 mg base) per day or more for 14 days may cause hemolytic anemia, especially in patients whose red cells are deficient in glucose-6-phosphate dehydrogenase. This deficiency is most common in blacks, Orientals, and Mediterranean peoples.
4. In falciparum malaria, if the patient has not shown a prompt response to conventional doses of chloroquine, parasitic resistance to this drug must be considered.
5. In the U.S.A., this drug is available from the Parasitic Disease Division, Center for Disease Control, Atlanta, Georgia 30333; telephone 404-329-3311.
6. Intravenous administration of quinine dihydrochloride can be hazardous, and it must be given slowly. Constant monitoring of the pulse and blood pressure is necessary to detect arrhythmia or hypotension. Oral quinine sulfate should be substituted as soon as possible accompanied by other drugs recommended for uncomplicated attack.
7. Chloroquine-resistant strains of *P. falciparum* have been reported from Bangladesh, Brazil, Burma, Cambodia, Colombia, Ecuador, French Guiana, Guyana, India, Indonesia, Laos, Malaysia, Nepal, Panama, Papua New Guinea, the Philippines, Surinam, Thailand, Venezuela, Vietnam, and, recently, East Africa (CC Campbell, Lancet, 2:1151, Dec 1, 1979).
8. Pyrimethamine plus sulfadoxine is available in a fixed-dose combination as Fansidar, but not in the U.S.A. (December 1979). Each tablet of Fansidar contains 25 mg of pyrimethamine and 500 mg of sulfadoxine.
9. Quinine alone will control an acute attack of resistant *P. falciparum*, but in a substantial number of infections, particularly with strains from Southeast Asia, it fails to prevent recurrence. Addition of pyrimethamine with sulfadiazine lowers the rate of recurrence.
10. Considered an investigational drug for this condition by the U.S. Food and Drug Administration.

Table 6-5. Treatment for malaria—cont'd

Infection	Drug	Adult dose*	Pediatric dose*
Treatment of severe illness, parenteral dosage—only if oral dose cannot be administered (regardless of severity) (all plasmodia except chloroquine-resistant *P. falciparum*)			
Drug of choice	Chloroquine HCl[4]	250 mg (200 mg base) IM q6h	5 mg/kg base IM q12h
Alternative	Quinine dihydro-chloride[5,6]	600 mg in 300 ml normal saline IV over at least 1 hr; repeat in 6-8 hr (max. 1800 mg/d)	25 mg/kg/d; administer half of dose in 1-hr infusion, then other half 6-8 hr later if oral therapy still cannot be started (max. 1800 mg/d)
Prevention of relapses ("radical" cure after "clinical" cure) (*P. vivax* and *P. ovale* only)			
Drug of choice	Primaquine phos-phate[3]	26.3 mg (15 mg base)/d × 14d or 79 mg (45 mg base)/wk × 8 wk	0.3 mg/kg base/d × 14d
P. falciparum (chloroquine-resistant)[4,7]			
Suppression or chemoprophylaxis			
Drug of choice	Pyrimethamine *plus* sulfadoxine[8]	1 tablet (25 mg pyrimethamine, 500 mg sulfadoxine) once every wk	*6-11 mo:* ⅛ tablet; *1-3 yr:* ¼ tablet; *4-8 yr:* ½ tablet; *9-14 yr:* ¾ tablet weekly
Treatment of uncomplicated attack[9] (chloroquine-resistant *P. falciparum*)			
Drug of choice	Quinine sulfate *plus* pyrimethamine	650 mg tid × 3d 25 mg bid × 3d	25 mg/kg/d in 3 doses × 3d *<10 kg:* 6.25 mg/d; *10-20 kg:* 12.5 mg/d; *20-40 kg:* 25 mg/d
	plus sulfadiazine	500 mg qid × 5d	100-200 mg/kg/d in 4 doses × 5d (max. 2 gm/d)
Alternatives	Quinine sulfate *plus* tetracycline[10]	650 mg tid × 3d 500 mg qid × 7d	25 mg/kg/d in 3 doses × 3d 10 mg/kg qid × 7d (max 2 gm/d)
Treatment of severe illness, parenteral dosage (chloroquine-resistant *P. falciparum*)			
Drug of choice	Quinine dihydro-chloride[5,6]	600 mg in 300 ml normal saline IV over at least 1 hr; repeat in 6-8 hr (max. 1800 mg/d)	25 mg/kg/d; administer half of dose in 1-hr infusion, then other half 6-8 hr later if oral therapy still cannot be started (max. 1800 mg/d)
Alternatives	None		

Adverse effects of antiparasitic drugs

Chloroquine HCl and Chloroquine phosphate USP (Aralen; and others)

Occasional: pruritus; vomiting; headache; confusion; depigmentation of hair; skin eruptions; hemolysis especially with G6PD deficiency; corneal opacity; irreversible retinal injury (especially when total dosage exceeds 100 grams); weight loss; partial alopecia; extraocular muscle palsies; exacerbation of psoriasis, eczema and other exfoliative dermatitis

Rare: discoloration of nails and mucous membranes of mouth; nerve-type deafness; blood dyscrasias; photophobia

Amodiaquine HCl USP (Camoquin)

Occasional: vomiting; diarrhea; vertigo

Rare: agranulocytosis; pancytopenia; corneal deposits; bluish gray pigmentation of fingernails, skin and hard palate; retinopathy; polyneuropathy; liver damage

Primaquine phosphate USP

Frequent: hemolytic anemia in G6PD deficiency

Occasional: neutropenia; GI disturbances; methemoglobinemia in G6PD deficiency

Rare: CNS symptoms; hypertension; arrhythmias

Quinine dihydrochloride and Quinine sulfate

Frequent: cinchonism (tinnitus, headache, nausea, abdominal pain, visual disturbance)

Occasional: blood dyscrasias; photosensitivity reactions; arrhythmias; hypotension

Rare: blindness; sudden death if injected too rapidly

Pyrimethamine USP (Daraprim)

Occasional: blood dyscrasias; folic acid deficiency

Rare: rash; vomiting; convulsions; shock

be well informed in this matter. The risk of acquiring malaria varies from country to country and within given countries. Areas where malaria is known to exist are parts of Mexico, Haiti, Central America, South America, Africa, the Middle East, the Indian subcontinent, Southeast Asia, Korea, Indonesia, and Oceania. All travelers to these areas risk acquiring malaria. It is the responsibility of the physician to inform the traveler of the general protective measures for reducing exposure to mosquitoes, such as staying indoors in well-screened areas during dusk to dawn hours, sleeping under mosquito netting, and wearing adequate clothing outdoors with the use of mosquito repellents over the exposed areas of the body. A specific program of malaria chemoprophylaxis (Table 6-4) dependent on many factors such as intensity of exposure, presence of chloroquine-resistant malaria, drug allergies or intolerance, and pregnancy in the female, should be developed for the traveler.

Chloroquine phosphate is the drug of choice for suppression (prevention of clinical symptoms by eliminating erythrocytic but not exoerythrocytic [E.E.] stages) of *P. vivax, P. malariae, P. ovale,* and sensitive strains of *P. falciparum* (Table 6-5). Oral therapy should begin 1 to 2 weeks before entering the malaria zone and continued for 6 weeks after the last exposure. The physician should emphasize to the traveler the importance of starting prophylaxis early and continuing it after returning home. In some cases of *P. falciparum* and *P. malariae* infection, delayed primary attacks can occur after the six-week period of prophylaxis is terminated, and travelers should be alerted by the physician that if a fever develops after returning home they should contact him immediately. Since exoerythrocytic stages of *P. vivax* and *P. ovale* persist in the liver (chloroquine is relatively ineffective), delayed initial attacks or relapses can occur up to 4 years after chloroquine suppression has been terminated. Again, the travelers should contact

the physician if symptoms appear. Primaquine, the drug of choice for E.E. stages, is not recommended for prophylaxis. Each case must be evaluated as to the intensity of the traveler's exposure to *P. vivax* and *P. ovale* and the risk of primaquine toxicity (G6PD deficiency). If used, primaquine may be started during the last 2 weeks of, or following, the chloroquine suppression regimen.

Panama, South America, the Indian subcontinent, Southeast Asia, New Guinea, and lately Africa have chloroquine-resistant strains of *P. falciparum.* Because of the complexity of the problem, recommendations for chemoprophylaxis must be made on an individual basis, but some general suggestions can be made. Since chloroquine suppresses *P. vivax, P. malariae, P. ovale,* and sensitive *P. falciparum,* this drug will provide some protection. Amodiaquine appears to be more effective than chloroquine against resistant *P. falciparum* and therefore may give additional but *not* absolute protection. The most effective drug probably is a fixed combination of pyrimethamine and sulfadoxine, a long-acting sulfonamide called Fansidar (not available in the United States). Most countries with the resistant *P. falciparum,* however, have it available. Travelers should start on chloroquine 1 to 2 weeks before entering the endemic area, as indicated previously, and continue prophylaxis until they can obtain pyrimethamine-sulfadoxine (Table 6-4). This drug combination is active primarily against erythrocytic stages and should be continued for 6 weeks after leaving the zone. It produces suppressive cure (destroys all parasites in the body) in *most* chloroquine-sensitive and resistant strains of *P. falciparum,* and effectively suppresses *P. malariae, P. ovale,* and strains of *P. vivax* sensitive to pyrimethamine. Some suggest adding chloroquine to suppress the pyrimethamine-resistant *P. vivax.* Patients with known allergies to sulfonamides should not receive this drug. Physicians should be aware of other potential serious reactions from sulfonamides. Long-term use of pyrimeth-amine-sulfadoxine should be avoided. Like chloroquine, this drug combination will not prevent delayed primary attacks or relapses resulting from persistent E.E. stages of *P. vivax* and *P. ovale* when suppression is stopped. As indicated, primaquine prophylaxis may be advisable under certain conditions. For details of treatment see Table 6-5.

Malaria eradication

A global eradication program was begun by WHO in 1956 after it was apparent that residual house-spraying with DDT would eliminate the transmission of malaria by the anopheline mosquito. At the peak of the campaign in 1962 some 100 million dwellings housing 575 million people were sprayed by 130,000 spraymen. As a result, eradication was achieved among some 370 million people by 1961 and some 745 million by 1972 or fully 40% of the 1.8 billion population at risk. Everything looked promising. Malaria transmission had been eradicated from Europe, the United States, the U.S.S.R., Taiwan, a great many of the Caribbean islands, parts of Mexico, South America, and the Middle East. Malaria was on its way out. The case estimate had fallen from over 300 million in 1943 to around 100 million by 1970. However, the tide began to turn around 1975. Self-complacency, the reluctance of government officials to spend money on necessary surveillance, and a shortage of technical personnel became apparent. Inflation and the energy crisis left their mark on the eradication program. Mosquitoes and parasites alike became resistant to insecticides and drugs. The incidence of malaria in India, which had fallen from 75 million in 1947 to 125 thousand in 1965, returned to over 4 million in 1975, and is now getting worse. Southeast Asia has reported the greatest increase. Bangladesh and Sri Lanka (Ceylon) have seen a resurgence near their former levels. The situation has become worse in Thailand. Turkey, not

long ago, reported a malaria epidemic, thus posing a threat to countries along the Mediterranean coast and to tourists as well. Migrant workers may spread the disease to other parts of Europe. Tropical Africa has serious problems. Countries that have eradicated malaria, such as England and the United States, are now importing cases. England and Wales had 1,624 published cases for 1978 and many others not officially recognized. The Federal German Republic reported 528 cases in 1978, an increase from 100 in 1974. Fifty persons have died from malaria in Germany since 1970. Around 2,000 cases, including 20 deaths, were estimated in France in 1978. Between 1970 and 1976 an estimated 887 American civilians (not military) brought back malaria from abroad with 19 deaths occurring. In Central America, particularly in Guatemala and El Salvador, *Anopheles albimanus*, the malarial vector in these regions, has become resistant to malathion and propoxur in addition to DDT and dieldrin. The incidence of malaria in these regions is increasing. Globally, in 1976 there were 2.3 times as many cases of malaria as in 1972. It is predicted that non-endemic countries can expect a continuous rise in imported malaria.

Vector resistance to a growing number of insecticides is becoming increasingly problematic, and although improvement is being made in control, the rate has progressed slowly in recent years and with considerable increase in costs. Virtually no eradication programs are going on in tropical Africa, where emphasis is being given to control rather than eradication. The same is true for many other areas, and, in addition, more attention is being given to alternate methods of control other than residual home spraying; the potential of biological and genetic approaches as well as other methods are under investigation. The use of temephos (Abate) as a larvicidal agent is increasing along with use of larva-eating fish such as *Gambusia*, a technique that is being tried in selected

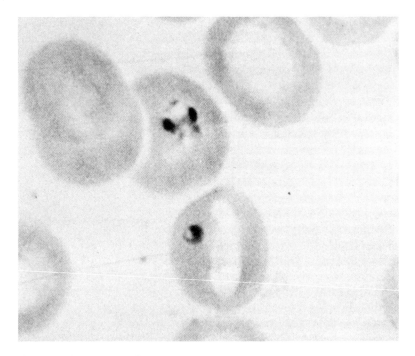

Fig. 6-17. Thin blood film showing *Babesia microti* in human red blood cells. Note the similarity to malarial parasites (AFIP 75-1178.)

areas of the world. The problem of chloroquine-resistant parasites has resulted in a search for newer antimalarial drugs; it must therefore be increasingly evident that complacency can have no place in malarial control and the problem of vector resistance is very serious.

BABESIOSIS

Species of the sporozoan parasite *Babesia* are parasites of ticks and mammals. Asexual reproduction takes place in the erythrocytes or other blood cells of mammals by binary fission. Sexual reproduction is unknown. Long known as an important disease of cattle in the United States, where babesiosis (piroplasmosis) became known as Texas cattle fever or redwater fever, in more recent times it has come into prominence as a disease in humans.

Since 1957, 24 cases in humans have been reported from Europe and North America.

Of these, six were known to have had splenectomies before infection, a factor known to increase the severity of infection in animals. Three of the six died after a rapidly progressive illness with high fever, jaundice, hemolytic anemia, and renal failure. Fourteen of the 24 were infected with *Babesia microti*, a parasite of meadow voles and other rodents, and were identified in the United States. None were splenectomized. Symptoms recorded were fever, chills, fatigue, general myalgia, and hemolytic anemia. One focus of infection was Nantucket Island, Massachusetts. Cases have also been reported from New York State on Shelter Island (near Long Island).

Babesiosis is a hemolytic disease similar to malaria. Transmission occurs by bite from the infected tick. There is no exoerythrocytic phase in the vertebrate, the parasite entering directly into the red blood cells. They are best observed after staining with one of the

Romanovsky stains, such as Giemsa, as for malaria (Fig. 6-17). They appear as teardrop-shaped small organisms but sometimes are ovoid, ameboid, or spherical. In undergoing schizogony they may appear in pairs or tetrads. The failure of chloroquine phosphate to have any effect on the height or duration of parasitemia in humans as well as similar action in animals, although symptomatic improvement is noted, suggests that the action of this drug is primarily anti-inflammatory rather than antibabesial. Successful treatment has been noted with diminazene aceturate, an experimental drug. However, neurologic complications (Landry-Guillain-Barré syndrome) following treatment were observed.

REVIEW QUESTIONS

1. Describe the life cycle of a typical coccidian parasite.
2. Discuss the possible relationship between *Isospora*, *Toxoplasma*, and *Sarcocystis*.
3. Discuss the pathology and prognosis of toxoplasmosis in the adult and in utero.
4. What is the chief method for the diagnosis of toxoplasmosis; the treatment?
5. In what age group is infection with *Pneumocystis carinii* most common?
6. How can other pneumonias be differentiated from interstitial plasma cell pneumonia?
7. What is the clinical and therapeutical significance of the E.E. stages of malaria?
8. How does the pathology explain the symptomatology of malignant tertian malaria?
9. What essential points should be kept in mind in the laboratory diagnosis of malaria?
10. Discuss the treatment of malaria from the standpoint of prophylaxis, uncomplicated attacks, severe illness, prevention of relapses, and drug resistance.
11. Discuss the significance of culturing malarial parasites in vitro.
12. What is the status of vaccination against malaria?
13. What is babesiosis? Discuss.

REFERENCES

Beaver, P. C., R. K. Gadgil, and P. Morera. 1979. *Sarcocystis* in man: a review and report of five cases. Am. J. Trop. Med. Hyg. **28**:819-844.

Benach, J. L., D. J. White, J. P. McGovern, and M. M. Jacovina. 1979. Immunological relationships of Long Island isolates of *Babesia microti*. Am. J. Trop. Med. Hyg. **28**:643-648.

Bennett, W. M., and others. 1977. Guidelines for drug therapy in renal failure. Ann. Intern. Med. **86**:754-783.

Bienzle, W., O. Ayeni, A. O. Lucas, and L. Luzzatto. 1972. Glucose-6-phosphate dehydrogenase and malaria. Greater resistance of females heterozygous for enzyme deficiency and of males with non-deficient variant. Lancet **1**:107-110.

Brandborg, L. L., S. B. Goldberg, and W. C. Briedenbach. 1970. Human coccidiosis: a possible cause of malabsorption. The life cycle in small bowel mucosal biopsies as a diagnostic feature. N. Engl. J. Med. **283**:1306-1313.

Brogger, R. C., and others. 1978. Changing patterns in the humoral immune reponse to malaria before, during, and after the application of control measures: a longitudinal study in the West African Savanna. Bull. WHO **56**:579-600.

Brown, A. W. A., J. Haworth, and A. R. Zahar. 1976. Malaria eradication and control from a global standpoint. J. Med. Entomol. **13**:1-25.

Camargo, M. E., and others. 1978. Immunoglobulin G and immunoglobulin M enzyme-linked immunosorbent assays and defined toxoplasmosis serological patterns. Infect. Immun. **21**:55-58.

Center for Disease Control, 1973, Babesiosis: Massachusetts. Morbidity and Mortality Weekly Report **22**:331-332.

Center for Disease Control. 1976. Parasitic disease drug service: pentamidine releases for *Pneumocystis* pneumonia. Morbidity and Mortality Weekly Report **25**:365-366.

Center for Disease Control. 1978. Malaria in participants of a natural history safari in Kenya, Africa. Morbidity and Mortality Weekly Report **27**:214.

Center for Disease Control. 1978. Chemoprophylaxis of malaria. Morbidity and Mortality Weekly Report **27**:80-81. (Supplement).

Clyde, D. F., V. C. McCarthy, R. M. Miller, and W. E. Woodward. 1975. Immunization of man against falciparum and vivax malaria by use of attenuated sporozoites. Am. J. Trop. Med. Hyg. **24**:397-403.

Cohen, S. 1979. Immunity to malaria. Proc. R. Soc. Lond. [Biol.] **203**:323-345.

Desmonts, G., and J. Courreur. 1974. Congenital toxoplasmosis: a prospective study of 378 pregnancies. N. Engl. J. Med. **290**:1110-1116.

Dutta, J. K., and S. K. Chadha. 1978. Toxoplasma antibody study in exanthematous states. Indian J. Med. Res. **68**:52-54.

Elsdon-Dew, R. 1975. Parasitic infections and the genitourinary tract. Practitioner **214**:75-79.

Faust, E. C., and others. 1961. Human isosporiasis in the western hemisphere. Am. J. Trop. Med. **10**:343.

Fayer, R. 1974. Development of *Sarcocystis fusiformis* in the small intestine of the dog. J. Parasitol. **60**:660-665.

Fayer, R., and A. J. Johnson. 1973. Development of *Sarcocystis fusiformis* in calves infected with sporocysts from dogs. J. Parasitol. **59**:1135-1137.

Fegies, M., and J. Guerrero. 1977. Treatment of toxoplasmosis with levamisole. Trans. R. Soc. Trop. Med. Hyg. **71**:178-179.

Feldman, H. A. 1974. Congenital toxoplasmosis, at long last. N. Engl. J. Med. **290**:1138-1140.

French, J. M., J. L. Whitby, and A. G. W. Whitfield. 1974. Steatorrhea in a man infected with coccodiosis *(Isospora belli):* case reports. Gastroenterology **47**: 642-648.

Frenkel, J. K. 1971. Toxoplasmosis. In R. Marcial-Rojas, Editor. Pathology of protozoal and helminthic diseases. The Williams & Wilkins Co., Baltimore, pp. 254-290.

Frenkel, J. K. 1971. Toxoplasmosis. Mechanisms of infection, laboratory diagnosis, and management. Curr. Top. Pathol. **54**:29-75.

Frenkel, J. K. 1973. Toxoplasmosis: parasitic life cycles, pathology, and immunology. Pages 343-410. In Hammond, D. M., and P. L. Long, Editors. The coccidia. University Park Press, Baltimore, Md.

Frenkel, J. K. 1974. Toxoplasmosis and pneumocystosis: clinical and laboratory aspects in immunocompetent and compromised host. Pages 203-259. In Prier, J. E., and H. Friedman, Editors. Opportunistic pathogens. University Park Press, Baltimore, Md.

Frenkel, J. K. 1974. Advances in the biology of sporozoa. A. Parasitenkol. **45**:125-162.

Frenkel, J. K., and J. P. Dubey. 1972. Rodents as vectors for feline coccodia, *Isospora felis* and *Isospora rivolta*. J. Infect. Dis. **125**:69-72.

Frenkel, J. K., and J. P. Dubey. 1973. Effects of freezing on the viability of toxoplasma oocysts. J. Parasitol. **59**:587-588.

Frenkel, J. K., and G. Perkarski. 1978. The demonstration of *Toxoplasma* and other organisms by immunofluorescence: a pitfall. J. Infect. Dis. **138**:265-266.

Frenkel, J. K., A. Ruiz, and M. Chinchilla. 1975. Soil survey of toxoplasma oocysts in Kansas and Costa Rica. Am. J. Trop. Med. Hyg. **24**:439-443.

Garnham, P. C. C. 1966. Malaria parasites and other haemosporidia. Blackwell Scientific Publications, Oxford.

Garnham, P. C., and others. 1969. Human babesiosis in Ireland: further observations and the medical significance of this infection. Br. Med. J. **4**:768-770.

Greenwood, B. M., D. Stratton, W. A. Williamson, and I Mohammed. 1978. A study of the role of immunological factors in the pathogenesis of the anaemia of acute malaria. Trans. R. Soc. Trop. Med. Hyg. **72**: 378-385.

Grossman, P. L., and J. S. Remington. 1979. The effect of trimethoprim and sulfamethoxazole on *Toxoplasma*

gondii in vitro and in vivo. Am. J. Trop. Med. Hyg. **28**:445-455.

Grunwaldt, E. 1977. Babesiosis on Shelter Island. N.Y. State. J. Med. **77**:1320-1321.

Hall, A. P. 1976. The treatment of malaria. Br. Med. J. **1**:323-328.

Hall, C. L., J. D. Haynes, J. D. Chulay, and C. L. Diggs. 1978. Cultured *Plasmodium falciparum* used as antigen in a malaria indirect fluorescent antibody test. Am. J. Trop. Med. Hyg. **27**:844-852.

Healy, G. R., A. Spielman, and N. Gleason. 1976. Human babesiosis: reservoir of infection on Nantucket Island. Science **192**:479-480.

Heineman, H. S. 1972. The clinical syndrome of malaria in U.S.A. Arch. Intern. Med. **129**:607-616.

Hoare, C. A. 1972. The developmental stages of *Toxoplasma*. J. Trop. Med. **75**:56-58.

Hughes, W. T. 1976. Treatment of *Pneumocystis carinii* pneumonitis. N. Engl. J. Med. **295**:726-727.

Hughes, W. T., S. Feldman, and S. K. Sanyal. 1975. Treatment of *Pneumocystis carinii* pneumonitis with trimethoprim-sulfamethoxazole. Can. Med. Assoc. J. **112**:475-505.

Hutchison, W. M., and others. 1970. Coccidian-like nature of *Toxoplasma gondii*. Br. Med. J. **1**:142-144.

Jopling, W. H. 1979. Malaria and the traveller. Lancet **1**:1340.

Kagan, I. G., and L. Norman. 1976. Serodiagnosis of parasitic diseases. Pages 382-408. In Rose, N. R., and H. Friedman, Editors. Manual of clinical immunology. American Society of Microbiology, Washington, D.C.

Kean, B. H. 1972. Clinical toxoplasmosis: 50 Years. Trans. R. Soc. Trop. Med. Hyg. **66**:549-567.

Kean, B. H., and R. C. Breslav. 1964. Cardiac sarcosporidiosis. Pages 74-83. In Parasites of the human heart. Grune & Stratton, Inc., New York.

Kean. B. H., and P. D. Reilly. 1976. Malaria: the mime. Recent lessons from a group of civilian travelers. Am. J. Med. **61**:159-164.

Krotoski, W. A., and others. 1980. Relapses in primate malaria: discovery of two populations of exoerythrocytic stages. Preliminary note. Br. Med. J. **280**:153-154.

Lake, K. B., J. J. Van Dyke, R. M. Abts, and D. R. Moyes. 1979. Lymphoglandular toxoplasmosis. Postgrad. Med. **65**:110-117.

Lau, W. K., and L. S. Young. 1976. Trimethoprim-sulfamethoxazole treatment of *Pneumocystis carinii* pneumonia in adults. N. Engl. J. Med. **295**:716-718.

Leak, D., and M. Meghji. 1979. Toxoplasmic infection in cardiac disease. Am. J. Cardiol. **43**:841-849.

Leonard, J. A. 1979. The "queen of diseases" strikes back. Harvard Magazine, July-August:20-24.

Markus, M. B. 1978. *Sarcocystis* and sarcocystosis in

domestic animals and man. Adv. Vet. Sci. Comp. Med. **22**:159-193.

Mason, S. J., and others. 1977. The Duffy blood group determinants: their role in the susceptibility of human and animal erythrocytes to *Plasmodium knowlesi* malaria. Br. J. Haematol. **36**:327-335.

McLeod, R., and J. S. Remington. 1977. Influence of infection with *Toxoplasma* on macrophage function and role of macrophages in resistance to *Toxoplasma*. Am. J. Trop. Med. Hyg. **26**:170-186.

Miller, Jr., F. H., A. V. Pizzuto, and H. McCauley. 1974. Human isosporosis: two cases. Am. J. Trop. Med. Hyg. **20**:23-25.

Molineaux, L., R. Cornille-Brögger, H. M. Mathews, and J. Storey. 1978. Longitudinal serological study of malaria in infants in the West African Savanna. Bull. WHO **56**:573-578.

National Cancer Institute. 1976. Monograph no. 43. Symposium on *Pneumocystis carinii* infection. U.S. Department of Health, Education, and Welfare, Public Health Service, National Institute of Health.

Nussenzweig, R. S., and others. 1972. Sporozoite-induced immunity in mammalian malaria: a review. Am. J. Trop. Med. Hyg. **21**:722-728.

O'Holohan, D. R., and J. Hugoe-Matthews. 1971. Malaria suppression in prophylaxis on a Malaysian rubber estate: sulformethoxine-primethamine single monthly dose vs. chloroquine single weekly dose. Southeast Asian J. Trop. Med. Public Health **2**:164-168.

Omanga, U. 1978. Possible pathogenic mechanism of hemolysis in malaria. Trop. Ped. Environ. Child Health **24**:230-232.

Pan American Health Organization. 1978. Malaria: growing alert. Editorial. Bull. Pan Am. Health Organ. **12**:271-272.

Pearlman, E. J., and A. P. Hall. 1975. Prevention of chloroquine-resistant falciparum malaria. Ann. Intern. Med. **82**:590-591.

Peters, W. 1971. Chemotherapy and drug resistance in malaria. Academic Press, Inc., New York.

Rodgers, B. M., F. Moazam, and J. L. Talbert. 1979. Thoracoscopy: early diagnosis of interstitial pneumonitis in the immunologically suppressed child. Chest **75**:126-130.

Roncoroni, A. J., and O. A. Martino. 1979. Therapeutic use of exchange transfusion in malaria. Am. J. Trop. Med. Hyg. **28**:440-444.

Ruebush, J. K., and others. 1979. Neurologic complications following the treatment of human *Babesia microti* infection with diminazene aceturate. Am. J. Trop. Med. Hyg. **28**:184-189.

Samuels, B. S., and R. L. Rietschel. 1976. Polymyositis and toxoplasmosis. J.A.M.A. **235**:60-61.

Scholtens, R. G., E. H. Braff, G. R. Healy, and N. Gleason. 1968. A case of babesiosis in man in the United States, Am. J. Trop. Med. Hyg. **17**:810-813.

Scott, R. J. 1978. Toxoplasmosis. Bureau Hyg. Trop. Dis. **75**:809-827.

Sheffield, H. G., and M. L. Melton. 1970. *Toxoplasma gondii*: the oocyst, sporozoite and infection of cultured cells. Science **167**:892-893.

Singh, P., T. D. Chug, and P. Garg. 1978. Toxoplasma IHA antibodies in human sera. Indian J. Pathol. Microbiol. **21**:125-129.

Sirotzky, L., V. Memoli, J. L. Roberts, and E. J. Lewis. 1978. Recurrent *Pneumocystis* pneumonia with normal chest roentgenograms. J.A.M.A. **240**:1513-1515.

Spira, D. J., and C. L. Greenblatt, Editors. 1978. International symposium on immunology and immunopathology of malaria: summing-up of the symposium. Isr. J. Med. Sci. **14**:712-717.

Sulzer, A. J., and M. Wilson. 1971. The indirect fluorescent antibody test for the detection of occult malaria in blood donors. Bull. WHO **45**:375-379.

Targett, G. A. T. 1970. Antibody response to *Plasmodium falciparum* malaria: comparisons of immunoglobulin concentrations, antibody titers and the antigenicity of different asexual forms of the parasite. Clin. Exp. Immunol. **7**:501-517.

Teutsch, S. M., and others. 1979. Epidemic toxoplasmosis associated with infected cats. N. Engl. J. Med. **300**:695-699.

Trier, J. S., P. C. Moxey, E. M. Schimmel, and E. Robles. 1974. Chronic intestinal coccidiosis in man: intestinal morphology and response to treatment. Gastroenterology **66**:923-935.

Walker, A. J. 1963. Manual for the microscopic diagnosis of malaria. Ed. 2. Pan American Health Organization Scientific Publication no. 87. U.S. Government Printing Office, Washington, D.C.

Wallace, G. D. 1973. The role of the cat in the natural history of *Toxoplasma gondii*. Am. J. Trop. Med. Hyg. **22**:313-322.

Wallace, G. D. 1974. Experimental transmission of *Toxoplasma gondii* by filth-flies. Am. J. Trop. Med. Hyg. **20**:411-413.

Walls, K. W. 1979. Immunoserology of parasitic diseases. In Friedman, H., T. J. Linna, and J. E. Prier, Editors. Immunoserology in the diagnosis of infectious diseases. University Park Press, Baltimore, Md.

Walzer, P. D., and others. 1974. *Pneumocystis carinii* pneumonia in the United States: epidemiologic, diagnostic and clinical features. Ann. Intern. Med. **80**:83-93.

Western, K. A., and others. 1970. Babesiosis in a Massachusetts resident. N. Engl. J. Med. **283**:854-856.

Western, K. A., D. R. Perera, and M. G. Schultz. 1970. Pentamidine isethionate in the treatment of *Pneumo-*

cystis carinii pneumonia. Ann. Intern. Med. **73:** 695-702.

Whitcomb, M. E., M. I. Schwarz, M. A. Charles, and P. H. Larson. 1970. Interstitial fibrosis after *Pneumocystis carinii* pneumonia. Ann. Intern. Med. **73:** 761-765.

Wilcox, A. 1960. Manual for the microscopic diagnosis of malaria in man. Public Health Series Publication no. 716, U.S. Department of Health, Education, and Welfare, Public Health Service, U.S. Government Printing Office, Washington, D.C.

Woodruff, A. W., Editor. 1974. Medicine in the tropics. Churchill Livingstone, Edinburgh and London.

World Health Organization. 1965. Resistance of malaria parasites to drugs. WHO Tech. Rep. Ser. no. 296. Geneva, Switzerland.

World Health Organization. 1973. Chemotherapy of malaria and resistance to antimalarials. WHO Tech. Rep. Ser. no. 529. Geneva, Switzerland.

World Health Organization. 1976. Information on malaria risk for International travelers. Weekly Epidemiological Record **51:**181-200.

World Health Organization. 1977. Information of the world malaria situation. Weekly Epidemiological Record **52:**70-73.

Yaeger, R. G. 1965. The detection and identification of *Pneumocystis carinii* in the host. Proceedings of the Second International Congress of Parasitology, International Congress Series no. 91, Excerpta Medica Foundation, pp. 128-129.

Zaman, V. 1968. Observations on human *Isospora*. Trans. R. Soc. Trop. Med. Hyg. **62:**556-557.

Zuckerman, A. 1977. Current status of the immunology of blood and tissue protozoa. II. *Plasmodium*. Exp. Parasitol. **42:**374-446.

PART TWO

Medical helminthology

CHAPTER 7

Introduction to the helminths

The helminths, or worms, unlike the protozoa, are macroscopic and multicellular. Like the higher vertebrates, they have digestive, excretory, reproductive, and nervous systems, though these may be lacking or highly modified in some species.

At one time almost any elongated creeping organism was considered a worm in the large phylum Vermes. As life histories became known, new phyla were defined; those of medical importance are as follows:

Nematoda—threadworms, or roundworms
Platyhelminthes—flatworms
Acanthocephala—spiny- or thorny-headed worms

Like the protozoa, the worms can be categorized according to their habitat in the host. Thus, there are intestinal roundworms, liver flukes, blood flukes, and others.

Geographic distribution. The late Norman Stoll in describing this "wormy world" once stated that there were enough worms, if evenly distributed, for every person in the world and a goodly number left over for a second-go-around. However, like money and brains, some people have more than others. According to 1979 estimates, approximately 180 million persons are infected with schistosomes, 650 million with Ascaris, 450 million with hookworms, and 270 million with filarial worms, not to mention a wide assortment of more worms of lesser prevalence or lesser significance. Because of their complicated life histories, many worms may be quite restricted in distribution. The schistosomes, for example, require certain species of snails as intermediate hosts, which in turn require

specific environments for survival. Hookworms, during their phase in the soil, require proper conditions of temperature, moisture, and soil texture, as well as skin contact, in order to survive and continue their life cycle. Although *Trichinella spiralis* and the pinworm (*Enterobius vermicularis*) are widely distributed without regard to climate, poverty, or poor sanitation, worms usually are more prevalent in warm climates with poor sanitation, where most of the ecologic niches required for worm propagation and survival can be found.

Life cycles. Despite apparent variations, a basic life pattern is common to all worms. The host harboring the adult or sexual stage of the worm is the final or definitive host. All worms produce eggs, which in turn develop larvae. With few exceptions, eggs (or their larvae) must pass outside of the body where growth and development result in larvae infective for the definitive host. Intermediate hosts may be required for development of all larval stages. In all instances, the cycle is complete when the infective larvae again reach a definitive host and become adults.

Modes of entrance and exit from the definitive host are varied. Eggs and larvae may be ingested in food and drink. Larvae may penetrate the skin from soil contact, or through the bite of an insect. Once inside the host, grand tours through the body via the circulation may be the choice of some, whereas others may reach their abode with minimal movement. The modes of exit may include the oral and anal routes, as well as the skin by rupturing of blisters or the bite of an insect. Their tours outside humans may be even more complicated and daring. Many worms follow pathways through life so complicated that one wonders how they manage to survive at all.

Host-parasite relationship. Many factors, such as location, numbers, toxic secretions, and immune response of the host, determine the pathogenicity of worms. Although the protozoa multiply within the host much as bacteria do and thus can overwhelm the host, each worm larva matures into but a single adult and pathogenicity usually is proportional to the number of adult helminths harbored. Pathogenicity caused by offspring from adult worms produced within the host varies.

Diagnosis and treatment. Clinical manifestations, as in the protozoa, are not pathognomonic of most worm infections. The recovery of eggs, larvae, or adults is usually necessary for diagnosis. Adjuncts such as history, immunoserology, and culture may be helpful. Since many worms produce large numbers of eggs recoverable in the feces, their identification becomes very important. Size, shape, color, nature of shell membranes, and stage of development become useful characteristics. Morphologic features of some larvae recovered in the feces, blood, or body tissues are used for identification, where adults may make diagnosis certain in others.

Unlike the protozoa, reduction in worm burden rather than complete eradication is usually adequate. A few worms, unable to multiply within the host, may be better tolerated than the anthelminthics used to kill them. When a state of "armed truce" exists betwen host and parasite, good judgement by the physician may suggest no treatment at all.

Significant efforts are now being made to utilize disciplines of pharmacology and biochemistry in the study of the chemotherapy of the helminths. Emphasis on the metabolic differences between worms and their host

has opened an avenue of investigation into the study of the inhibition of enzyme systems crucial to the parasite but not the host. While research in the area of cellular regulatory biology has enhanced our knowledge of many basic principles in enzyme and hormone control in various organisms, progress in parasitology has been impeded, in part, by the difficulties in culturing many of these organisms in well-defined media.

Well-coordinated and rhythmic movements characterize the various helminths and play a significant role in enabling the parasite to remain in situ, whether exposed to peristalsis in the gastrointestinal tract or the movement of blood and lymph in the circulation. Studies indicate that piperazine, for example, increases the resting potential of *Ascaris* muscle and suppresses its pacemaker activity, resulting in flaccid paralysis and expulsion. Evidence indicates that the cellular regulatory sites that control mobility, metabolism, chemotaxis, and egg formation of the helminths are affected by many chemotherapeutic agents. The great success achieved against bacterial infections offers hope that the combined efforts of pharmacologists, biochemists, molecular biologists, and parasitologists will bring about the development of more and better anthelminthics.

REVIEW QUESTIONS

1. Contrast the helminths with the protozoa as to the following:
   a. Morphology
   b. Life cycle
   c. Georgraphic distribution
   d. Host-parasite relationship
   e. Treatment
2. The statements in this chapter are generalizations about helminths. As you study the following chapters, ask yourself which helminths are exceptions:
   a. Which are worldwide rather than producing primarily tropical diseases associated with poverty and poor sanitation?
   b. Which are capable of autoinfection without passing part of their life cycle separate from the host?
   c. Which may have major pathologic changes related to the larval stage?

    d. Which are at a dead end in their life cycle when they infect humans?

    e. Which should be completely eradicated with treatment?

3. What is the current approach in the treatment of the helminths? Discuss.

REFERENCES

Barrett-Connor, E. 1975. Recent advances in the treatment of common intestinal helminths. Am. J. Gastroenterol. **63**:105-116.

Beaver, P. C. 1975. Biology of soil-transmitted helminths: the massive infection. Health Lab. Sci. **12**:116-125.

Belding, D. L. 1965. Textbook of clinical parasitology. Ed. 2. Appleton-Century-Crofts, New York.

Chandler, A. C., and C. P. Read. 1961. Introduction to parasitology. Ed. 10. John Wiley & Sons, Inc., New York.

Faust, E. C., P. F. Russell, and R. C. Jung. 1970. Clinical parasitology. Ed. 8. Lea & Febiger, Philadelphia.

Garcia, E. G. 1978. Treatment of multiple intestinal helminthiasis with oxantel and pyrantel. Drugs **15** (suppl. 1):70-72.

Keystone, J. S., and J. K. Murdoch. 1979. Diagnosis and treatment. Five years later: mebendazole. Ann. Intern. Med. **91**:582-586.

Medical protozoology and helminthology. 1965. Revised ed. U.S. Naval Medical School, National Naval Medical Center, Besthesda, Md.

Mettrick, D. F., and R. B. Podesta. 1974. Ecological and physiological aspects of helminth-host interactions in the mammalian gastrointestinal canal. In Dawes, B., Editor. Advances in parasitology. Vol. 12. Academic Press, New York.

Schmidt, G. D., and L. S. Roberts. 1977. Foundations of parasitology. The C. V. Mosby Co., St. Louis.

Sirisinha, S. 1978. Humoral immune response in parasitic infections. Southeast Asian J. Trop. Med. Public Health 9:142-152.

Stoll, N. R. 1947. This wormy world. J. Parsitol. 33:1-18.

Welch, J. S., and C. Dobson. 1978. Immunodiagnosis of parasitic zoonoses: comparative efficacy of three immunofluorescence tests using antigens purified by affinity chromatography. Trans. R. Soc. Trop. Med. Hyg. **72**:282-288.

THE ROUNDWORMS
(Nematoda)

■ All of the roundworms parasitic in humans occur in the phylum Nematoda. However, a member of class Gordiacea in another phylum, parasitic during the larval stages in insects but free living as adults, at times may be found in the patient's toilet bowl, bathtub, or sink, and brought to the doctor's office. This situation occurs in tropical climates where insects are virtually household pets. They are commonly referred to as "horsehair worms" because of their gross resemblance to a long horse hair. The adult worm measures 4 to 5 inches in length and is slender and black. It is uniform in diameter and quite active in freshwater. The worms are harmless but frightening, nevertheless. Accidental ingestion in drinking water has been reported but probably is rare. The worm is either vomited quickly or destroyed in the stomach by gastric juice.

The nematodes (threadworms, roundworms) are characterized by a cuticle-covered cylindrical body containing a pseudocoelom, or body cavity, with a complete digestive system with mouth and anus, as well as a nervous, an excretory, and a genital system. The sexes are separate.

Species differ as to morphology, hosts infected, and the stages found within those hosts and in the external environment. A typical life pattern, common to all nematodes, is represented diagrammatically as follows:

$$♀ \, \Big> \quad \text{Eggs} \; \rightarrow \; \text{Larvae} \; \rightarrow \; \text{Infective larvae} \xrightarrow{\text{In definitive host}} \begin{array}{c} ♀ \\ ♂ \end{array}$$

For convenience, the nematodes may be studied in groups according to the area of the body inhabited, that is, intestinal and tissue roundworms.

CHAPTER 8

The intestinal roundworms

The intestinal roundworms include all nematodes with their adult stage in the intestinal tract even though the larval stages may be located elsewhere in the body. With the exception of *Trichinella spiralis*, the larvae of which become encysted in the skeletal muscles, the intestinal nematode infections may be diagnosed by recovery and identification of the egg and larval stages from the intestinal canal. In some instances, adults may also be recovered. The laboratory diagnosis can be made by routine stool analysis as described for the intestinal protozoa, except for *Enterobius vermicularis* and *Trichinella spiralis*.

The following nematodes parasitize the intestinal tract of humans:

Enterobius vermicularis	*Trichinella spiralis*
Trichuris trichiura	*Necator americanus*
Trichostrongylus sp	*Ancylostoma duodenale*
Ascaris lumbricoides	*Strongyloides stercoralis*

The intestinal nematodes are presented in this order because it represents a series, each succeeding species of which becomes more complicated in its life cycle. This sequence has no evolutionary significance and is used only to facilitate the understanding of the life histories of these parasites. *Trichinella spiralis*, somewhat aberrant in the series, is most conveniently placed in the position as shown for study.

Enterobius vermicularis

Geographic distribution. The pinworm, or seatworm, is one of the more common worm infections of humans. Though cosmopolitan in distribution, it is more prevalent in temperate than tropical climes. The incidence in North American white children approximates 40%, whereas blacks show about one third that number. In some European communities, 80% of the children are infected.

Morphology. The adult female averages 10 mm in length, with maximum width about 0.4 mm. The fusiform body terminates in a long, thin, tapering tail. The anterior end tapers and is flanked on each side by cuticular swellings called "alae." The esophagus is slender, terminating in a prominent posterior bulb that can be readily seen through the semitransparent cuticle. Males average 3 mm in length and about 0.15 mm maximum width. They are rarely seen since they are apparently short lived after copulation. In appearance the male resembles the female, except for the curled tail with its copulatory apparatus (Fig. 8-1).

The eggs are oval, 50 to 60 μm by about 25 μm, and are flattened on one side. Each is clear, colorless, possesses a doubly refractive wall, and, when oviposited, contains an undeveloped larva, referred to by some as the "tadpole" larval stage (Fig. 8-2).

Life cycle. The elapsed time from the ingestion of the infective larval stage to the presence of a gravid female may be as little as 2 to 4 weeks but is usually longer. The adult female has a life span of 1 to 2 months. The adult worms live in the cecum and colon where they hold on to the mucosa with their lips. Although they occasionally migrate into the stomach and are regurgitated into the mouth, usually the gravid female migrates to-

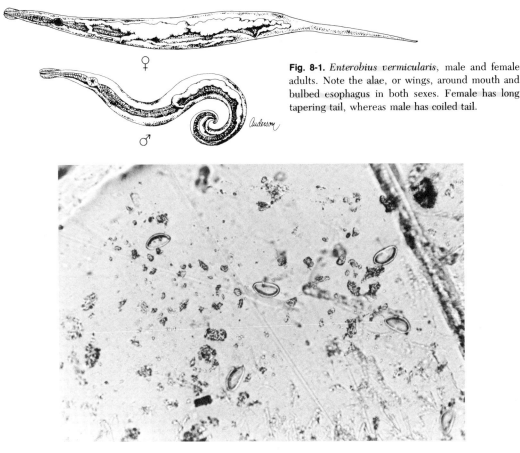

Fig. 8-1. *Enterobius vermicularis*, male and female adults. Note the alae, or wings, around mouth and bulbed esophagus in both sexes. Female has long tapering tail, whereas male has coiled tail.

Fig. 8-2. Cellophane tape impression showing pinworm eggs. (Courtesy Department of Pathology, University of Miami, School of Medicine.)

ward the anus and emerges nocturnally on the perianal skin where drying worms extrude large showers of eggs. One pinworm may release over 10,000 eggs. When deposited, these eggs are in the "tadpole" embryonated stage, but within 6 hours they become infective for the same or other persons. To a limited extent, retroinfection may occur when hatched larvae reenter the intestinal tract through the anal route. Most of the eggs, however, do not hatch but are scattered in the environment or retained in the perianal region of the host. Scratching leads to contamination of the hands and nails, and hand-to-mouth contact results in reinfection. Ova also contaminate food and drink,

bed linen, and dust throughout the home. Ingested eggs hatch and the liberated larvae develop in the small intestine. Mating probably takes place in the cecum, and the adults become established there and in the remainder of the colon.

Epidemiology. The prevalence of infective eggs in a contaminated household or orphanage is appalling. Viable eggs can be recovered from bed linens, towels, furniture, windowsills, doorjambs, and dust about the house. While conducting a pinworm study in a local children's home, investigators discovered that the cleaning of used cellophane tape slides resulted in the contamination of stock protozoan cultures, subcultured on alternate days, with pinworm eggs. In a cool, moist atmosphere (20° to 25° C) the eggs will survive up to a week. At temperatures above 25° C and in dry air, they will perish within a day. The opportunities for dissemination and transmission to members of the household are ever present, and pinworms thus become a family infection. Hand-to-mouth contact, inhalation, and contamination of food and drink result in the maintenance of the high incidence rate throughout the world, which, in European white children, may reach levels of over 80%. In the rural tropics, where people wear less clothing and live mostly in the open in the sunshine and dry heat, survival and transmission of eggs are more difficult, and the resultant incidence becomes lower.

E. vermicularis is the common pinworm found in humans. *Syphacea obvelata*, the pinworm of rats and mice, has been reported once in a child in the Philippines, but, with this exception, *E. vermicularis* is the only oxyurid found in humans. This is important because veterinarians become justifiably disturbed when patients tell them that their physician blames their pet cat or dog for the family pinworm problems. Enterobiasis is most common where people live under crowded conditions such as in orphanages, mental institutions, and large families. Though personal hygiene is to be commended and the wearing of tight underpants by the children with the anus well covered with petrolatum is very helpful, for the most part the meticulous care so often exercised by diligent mothers goes for naught and repeated reinfections can usually be expected sooner or later. In the long run only repeated treatment will solve the problem.

Symptomatology and pathology. About one third of pinworm-infected persons are asymptomatic. The adult worms may cause slight irritation of the intestinal mucosa, and mild nausea, vomiting, and diarrhea have been attributed to their presence. Anemia, eosinophilia, and systemic symptoms are rare. The worm has been found in both normal and diseased appendixes and is not considered an important factor in appendicitis. Major symptoms are associated with the nocturnal migration of the gravid females from the anus and deposition of eggs in the perianal folds of the skin. Restlessness, nervousness, and irritability, probably resulting from poor sleep associated with *pruritus ani* (hypersensitivity reaction), are common in children. Intense scratching may lead to secondary infection. In young girls migration of the worms may produce vaginitis and rarely salpingitis or granulomas of the peritoneal cavity. For the most part, despite its overwhelming prevalence, this parasite is relatively nonpathogenic.

Diagnosis. Less than 5% of positive cases ever show eggs in the feces. The eggs, and sometimes the female adults as well, can be removed from the folds of the skin in the perianal regions by the use of the cellophane tape method as depicted in Fig. 8-3. Cellophane tape impressions are best taken in the morning before the child has bathed or gone to the toilet. Such impressions in the physician's office are less useful because the mother usually has bathed the child before the visit. An examination of the perianal region during the early hours after retiring will frequently reveal the migrating female worms. Seven consecutive early-morning cellophane tape impressions should be examined before concluding that the patient is free of the eggs. Because of the time factor involved, this relatively simple technique must be learned by the mother or person in attendance in the household. Preparations may be examined at leisure; positive slides can be identifiable many years later!

Treatment. A variety of compounds have shown activity against the pinworm. Since the life span is less than 2 months, the major problem is prevention of reinfection. Major hygienic efforts usually are ineffectual, and repeated treatment is the only course available. Many drugs, efficacious for pinworms,

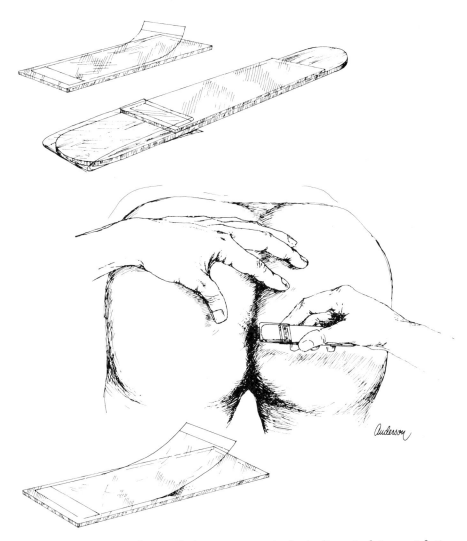

Fig. 8-3. Technique for making a cellophane tape impression for the diagnosis of pinworm infection.

have met with disfavor because of the necessity of repeated treatment 2 or 3 times a day, for several days or longer. For details of treatment see Table 8-1. In institutions and large families where pinworms are perennial guests it is now feasible to deworm the entire household several times a year.

Trichuris trichiura

Geographic distribution. The nematode *Trichuris trichiura*, commonly known as the whipworm because of its resemblance to a buggy whip, occurs extensively throughout the tropics and subtropics. In the United States it is prevalent throughout the warm, moist South, occurring extensively south of the Piedmont Plateau, in the foothills of the southern Appalachian range, in southwest Louisiana, and the fringes of many southern cities where living conditions are crowded and sanitation is poor.

Morphology. The female worm, averaging 40 mm in length, has a long, slender esophageal region that accounts for about

Table 8-1. Treatment for intestinal roundworms

Infection	Drug	Adult dose*	Pediatric dose*
Enterobius vermicularis[1] (pinworm)			
Drug of choice	Pyrantel pamoate	A single dose of 11 mg/kg (max. 1 gm); repeat after 2 wk	A single dose of 11 mg/kg (max. 1 gm); repeat after 2 wk
	OR		
	Mebendazole	A single dose of 100 mg; repeat after 2 wk	A single dose of 100 mg for children > 2 years; repeat after 2 wk
Alternative	Piperazine citrate	65 mg/kg (max. 2.5 gm)/d × 7d; repeat after 2 wk	65 mg/kg (max. 2.5 gm)/d × 7d; repeat after 2 wk
	Pyrvinium pamoate	5 mg/kg single dose (max. 350 mg); repeat after 2 wk	5 mg/kg single dose (max. 350 mg); repeat after 2 wk
Trichuris trichiura (whipworm)			
Drug of choice	Mebendazole	100 mg bid × 3d	100 mg bid × 3d
Alternative	None		
Trichostrongylus species			
Drug of choice	Thiabendazole[2]	25 mg/kg bid × 2d	25 mg/kg bid × 2d
Alternative	Pyrantel pamoate[2]	A single dose of 11 mg/kg (max. 1 gm)	A single dose of 11 mg/kg (max. 1 gm)
Ascaris lumbricoides (roundworm)			
Drug of choice	Pyrantel pamoate	A single dose of 11 mg/kg (max. 1 gm)	A single dose of 11 mg/kg (max. 1 gm)
	OR		
	Mebendazole	100 mg bid × 3	100 mg bid × 3d for children > 2 yr
Alternative	Piperazine citrate	75 mg/kg (max. 3.5 gm)/d × 2d	75 mg/kg (max. 3.5 gm)/d × 2d
Trichinella spiralis			
Drug of choice	Steroids for severe symptoms *plus* Thiabendazole[3]	25 mg/kg bid × 5d	25 mg/kg bid × 5d
Alternative	Mebendazole[2]	200-400 mg tid × 3d, then 400-500 mg tid × 10d	
Necator americanus (hookworm)[1,4]			
Drug of choice	Pyrantel pamoate[2]	A single dose of 11 mg/kg (max. 1 gm)	A single dose of 11 mg/kg (max. 1 gm)
	OR		
	Mebendazole	100 mg bid × 3d	100 mg bid × 3d for children > 2 yr
Alternative	Thiabendazole	25 mg/kg bid (max. 3 gm/d) × 2d	25 mg/kg bid (max. 3 gm/d) × 2d

From The Medical Letter, Inc., 56 Harrison Street, New Rochelle, N.Y.
*The letter d indicates day.

1. Pyrantel pamoate and mebendazole are equally effective and equally safe. Mebendazole should not be used in pregnancy because it is teratogenic in animals, but the safety of pyrantel pamoate in pregnancy is not established either. Mebendazole is available in the U.S.A. only in tablets that should be chewed for best effect; pyrantel pamoate is available as a suspension. The patient's family should also be treated for pinworm infection to prevent recurrence.
2. Considered an investigational drug for this condition by the U.S. Food and Drug Administration.
3. The efficacy of thiabendazole for trichinosis is not clearly established. It appears to be effective during the intestinal phase but its effect on larvae which have migrated is questionable.
4. Light hookworm infections need not be treated in the absence of symptoms or anemia.
5. In disseminated strongyloidiasis, thiabendazole therapy should be continued for at least 5 days.

Table 8-1. Treatment for intestinal roundworms—cont'd

Infection	Drug	Adult dose	Pediatric dose
Ancylostoma duodenale[4] (hookworm)			
Drug of choice	Mebendazole	100 mg bid × 3d	100 mg bid × 3d for children > 2 yr
	OR		
	Pyrantel pamoate[2]	A single dose of 11 mg/kg (max. 1 gm)	A single dose of 11 mg/kg (max. 1 gm)
Strongyloides stercoralis			
Drug of choice	Thiabendazole	25 mg/kg bid (max. 3 gm/d) × 2d[5]	25 mg/kg bid (max. 3 gm/d) × 2d[5]
Capillaria philippinensis			
Drug of choice	Mebendazole[2]	200 mg bid × 20d	200 mg bid × 20d
Alternative	Thiabendazole[2]	25 mg/kg/d × 30d	25 mg/kg/d × 30d

Adverse effects of antiparasitic drugs

Pyrantel pamoate (Antiminth)
  Occasional: GI disturbances; headache; dizziness; rash; fever
Mebendazole (Vermox)
  Occasional: diarrhea; abdominal pain
Piperazine citrate USP (Antepar; others)
  Occasional: dizziness; urticaria; GI disturbances
  Rare: exacerbation of epilepsy; visual disturbances; ataxia; hypotonia
Pyrvinium pamoate USP (Povan)
  Frequent: turns stool red
  Occasional: vomiting; diarrhea
  Rare: photosensitivity skin reactions
Thiabendazole USP (Mintezol)
  Frequent: nausea; vomiting; vertigo
  Occasional: leukopenia; crystalluria; rash; hallucinations; olfactory disturbance
  Rare: shock; tinnitus; Stevens-Johnson syndrome

two thirds the total length. The name *Trichuris* means "threadtail," the name given under the mistaken impression that the slender part was the tail and not the head end. Later the more appropriate name *Tricocephalus*, "threadhead," was adopted by some, but priority goes to *Trichuris* even though it reflects the inaccuracy of its originator. Many people in Latin America use *Tricocephalus*, nevertheless. The posterior one third consists of a fleshy, robust portion containing the body organs. The male is smaller and can be readily recognized by the curled tail containing the copulatory apparatus (Fig. 8-4).

The eggs are typically barrel shaped, averaging 50 μm × 20 μm and are stained with bile pigments when passed in the feces. They contain two shell membranes, translucent polar plugs, and an unsegmented ovum (Fig. 8-5).

Life cycle. The adult worms live primarily in the cecum but, in heavy infections, can be found in the entire colon, including the rectum. They live for several years, during which time eggs are produced and discharged in feces. In a moist, warm environment, these embryos develop into the infective larval stage within the eggshell in 3 to 6 weeks. Under adverse conditions, development may be delayed several months or even years. After ingestion, the fully developed larva hatches in the jejunum and penetrates the intestinal villus where it undergoes development for 3 to 10 days. The adolescent worm then moves into the cecum and

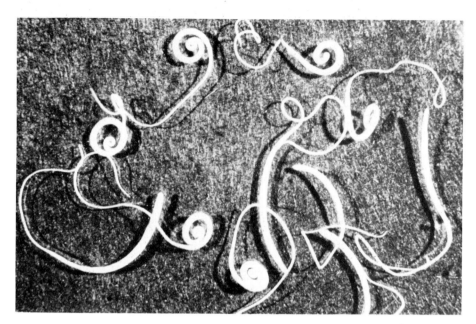

Fig. 8-4. *Trichuris trichiura* male and female adults. Note the long slender esophagus and fleshy body resembling a buggy whip. Males have coiled tails. (From a nonprofit cooperative endeavor by numerous colleagues under the editorship of Dr. Herman Zaiman, Valley City, N.D.)

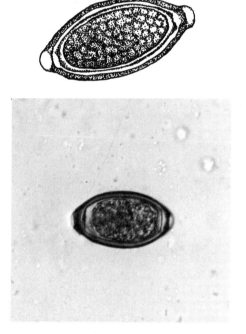

Fig. 8-5. Egg of *Trichuris trichiura*, with drawing. (Photomicrograph courtesy Department of Pathology, University of Miami, School of Medicine.)

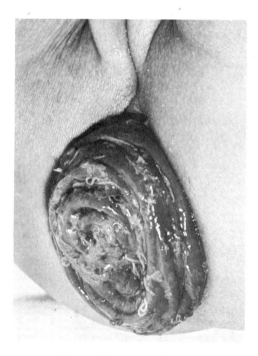

Fig. 8-6. Prolapse of the rectum due to whipworm infection. (Courtesy Department of Pathology, University of Miami, School of Medicine.)

becomes an adult. The period of development from the time of ingestion to a fully developed gravid female is approximately 90 days. In the cecum and colon the adult worm buries its long, slender neck into the folds of the mucosa and with the aid of a small spear attaches itself into the mucosa much like a needle and thread in a piece of cloth.

Epidemiology. Infections occur most abundantly in areas where humidity is high and a hard clay soil holds moisture. Dense shade and a warm climate are necessary. Such conditions are best met in the tropics. Dooryard pollution and no sanitation result in heavy infections. The incidence is highest among children because this group is closest to soil pollution, which readily affords hand-to-mouth contact, as well as contamination of food and drinks. Infections are usually co-extensive with *Ascaris lumbricoides*, which requires a similar environment. Distribution, however, may be more spotty because of the lesser resistance of the eggs of *T. trichiura* to environmental changes.

Symptomatology and pathology. Light infections, seen most commonly in the United States, are frequently asymptomatic. Abdominal pain (sometimes suggesting appendicitis), vomiting, constipation, fever, distention and flatulence, headache, backache, anorexia, and weight loss have been attributed to this parasite. The stitching of the anterior end in the mucosa may pave the way for the entrance of bacteria. Epithelial cells in the area are compressed and the crypts beneath may become dilated with mucus, fibrin, and neutrophils. A chronic inflammatory reaction may occur with small, subepithelial hemorrhages. In heavy infections, bloody diarrhea and emaciation may occur. Prolapse of the rectum caused by extreme tenesmus is associated with heavy worm burdens (Fig. 8-6). Eosinophilia, noted in acute cases, is usually absent in chronic cases. Rare fatalities occur in malnourished and neglected children, with edema of the face, dyspnea, cardiac dilatation, and convulsions being observed.

Diagnosis. Diagnosis is made by recovery and identification of the typical bile-stained, barrel-shaped ova with translucent polar plugs. Since the adults are firmly attached to the mucosa, they are rarely seen in the feces, except in overwhelming infections or after effective treatment. When rectal prolapse occurs, myriads of tiny white adult worms with their free undulating ends can be seen on the rectal mucosa (Fig. 8-6).

Treatment. Trichuriasis is a difficult infection to treat because of the firmness with which the adults are fastened to the intestinal wall. Uncomplicated light infections require no therapy. In certain tropical areas where the wild fig trees *Ficus glabrata* and *F. dolaria* grow, the latex, *leche de higuerón*, is efficacious when used fresh. Its instability, however, along with its unpalatability, limits its use.

The latest of the broad spectrum anthelminthics is mebendazole (Vermox) and is considered the drug of choice for trichuriasis in the dosage of 100 mg twice daily for 3 days (Table 8-1). Mebendazole is also active against *A. lumbricoides*, the hookworms, *S. stercoralis*, and the pinworm *E. vermicularis*.

Trichostrongylus

A variety of members of this genus, normally parasitic in the digestive tract of various herbivores, also occur as incidental parasites of humans through the ingestion of contaminated food and drink containing infective larvae. Infections are most common in the Middle East, the Far East, and the tropics, where a close association of humans and animals is common. In southeast Iran and in a village in Egypt infection rates approximating 70% have been reported. The adults are slightly smaller than the hookworms and likewise live in the small intestine where they burrow into the mucosa. They are recognized by the finely drawn-out head without a buccal capsule. Eight to ten species, normally parasitic in sheep, goats, or camels, have been reported in man. In heavy infections the burrowing worms damage the intestinal mucosa, and hemorrhage, mild anemia, and emaciation may occur. Most infections are light and not especially symptomatic. The eggs produced closely resemble hookworm ova (Fig. 8-7) and are frequently so identified by the experienced. Since hookworm chemotherapy is

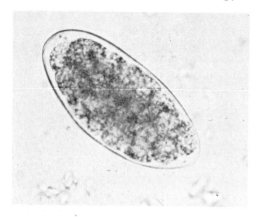

Fig. 8-7. *Trichostrongylus* ovum from human stool. Characteristically longer than hookworm ova. (From a nonprofit cooperative endeavor by numerous colleagues under the editorship of Dr. Herman Zaiman, Valley City, N.D.)

ineffective against these worms, diagnosis is important to prevent prolonged and useless therapy (Table 8-1). The eggs are larger (75 to 95 μm in length), more slender, and more pointed at one end than are hookworm ova.

Ascaris lumbricoides

Geographic distribution. *Ascaris lumbricoides* has been a parasite of man down through the Stone, Copper, and Iron Ages. Probably the domestication of the pig and the bringing of this animal into the home made possible the development of a strain suitable to man, which, over time, became host specific. Today, however, modern plumbing may sever this relationship between the parasite, the pig, and man—at least where modern toilet facilities are available.

Ascaris lumbricoides is one of the largest of the intestinal nematodes parasitizing humans and is commonly referred to as the "roundworm of man." It is most prevalent throughout the tropics and subtropics around the world but extends also into temperate regions. Next to the pinworm it is probably the most common nematode in man. In the United States it is coextensive with *T. trich-*

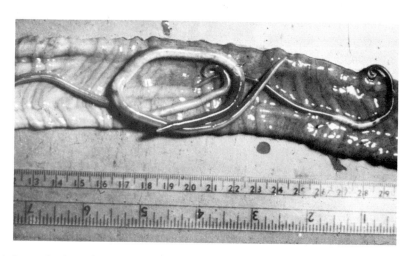

Fig. 8-8. *Ascaris lumbricoides* male and female adults. Note the coiled tail in the male. (Courtesy Dr. Rodolfo Céspedes, Department of Pathology, Hospital San Juan de Dios, San José, Costa Rica.)

iura, occurring predominantly in the mountainous areas of the southeastern states and the fringes of many southern cities. *Ascaris*, the hookworm, and the whipworm make up the "unholy three."

Morphology. The adult female averages 30 cm in length and about 5 mm in diameter. It is long, slender, and uniform in girth except for a slightly attenuated tail. The male is smaller, averaging 20 cm in length and distinctly more slender than the female. The typical curled tail with the copulatory apparatus readily distinguishes its sex. *A. lumbricoides* is the most "wormlike" of the worms, somewhat resembling the earthworm in superficial gross appearance (Fig. 8-8).

The eggs produced by the female may be fertile or infertile. The fertile eggs are round to oval, measuring about 45 μm $\times$ 65 μm. They have an outer warty, albuminous coat, stained yellowish to brown with bile pigments, and a thick inner hyaline shell coat that surrounds the unsegmented ovum. Unsegmented ova passed in the feces become embryonated upon standing, even in many fixative solutions such as 5% formalin. In fertile eggs also are oviposited by the female (probably because of faulty fertilization, egg-laying before fertilization, or the absence of males entirely). These eggs contain the same shell layers as the fertile eggs but with much thinner and often indistinct coats. They are usually elongated and somewhat barrel shaped, measuring 80 μm in length, but may also assume various shapes. They are amorphous within and their general appearance makes them easily confused with some vegetable cells (Fig. 8-9).

Life cycle. The adults live free and unattached in the small intestine, nipping at the mucosa with their three fleshy lips. One adult female can produce approximately 200,000 eggs per day. Eggs pass out in the feces unsegmented. In the soil, cleavage takes place, with the infective larva appearing within the eggshell in about 3 weeks under ideal conditions. After ingestion, hatch-

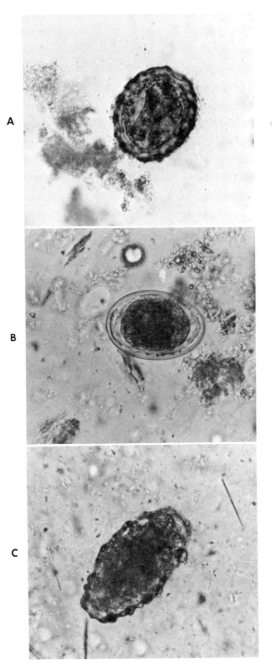

Fig. 8-9. *Ascaris lumbricoides* eggs. A, Fertile egg showing larva within. B, Decorticated egg sometimes confused with hookworm eggs. C, Infertile egg sometimes confused with vegetable cells. (Courtesy Department of Pathology, University of Miami, School of Medicine.)

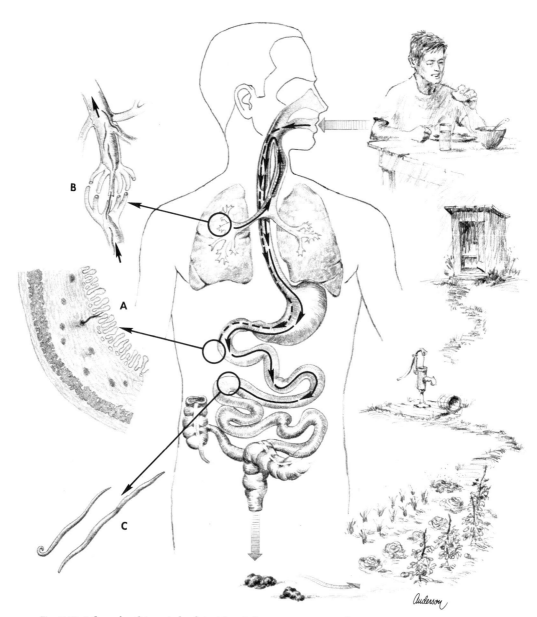

Fig. 8-10. Life cycle of *Ascaris lumbricoides*. Infective eggs, ingested in contaminated food and water, hatch in the small intestine where penetration of the mucosa, **A,** results in invasion of the bloodstream by the larvae, which are carried to the lungs. The larvae, too large to cross the capillary bed, break out into the alveolar spaces, **B,** are carried up the bronchial tree, are swallowed, and reach the small intestine where they become adult worms, **C.**

ing takes place in the small intestine where the infective larva burrows into the mucosal wall, enters the circulation, and is carried through the heart to the lungs from 1 to 7 days after infection. In the lungs over a period of about 10 days to 2 months further development takes place before the larva passes up the bronchial tree. Because of its large size, the larva is unable to pass across the capillary bed, breaks into the alveolar spaces and bronchioles, is carried via the bronchial tree and trachea to the pharynx, and is swallowed. After the larva is swallowed, development to the adult stage takes place. Gravid females are present approximately 5 to 8 weeks after infection. Adults, both male and female, are short lived and survive a year at most before passing out of the intestinal tract (Fig. 8-10).

Epidemiology. Because of the heavy shell layers, the eggs in the soil are very resistant to environmental changes, although heat and desiccation are disastrous to *Ascaris* ova. When sandy soil provides good drainage, drying of the top layer occurs and eggs are readily destroyed by the sun. They thrive best where there is a clay soil, dense shade, heavy rainfall, and a warm climate. In such an environment, careless defecation habits seed the soil with viable eggs, which can remain infective for 5 years. Children, playing in yards close to the house, frequently show a high incidence in endemic areas because of the contact of invariably dirty hands with the mouth. In areas where night soil is used for fertilizer, infections are contracted from eating raw vegetables. Pollution of wells through improper drainage of surface waters may result in water transmission. Prophylaxis depends chiefly on the use of privies or inside toilets, instead of promiscuous defecation close to the home.

Symptomatology and pathology. The migration of larvae from the intestinal tract through the lungs may be associated with fever, cough occasionally productive of bloody sputum, and radiographic changes of fleeting pneumonitis. This symptomatic pulmonary phase is most likely to occur with a heavy infection. It is associated with eosinophilia and, in some patients, urticaria and is believed to be an allergic response. Increased levels in serum IgE are noted. Pneumonitis and bronchopneumonia, sometimes fatal, occur in endemic areas. It is important to note that at this stage of infection (*Ascaris* pneumonia) no eggs will be seen in the stool since the immature worms have not, as yet, reached the intestinal tract.

Most patients have recognized symptoms only in association with adult worms in the intestinal tract. A heavy worm burden can result in protein malnutrition, particularly in growing children on a poor diet. A group of worms may ball up and cause intestinal obstruction, again usually in children. The ascarid has a peculiar affinity for small orifices, so that even a single worm can be dangerous if it migrates into the common bile duct or pancreatic duct, or blocks the airway by migrating into the larynx or trachea (Fig. 8-11). This preference for narrow passages is reflected by the finding of worms caught in ingested objects with small openings, and the observation that the worm not infrequently enters nasogastric tubes. Worms may also penetrate surgical anastomoses and enter the peritoneum; they have been found in the fallopian tubes, fistulas, and the urinary bladder. Such migrations may occur spontaneously but are also potentiated by intercurrent illness in the host, anesthesia, and the use of tetrachloroethylene in the treatment of hookworm. Adult worms may migrate out of the anus or into the stomach and be vomited; such an event may be the first recognition by the patient that he harbors a parasite.

Death caused by ascariasis may follow severe pulmonary invasion or an unrecognized migration resulting in asphyxia or obstruction of some essential organ. Fatal peritonitis occurs rarely.

Diagnosis. Although symptoms may be

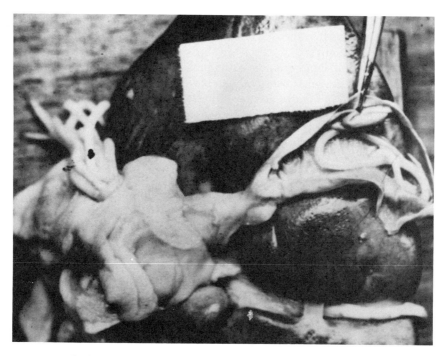

Fig. 8-11. *Ascaris lumbricoides* adults in gallbladder and common bile duct. (Courtesy Dr. Rodolfo Céspedes, Department of Pathology, Hospital San Juan de Dios, San José, Costa Rica.)

quite pronounced, none are pathognomonic of infection. The final diagnosis depends on the recovery and identification of the fertile and infertile eggs in the feces. Since infertile eggs do not float in zinc sulfate, a sedimentation procedure for concentration must be employed. The female worm is a prolific egg producer and the ova are readily recovered in the feces. A single worm is potentially dangerous because of its migratory nature; if the worm is a male, stool examination for ova is negative. Adults may be recovered from the anus, mouth, or nose. Marked cross-reaction is observed with *Toxocara*, and until recently both the indirect hemagglutination (IHA) test and the bentonite-flocculation test (BFT) were employed, the BFT being less sensitive than the IHA test but more specific. Consequently diagnosis depended on both tests being positive. The enzyme-linked immunospecific assay (ELISA) is now used, being superior in both sensitivity and specificity.

Treatment. During the period of lung migration, only supportive therapy can be used. Intestinal obstruction from the ascarids may require intubation and drainage. Severe obstruction or ectopic parasites require surgery. For details of treatment see Table 8-1. Stool examination in 1 to 2 weeks determines the efficacy of treatment. When other intestinal helminths are also present, *Ascaris* should be treated first to avoid possible stimulation to migration by the drugs employed.

Trichinella spiralis

Geographic distribution. Unlike other nematodes parasitic in humans, *Trichinella spiralis* has an extensive distribution throughout a wide range of mammalian hosts. Infection in humans is found from the arctic region to the tropics. In Africa small epidemics usually follow the eating of infected meat of game animals such as bushpigs and warthogs. The eating of infected bear meat results in epidemics in the Arctic. Conservative estimates at one time gave the incidence in the United States as about 20%, over three times as much as the rest of the world. Prevalence today, based on current autopsy studies, is about 4%.

Morphology and life cycle. The adult female worm measures 3 to 4 mm in length, is ovoviviparous, and has an esophagus about one half as long as the body. The male averages 1.5 mm in length, with a posterior extremity having a conical projection on either side of a protrusile cloaca. The females have a life span of 2 to 3 months; the males, considerably less.

Infection in humans occurs by the ingestion of meat (skeletal muscle), chiefly pork, containing the infective larval stage encysted in the muscle. In the small intestine (jejunum, mainly) the larvae are liberated by digestion of the cyst wall and become attached to the mucosa and grow. Within approximately 2 days they become sexually mature and copulate within the folds of the mucosa. The females, burrowed deep in the mucosa, give birth to living larvae, many of which are deposited directly into lacteals and lymphatics. They are carried through the circulation to the capillary beds of various organs. By preference they penetrate the sarcolemma of skeletal muscle fibers in which they coil up and become encysted. Encystment takes place only in skeletal muscle, although rupture of capillaries with petechial hemorrhages may occur in any tissue. Coiling in skeletal muscle takes place about the seventeenth day after infection, with maximum growth occurring at about the beginning of encapsulation 35 days after infection. Calcification of the cyst usually takes place from 6 to 18 months later. Infective larvae remain dormant for many years. For completion of the cycle, encysted larvae must be ingested by a suitable definitive host (Fig. 8-12).

Epidemiology. Trichinosis from a medical point of view is primarily a disease of humans and pigs. Human infection usually results from ingestion of infected, inadequately cooked pork or pork products. Beef hamburger contaminated by a meat grinder also used for pork has resulted in human disease. Occasional outbreaks have followed ingestion of bear or walrus meat. Rats perpetuate the infection in nature, feeding on the carcasses of other infected rats. Hogs feeding in such environment also become infected.

The high incidence previously reported in the United States was partly caused by the failure to control disease in hogs. The feeding of uncooked garbage to swine, such garbage containing infected pork scraps, resulted in perpetuation of hog infection. This practice was prohibited in the mid-1950s, and this prohibition, along with the increasing use of commercial feeds, is probably responsible for much of the decline in trichinosis today. The use of frozen foods has also been important; freezing at $-18°$ C kills larvae within 3 days. Consumer education has also been important; most housewives know that pink pork is not adequately cooked. An oven temperature of at least 350° F and a cooking time of at least 35 minutes per pound is recommended. With a large roast even this cooking interval may not destroy larvae in the center of the meat.

It is important that the public recognize that the meat inspection stamp does *not* pertain to trichinosis and therefore is no protection against infection. Failure to realize that smoking, pickling, and heavy seasoning or spicing do not make pork products safe without cooking has resulted in many of the recent cases, often associated with homemade sausage.

The high standard of living in the United States has been related ironically to the high incidence of disease. Trichinosis is relatively rare among the poor in the tropics, where pork is a luxury and garbage is minimal or nonexistent.

Clinical picture. Trichinosis, like syphilis, has been called the great imitator, mim-

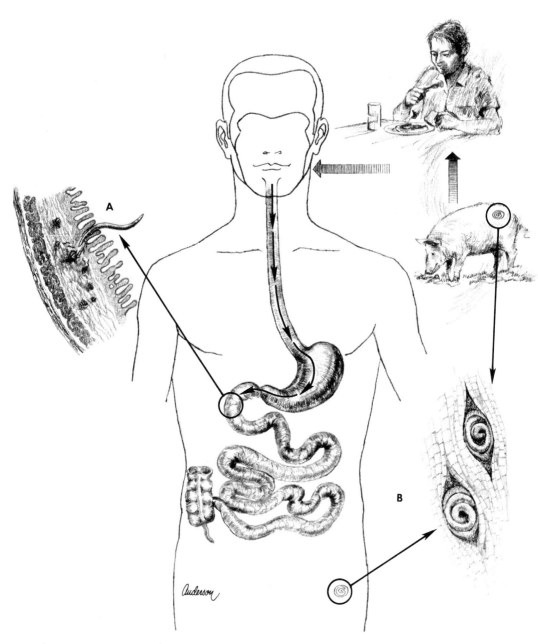

Fig. 8-12. Life cycle of *Trichinella spiralis*. Infective larvae, encysted in pork and other meat, when ingested, become adult worms in the small intestine. The female burrows into the mucosa and deposits larvae into lacteals and blood vessels, **A.** Circulating larvae eventually penetrate skeletal muscle and become encysted, **B.** In man these larvae are at a dead end, but in the pig and other animals they become a source of infection.

icking over 50 other human diseases. The presentation of the disease varies from asymptomatic cases to severe fulminating infections resulting in death. The incubation period averages 7 to 10 days but may vary from 1 to 28 days. It is usually inversely related to the severity of infection. Symptomatology may conveniently be divided into three stages—intestinal, muscle invasion, and convalescence.

During the initial stages, when the adult worms are maturing in the intestinal mucosa, symptoms occur in about half the cases, sometimes within the first 24 hours after infection. Symptoms are malaise, mild fever, anorexia, and gastrointestinal complaints, particularly diarrhea. This stage is self-limited and often is recognized only on repeated questioning.

The second stage of muscular invasion and encystment (Fig. 8-13) usually begins about a week after infection and lasts up to 2 months. The symptoms depend on the muscles involved. Muscular pain and tenderness extending throughout the body are frequent.

Dyspnea and pain on respiration may be prominent, with heavy involvement of the respiratory muscles. Pain on eye motion is a particularly suggestive symptom.

Encystment occurs only in skeletal muscle, but larval migrations and death in other tissues can result in focal lesions elsewhere. Edema of the eyelids, retinal hemorrhage, conjunctivitis, rash, splinter hemorrhages, meningitis and focal cerebral signs, and arthralgias may be prominent. Pulmonary hemorrhages mimic pneumonitis. Penetration of cardiac muscle, although encystment does not occur, may lead to death from myocarditis, usually between the fourth and eighth weeks following infection. Patients who survive the first 3 months generally recover completely.

Pathology. Pathologic changes in the gastrointestinal tract are usually mild, but in fatal cases mucosal hyperemia, punctate hemorrhages, and edema may be present. Mesenteric lymph nodes are regularly enlarged, and larvae are sometimes present. Major pathologic changes are associated

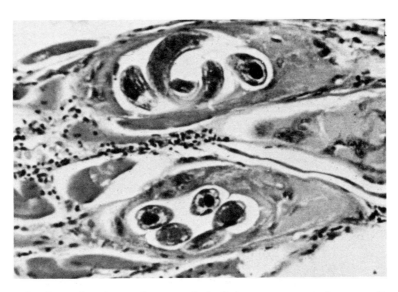

Fig. 8-13. *Trichinella spiralis* in human showing marked inflammatory reaction in the surrounding muscle. (From a nonprofit cooperative endeavor by numerous colleagues under the editorship of Dr. Herman Zaiman, Valley City, N.D.)

chiefly with muscle invasion. The extraocular muscles (Fig. 8-14), masseters, tongue diaphragm, intercostals, and muscles of the neck region are most commonly and extensively affected. Larvae are most numerous at the sites of muscular attachment to tendons. Edema of the muscle fibers, followed by shrinkage, eventual replacement of degenerated fibers by an irregular network of fine granular threads, and collapse of the muscle wall, occur. Granulocytic and lymphocytic infiltration reaches a peak at the fifth or sixth week when encapsulation takes place. Inflammation subsides and scar tissue forms.

Hemorrhagic extravasation of the epicardium may be present, with thrombi in the endocardium. The myocardium becomes edematous and hemorrhagic and shows scat-

tered foci of focal necrosis in the muscle fibers.

The lungs, likewise, show hemorrhagic foci in the bronchioles and alveoli. Pressure in the cerebrospinal fluid may be increased because of the presence of larvae, and the meninges as well as the brain may be hyperemic and edematous and show scattered punctate hemorrhages. The bone marrow shows marked eosinophilia. Peripheral eosinophilia usually begins during the second week of infection, reaches its height during the third and fourth weeks, and gradually declines over several months. Although other helminth infections frequently are associated with an eosinophilia, usually mild, this is very often the most significant sign that the patient presents in trichinosis. It is usually the first sign that arouses suspicion.

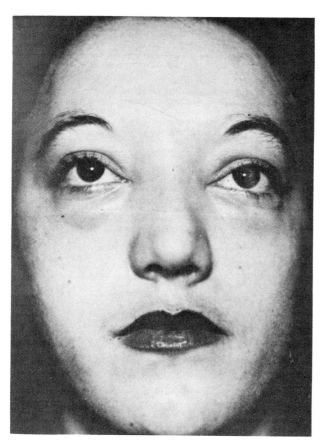

Fig. 8-14. Patient with trichinosis. Note the bilateral periorbital edema. (AFIP 52-8038).

The highest eosinophilia on record is 89%. In fulminating cases death may ensue before eosinophilia appears.

Diagnosis. Recovery and identification of adult worms from the feces or larvae from the circulation have not proved to be satisfactory means of diagnosis. The surest method of diagnosis is muscle biopsy of the deltoid, biceps, gastrocnemius, or, indeed, any tender muscle. A negative biopsy finding does not exclude the possibility of infection. Serologic tests such as the precipitin, complement-fixation, bentonite-flocculation, and fluorescent antibody tests usually show demonstrable titers 3 to 4 weeks after infection. The bentonite-flocculation test (BFT) is probably the most desirable because it more closely approximates the desired features of a positive reaction only during the acute stage and yet is sensitive and reproducible enough to measure a rise or fall in titer. The test results of nearly all patients are negative after 2 to 3 years. Titers of 1:5 are considered significant by the Center for Disease Control diagnostic laboratory. The indirect fluorescent antibody (IFA) test is equally as sensitive as the BFT. Other tests such as the latex, cholesterol-lecithin flocculation, and the complement-fixation (CF) are also good and, because of their simplicity and the availability of reagents, are preferred by many small laboratories. The skin test, which becomes positive in about 3 weeks, may show demonstrable titers persisting for 7 to 10 years and is most useful for detecting remote infection.

A history of having recently eaten pork, febrile myalgia, bilateral periorbital edema (Fig. 8-14), and rising eosinophilia are highly suggestive of infection and warrant a presumptive diagnosis. Similar symptoms in other members of the family or friends dining at the same place further substantiate the diagnosis.

Treatment. There is no satisfactory treatment for trichinosis. Both piperazine and purgation have theoretic value for early in-

fection, but the diagnosis is seldom made when major pathologic changes are limited to the gastrointestinal tract. Treatment of the myositis and other sequelae of systemic invasion is primarily symptomatic. In severely ill patients corticosteroids have been advocated, but a comparable therapeutic response is probably, and usually if not always, obtained with aspirin; in addition, there is some evidence that corticoids may prolong the life of the adult worm. Thiabendazole (Mintezol) has been shown to destroy some of the larvae after muscle penetration; evaluation of its clinical efficacy is difficult because of the variable course of untreated disease. The dosage is 25 mg/kg twice daily until symptoms subside or toxicity occurs (Table 8-1). Thiabendazole frequently causes nausea, vomiting, and vertigo. Occasionally leukopenia, crystalluria, hallucination, rash, and disturbance of color vision occur. Tinnitus and shock are rare. Corticosteroids should be administered concomitantly with therapy.

Hookworms

Two species of hookworms, *Necator americanus* and *Ancylostoma duodenale*, are parasitic in the human intestinal tract. Because the hookworms of humans cannot be differentiated in the egg and larval stages, the diagnosis "hookworm infection" alone usually is made.

Geographic distribution. Both species occur predominately in the tropics and subtropics between 36° north and 30° south latitude. *A. duodenale* occurs also in more temperate regions and has been reported in the mining areas of Europe as far north as Belgium and England. This species is found in the United States, but, as the name "Old World hookworm" implies, it occurs mainly in Europe, Asia, Africa, and also the Pacific Islands. *N. americanus*, the "New World hookworm," is the predominate species in the United States, with its origin in Africa, but it also occurs around the world. It was probably introduced into the United States during the slave-trading days. *Necator americanus* means "American killer." Evidence of human migrations is revealed in a study of the hookworm fauna of various populations. *Ancylostoma ceylanicum*, normally a parasite of carnivores, has been reported in humans in the Philippines. *Ancylostoma malayanum*, a parasite of bears in Malaysia and India, has been reported once in a human.

Morphology and life cycle. The female species of *N. americanus* averages about 10 mm in length and has the head end curved dorsally in a hooked position. The mouth capsule contains typical cutting plates by which the organism attaches to the mucosa (Fig. 8-15). The male is usually smaller, and differs only in that the posterior extremity is modified to form a copulatory bursa.

The female species of *A. duodenale* is slightly larger and more robust than *Necator*, with a mouth capsule containing two pairs of well-developed teeth, one pair on each plate (Fig. 8-16). The head is not curved dorsally. The male of the species, like *Necator*, is usually smaller than the female and terminates posteriorly in a copulatory apparatus or bursa. Although *Necator* is primarily a parasite of humans, capable of developing in apes and monkeys, *A. duodenale* has been found in pigs and experimentally will develop in cats, dogs, and monkeys.

The hookworms live in the small intestine of the definitive host with a firm grasp on the intestinal wall (Fig. 8-17). A single female can produce over 50 eggs per gram of feces that are passed in a normal bowel movement in the 2- to 8- cell stage of cleavage. They average 40 to 70 μm in length by about 40 μm in diameter and have a thin, clear, colorless shell wall. *Necator* eggs are usually larger than those of *A. duodenale* (Fig. 8-18).

On oxygenation, embryonation takes place and eggs hatch, in suitable soil, in 5 days. Under ideal conditions of moisture and warmth a rhabditiform larva may hatch within 24 hours; in less favorable conditions, in 5 weeks. The hatched larvae measure about

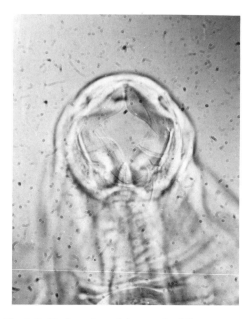

Fig. 8-15. En face view of the mouth of *Necator americanus*. Note the broad cutting plates. (From Schmidt, G. D., and Roberts, L. S.: Foundations of parasitology, 1977, St. Louis, The C. V. Mosby Co.)

275 μm in length, with a diameter of about 16 μm. They have a buccal cavity, more or less equal in length to the width of the worm (Fig. 8-19), in contrast with rhabditiform larvae of *Strongyloides stercoralis*, in which the buccal cavity is short and roughly equal to about half the width of the worm. The esophagus is typically hourglass shaped, a feature more or less characteristic of all rhabditiform larvae. Midway along the length of the intestinal tract, the small genital primordium, a cluster of cells that is the anlage of the adult genital system, may sometimes be seen. Frequently it is hidden by the intestinal tract. Hookworm rhabditiform larvae feed on bacteria and organic debris in the subsoil. After 2 days the larvae molt, continue their growth, and in about 5 days molt again, retaining the shed skin as a sheath. They reach a length of over twice their original size and become slender, nonfeeding filariform larvae, infective for the definitive host. In this stage the buccal cavity is closed

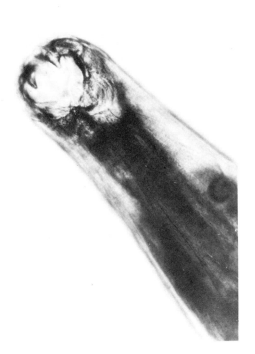

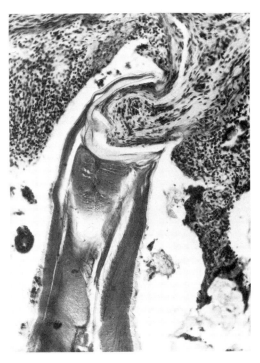

Fig. 8-16. *Ancylostoma duodenale*, dorsal view showing ventral teeth. (AFIP N-41730-2. From Schmidt, G. D., and Roberts, L. S.: Foundations of parasitology, St. Louis, 1977, The C. V. Mosby Co.)

Fig. 8-17. View showing firm grasp of a hookworm on the intestinal wall. Note the ventral tooth in the depth of the buccal capsule lacerating the intestinal mucosa. (AFIP N-33818. From Schmidt, G. D., and Roberts, L. S.: Foundations of parasitology, St. Louis, 1977, The C. V. Mosby Co.)

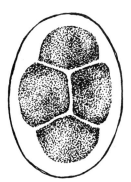
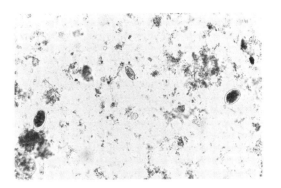
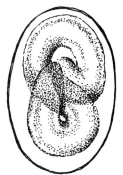

Fig. 8-18. Hookworm eggs. Note the *Trichuris trichiura* egg also present. (Photomicrograph courtesy Department of Pathology, University of Miami, School of Medicine.)

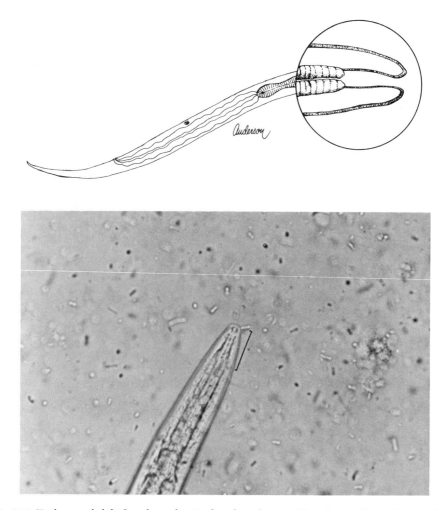

Fig. 8-19. Hookworm rhabditiform larva showing long buccal cavity. Note the small genital primordium midway up the body (see drawing). (Photomicrograph courtesy Department of Pathology, University of Miami, School of Medicine.)

by the retained molted cuticle and the esophagus becomes elongated, with a poorly defined terminal bulb. Hookworm filariform larvae are further characterized by slender, pointed tails, in contrast to *Strongyloides* filariform larvae, which have notched tails (Fig. 8-23).

The filariform larvae climb up on the moist dirt and vegetable particles and wave in the breeze, and there they may survive for several weeks, waiting for a warm-blooded host. Upon contact they penetrate the skin, invade

the circulatory system, and are carried into the lungs where, because of their large size, they are unable to pass across the capillary bed. They break out into the alveolar spaces and bronchioles and are carried up the bronchial tree to the pharynx where many are swallowed. In the small intestine another molt is completed and the young worms cling to the mucosa. After a fourth molt, the worms become mature (Fig. 8-20), fertilization takes place, and eggs appear in the feces. The complete cycle, from the time of infec-

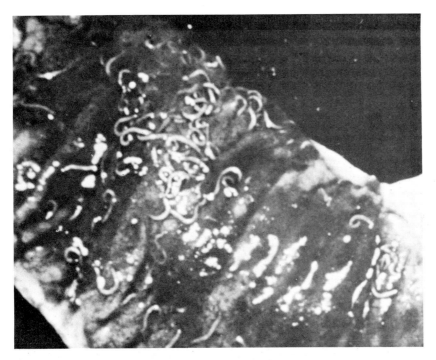

Fig. 8-20. *Ancylostoma duodenale* adults attached to the duodenal mucosa. (AFIP 75-14422.)

tion until the presence of eggs in the bowel, takes from 3 to 6 weeks in humans. The life span of the adult hookworm may be 5 years or longer (Fig. 8-21).

Epidemiology. Temperature and rainfall are among the most important environmental factors influencing the hookworm prevalence. Localities having less than 40 inches of rainfall a year never have heavy infections. The seasonal variation is also important since the filariform larvae cannot withstand desiccation or excessive rainfall. Temperatures above 85° F are destructive to the larvae, whereas those lower than 70° F result in retarded growth or death. Frost destroys all eggs and larvae. The nature of the soil is also very important in hookworm transmission for, although hard clay soil is detrimental, a sandy, loamy soil with good drainage and vegetation for shade affords an excellent culture medium. Many animals such as dogs and pigs can act as disseminators of eggs from fresh feces by the passage of eggs

through the intestinal tract unharmed. Dung beetles similarly aid in this dissemination, whereas chickens and cattle destroy the eggs after ingestion.

All ages and races are susceptible. Occupation plays an important role because farmers and others in the field are more likely to be exposed than are city dwellers. Dooryard defecation habits influence the incidence, particularly in children. The wearing of shoes markedly reduces the incidence of hookworm infection; in many areas, high rates occur only in children of barefoot age. The habit of frequent expectoration also decreases the worm burden in the Orient, where betel-nut chewing and expectoration is common. The incidence of infection may be high, but few worms are swallowed and clinical manifestations are rare. The virtues of tobacco chewing might be extolled from this point of view as well.

Symptomatology and pathology. Invasion of the skin by the filariform larvae may cause

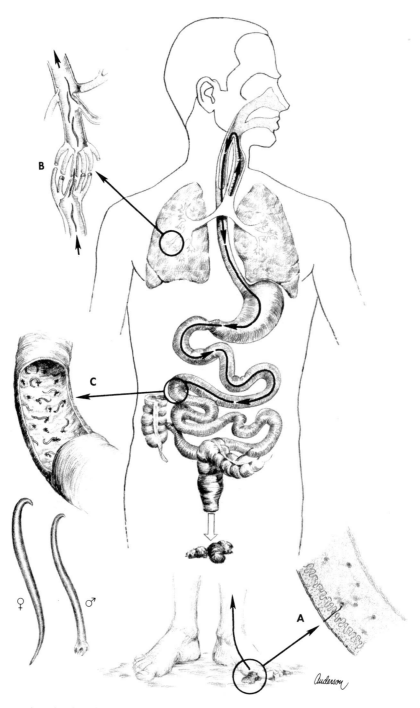

Fig. 8-21. Life cycle of the hookworm. Filariform larvae in the soil penetrate the skin, **A,** are carried via the circulation to the lungs where they break out of the capillary bed into the alveolar spaces, **B,** then are swept up the bronchial tree, are swallowed, and become adult worms in the small intestine, **C.**

a pruritic papular dermatitis (ground itch, water sore). This is more characteristic of infection with *Necator americanus* than of infection with *Ancylostoma duodenale*. Scratching may result in secondary infection.

The period of larval migration through the lungs is usually asymptomatic unless a large infection during a short period of time results in many larvae passing through the lungs simultaneously. Such patients may experience fever, headache, nausea, dyspnea, and a dry cough. Occasionally blood-streaked sputum is reported; examination of this sputum may show an excess of eosinophils and, rarely, larvae. Patchy pulmonary infiltrates or lung consolidation ensues. Symptoms, usually worse at night, may persist for several weeks. This phase results from the rupture of larvae through the capillary bed and their dissemination throughout the bronchial tree. Pathologic studies show leukocytic infiltration and petechial hemorrhages, followed later by fibroblast formation in some cases.

As the larvae enter the intestinal tract and mature to adults, nonspecific gastrointestinal symptoms (nausea, vomiting, flatulence, diarrhea or constipation, low-grade fever) may be noted. Sometimes symptoms are strongly suggestive of duodenal ulcer. An eosinophilia up to 60% may characterize the first two stages; usually it reaches its peak within 3 months and then gradually falls toward normal, despite the persistence of adult worms. A leukocytosis may also occur early in infection.

The major pathologic condition of hookworm infection is anemia and its sequelae. Worms are attached to the mucosa (Fig. 8-20) and suck blood. A single adult worm can extract 0.05 ml of blood per day; thus a not uncommonly heavy hookworm infection can result in the loss of over 100 ml of blood per day. The amount of iron lost in this way is proportional to the hemoglobin of the patient. Red blood cells are passed intact from the worm, and probably up to 60% of the

iron lost in this way is reabsorbed for incorporation into new erythrocytes. Nevertheless, over a period of time, a large worm burden can deplete the patient's iron stores and result in the microcytic hypochromic anemia of iron deficiency. The interval between infection and anemia is dependent on the number of worms (blood loss) and the amount of iron in the diet. An iron-poor diet and relatively few worms may result in severe anemia, particularly in the face of the increased demands for iron in childhood and pregnancy, whereas a heavy worm load may produce no anemia when iron intake is sufficient. Malnutrition may confuse the picture: a high carbohydrate diet, common in underdeveloped areas, may contain excessive iron-binding phytates that prevent optimal iron absorption and accelerate the anemia; a concomitant dietary folic acid deficiency may result in a megaloblastic macrocytic anemia that masks the iron deficiency. Worms also produce an anticoagulant to facilitate the sucking of blood and browse along the mucosa to new attachments; oozing bleeding sites may contribute to blood loss.

Severe hookworm anemia may result in symptoms of heart failure with an enlarged, flabby heart, tachycardia, and poor growth and development. Milder anemia results mainly in weakness and lassitude, which, like malaria, contributes to further malnutrition by preventing full use of the natural resources of the patient and his environment. (A farmer with a hemoglobin of 7 grams percent is obviously a less efficient provider than one functioning at full capacity, that is, with a hemoglobin of 14 grams percent.)

In addition to red blood cells, the hookworm also removes protein from the serum. With borderline nutrition, severe hypoalbuminemia may result. In patients with hookworm anemia it may be difficult to separate the edema resulting from hypoalbuminemia from that of heart failure secondary to anemia.

Diagnosis. The diagnosis of hookworm infection is chiefly dependent on the recovery and identification of the eggs in the feces. Eggs are present consistently in the stool, although numbers vary from time to time. Methods for determining the egg count per gram of feces (see Appendix A) are unnecessary for diagnosis, but they are useful in studying the relation of worm load (one worm yields 500 eggs per gram of feces) to anemia and in studies of efficacy of new treatment. Delay in the examination of the fecal specimen or the examination of a stool from a constipated individual may reveal hatched rhabditiform larvae, which must be differentiated from *Strongyloides* by the criteria previously mentioned. By spreading a thin film of feces over the middle portion of a strip of filter paper (Harada-Mori method, see Appendix A) and placing it in a 15-ml conical-tip centrifuge tube containing enough water to maintain contact with the tip of the paper pressed against the side of the tube, infective larvae may be collected in the bottom of the tube in a week to 10 days. The culture is kept in the dark at room temperature. Differentiation from *Strongyloides stercoralis* is readily made. If species identification is desired, adult worms must be recovered by satisfactory treatment. This recovery is seldom necessary unless sophisticated studies of anemia or therapy are proposed. The serodiagnosis of the hookworms is far from being satisfactory. While the indirect hemagglutination test is the method of choice, it has many shortcomings and is not recommended as a routine laboratory procedure. Infection with *Necator americanus* induces a marked elevation in serum IgG but whether or not antibodies are directed specifically against parasite antigens is uncertain.

Treatment. Differentiation between "hookworm infection" and "hookworm disease" affords an intelligent approach to the handling of the hookworm problem. Hookworm infection means the presence of worms without clinical manifestations. Individuals maintained on a diet rich in proteins, iron, and

vitamins and not having a worm burden great enough to elicit any clinical manifestations require no treatment. Prevention of reinfection by the wearing of shoes or by departure from the endemic area, along with adequate nutrition, is sufficient. In areas where malnutrition, hookworms, and other intestinal parasites coexist, hookworm infection is rare whereas hookworm disease is quite common. In such cases, chemotherapy is essential, along with adequate supportive treatment, including proper diet, iron therapy, and blood transfusions, if necessary.

By far the most important factor in the development of hookworm anemia is the iron content of the diet. Treatment with iron, with hookworms in place, will correct the anemia. Worming without iron replacement will not. Patients who are very ill with severe anemias should have their anemia corrected prior to therapy for the worms. The anemia, not the worms per se, causes death, and many forms of treatment are more toxic in the anemic patient. In contrast, hypoalbuminemia caused by worms and a low-protein diet will not be corrected by diet alone, and reduction in the worm burden is essential in such cases.

The drugs of choice in the treatment of the hookworms are given in Table 8-1.

Strongyloides stercoralis

Geographic distribution. *Strongyloides stercoralis* is found throughout the world and follows a distribution pattern similar to hookworm throughout the tropics and subtropics but is restricted more to warm, moist climates because of a greater frailty of the filariform larvae.

Life cycle and morphology. A difference of opinion exists as to the nature of the life cycle of this parasite. Many believe that only parthenogenetic females are parasitic in humans, whereas others maintain that both sexes exist, the male having a short life span and not observed in humans but reported in animals. *S. stercoralis* is primarily a human parasite; experimental infections have been produced in dogs, cats, and apes. Filariform larvae, like those of the hookworm, penetrate human skin. Once in the circulation they reach the lungs, escape from the capillaries into the alveolae, and pass up the bronchial tree to the pharynx where they are swallowed and become adults in the small intestine. Occasionally larvae mature into adults in the bronchial tree.

The parasitic female is slender and small, measuring about 2 mm in length by approximately 45 μm in diameter. It is one of the smallest nematodes of humans. The parasite burrows into the mucosa of the duodenum and upper jejunum; in heavy infections this may occur throughout the small and large intestines. The eggs are similar to, but smaller than, hookworm eggs, measuring about 50 μm $\times$ 32 μm, with a clear, thin shell. Deposited in the mucosa, they undergo development and hatch rapidly. The entire cycle in humans takes about 1 month. The rhabditiform larvae work their way into the lumen of the intestine and pass out in the feces. Like the rhabditiform larvae of the hookworm, they are about 275 μm in length by 16 μm in diameter with the typical hourglass esophagus. Unlike the hookworms, however, the buccal cavity (Fig. 8-22) is short, measuring approximately half the width of the larva, whereas the genital primordium is large and discernible about halfway down the length of the intestinal tract. Within 24 hours or longer the rhabditiform larvae molt and transform into the filariform stage, retaining the molted skin as a sheath. This stage (Fig. 8-23) is infective for the definitive host.

Rhabditiform larvae passed in the feces may also develop in the soil into free-living adults. They mate and produce eggs that hatch into rhabditiform larvae. This cycle may be repeated indefinitely, or filariform larvae infective for the definitive host may be formed.

Rhabditiform larvae delayed in passage down the intestinal canal may transform into filariform larvae before leaving the host. Penetration of the colonic mucosa or perianal skin may take place, resulting in autoinfection; in this way, a given individual may remain infected for more than 30 years.

Epidemiology. The pattern of transmission is similar to that of the hookworm. Unlike the hardier hookworms, the filariform stages of S. *stercoralis* show only slight resistance to temperature changes and desiccation. Although coextensive with hookworms throughout the tropics, they are spotty in distribution, being restricted to optimal living conditions. The presence of a free-living cycle assures the perpetuation of this parasite during the absence of a suitable host. Adverse environmental changes predispose the worms toward the direct route. Autoinfection explains the persistence of the parasite in an individual for years after leaving an endemic area and is also responsible for massive infections, which are sometimes encountered.

Symptomatology and pathology. Skin invasion usually causes a reaction that is less severe than the ground itch of hookworm, but previously sensitized persons may show marked urticaria. Creeping eruption caused by migration of larvae in the skin is common in chronic strongyloid carriers. Deep-tissue invasion, producing a picture like visceral larva migrans, has been reported. Migration through the lungs may elicit the same symptoms as the pulmonary phase of hookworm invasion with fever, cough, dyspnea, and malaise. In heavy autoinfection, inflammation, eosinophilia, pneumonitis, and severe allergic reactions with Loeffler's syndrome may occur. Sputum examination may show adult worms, as well as larvae, although this evidence is uncommon.

Although intestinal infection with adult worms is frequently asymptomatic, abdominal pain, nausea, vomiting, and diarrhea alternating with constipation may occur. Rarely, hematemesis or extreme diarrhea

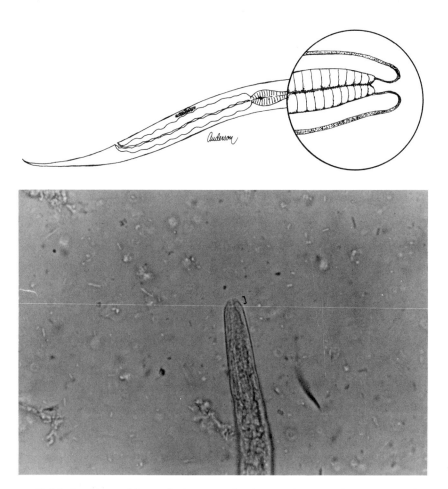

Fig. 8-22. Rhabditiform larva of *Strongyloides stercoralis* showing short buccal cavity. Note the large genital primordium midway up the body (see drawing). (Photomicrograph courtesy Department of Pathology, University of Miami, School of Medicine.)

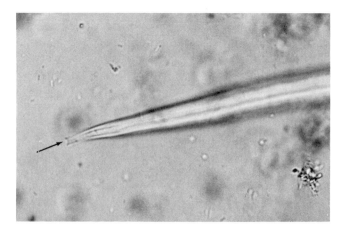

Fig. 8-23. Filariform larva of *Strongyloides stercoralis* showing notched tail. (Courtesy Department of Epidemiology and Public Health, University of Miami, School of Medicine.)

with tenesmus and bloody stools is noted. A clinical picture indistinguishable from duodenal ulcer or regional enteritis has been reported. Hepatitis, cholecystitis, or malnutrition with or without malabsorption may result. Death from bowel-wall penetration is rare. The peripheral eosinophilia averages up to 15%, but levels comparable with trichinosis may occur. Patients with severe autoinfection and fatal outcome may have no eosinophilia.

In fatal cases larvae have been found in almost every organ of the body. Usually the most noticeable pathologic condition is found in the small intestine (Fig. 8-24) where myriads of adult worms and a honeycombed appearance may be noted easily. Ulcers may be seen. Microscopic examination of the duodenum shows flattened villi, atrophy of the mucosa, and many larvae, eggs, and adults in the mucosal crypts. The lymphatic spaces may be filled with larvae. Occasionally granulomatous colitis is seen.

Diagnosis. Diagnosis depends on recovery and identification of the larval stages in the feces. The presence of larvae in freshly passed stools strongly suggests strongyloidiasis; the presence of eggs suggests hookworm infection. Rarely, with severe diarrhea, embryonated eggs of *Strongyloides* may be seen. Hookworm larvae are seen in stools that have been left standing, and they can be differentiated by morphology from *S. stercoralis* larvae, since *S. stercoralis* larvae have a short buccal cavity roughly equal to or less than half the width of a larva and a large genital primordium (Fig. 8-22). By spreading a thin film of feces in the middle portion of a strip of filter paper (Harada-Mori method, see Appendix A) and placing it in a 15-ml conical-tip centrifuge tube containing enough water to maintain contact with the tip of the paper pressed against the side of the tube, infective larvae may be collected in the bottom of the tube in a week to 10 days. The culture is kept in the dark at room temperature. Differentiation from hookworm larvae is readily made. Patients with autoinfection may have negative stool specimens and only duodenal aspiration will reveal the rhabditiform larvae. In cases of constipation or in stools left standing before examination, the filariform larvae with the typically notched tail may be found (Fig. 8-23). The nature of the stool specimen and the time of passage are helpful in differential diagnosis. Elevation of nonspecific serum IgE occurs as in many other helminth infections.

Treatment. Strongyloidiasis has been one of the more difficult helminth infections to treat. The risk of autoinfection and its complications requires not a reduction in worm burden, as in most other helminth infections, but an eradication of the infection. Thiaben-

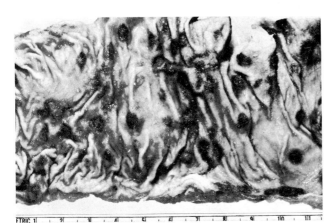

Fig. 8-24. Lesions of the intestinal mucosa from *Strongyloides stercoralis*. (From Anderson, W. A. D., and Scotti, T. M.: Synopsis of pathology, ed. 9, St. Louis, 1976, The C. V. Mosby Co.)

dazole (Mintezol) is the drug of choice with a dose of 25 mg/kg twice daily for 2 days (Table 8-1). As an alternative pyrvinium pamoate at the dosage of 5 mg/kg (250 mg maximum) for 5 to 7 days is recommended by some. Thiabendazole frequently causes nausea, vomiting, and vertigo. On occasions, leukopenia, crystalluria, rash, disturbance of color vision, and hallucinations may occur. Shock and tinnitus are rare. Pyrvinium pamoate (Povan) may occasionally cause vomiting and diarrhea. Photosensitivity skin reactions are rare. The stool becomes red.

Oesophagostomum

Geographical distribution and life cycle. Species of *Oesophagostomum*, or nodular

worms, are close relatives of *Ternidens deminutus*. Normally parasitic in monkeys, pigs, sheep, goats, cattle, and apes, occasionally infections occur in humans. Approximately 50 cases have been reported. Except for some isolated reports from Brazil and Indonesia, all others have occurred in tropical Africa. The adults resemble hookworms and likewise have a similar life cycle, except that the infective larvae of most species do not penetrate the skin but are ingested with vegetation. In their normal hosts, development after another molt occurs in the submucosa of the small or large intestine. Eggs appear in the feces 30 to 40 days after infection. In humans, however, ingested larvae do not become adults. Complete development

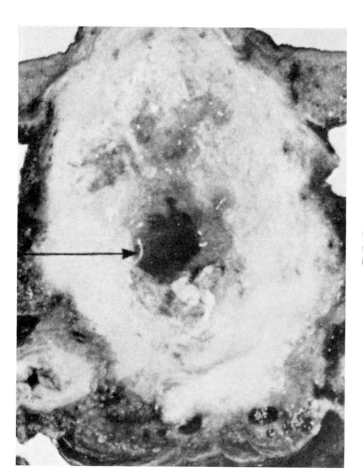

Fig. 8-25. Resected nodule of oesophagostomiasis showing the worm *(arrow)* protruding into the cavity. (AFIP 76-2110.)

does not occur except in a rare instance when stunted adults appear. If perchance any eggs do appear in the feces they resemble hookworm ova and would be so identified in all probability. Mature worms in their natural hosts are 8 to 30 mm in length by 310 to 900 μm in diameter.

Symptomatology and pathology. The most constant symptom is abdominal pain with localized tenderness, usually in the right lower quadrant. There may be a low-grade fever, but nausea, vomiting, anorexia, and diarrhea are noticeably absent. Usually a mass in the abdominal cavity adhering to the abdominal wall (Fig. 8-25) is revealed on physical examination and may be confirmed by radiologic examination. Perforation of the bowel wall is very rare. There may be extensive adhesions to neighboring structures with enlarged mesenteric lymph nodes and foci of fat necrosis in the mesentery.

Diagnosis and treatment. Differentiation from intestinal tuberculosis, ameboma, and schistosomal granuloma is necessary. Surgical removal is curative and will reveal the worms. Laboratory tests reveal very little and, since these patients come from areas where other worms are common, eosinophilia means very little also.

Physaloptera caucasica

Physaloptera caucasica is a large worm, the female measuring 3 to 10 cm in length by 1.2 to 2.8 mm in diameter. The males are about half that size. Superficially they resemble *Ascaris*. Characteristic features are a collarette surrounding the anterior end and a pair of trilobed lips. They are found in humans most frequently in the stomach but also in the small intestine to the mid-level of the ileum. Occasionally they are found in the liver. They live with the anterior end burrowed in the mucosa causing sores and ulcerations. Normally the worms are parasitic in African monkeys and are not uncommon among the natives of tropical Africa. The life cycle is unknown but probably involves insects as intermediate hosts. Infections reported from Central and South America, India, and the Middle East, in some instances, have been questionable.

Diploscapter coronata

Diploscapter coronata, a nematode previously known only as an inhabitant of the soil and sewage, were recovered in aspirated stomach contents from a group of patients some years ago in a Houston, Texas clinic. All patients had severe achlorhydria. Similar cases were frequently misdiagnosed as *Strongyloides* infections. Reexamination of one patient 4 days later revealed worms still established in the stomach. Very little is known about these infections.

Ternidens deminutus

Ternidens deminutus belongs to the Strongylidae family whose members have life cycles similar to the hookworms except that the infective larvae of most do not penetrate the skin but are ingested with vegetation. *T. deminutus* lives with the anterior end burrowed in the intestinal mucosa causing cystic nodules or crateriform ulcers. Perforation with peritonitis has been noted on occasion. They resemble hookworm ova but are larger, averaging 84 μm by 50 μm and are usually in the 8-celled stage of cleavage when passed. Pyrantel pamoate and bephenium hydroxynaphthoate are effective in treatment. Infections in humans have been reported from Rhodesia, where monkeys are also infected. Human infections have also been reported from Malawi and Mozambique.

Capillaria philippinensis

Geographical distribution and life cycle. *Capillaria philippinensis* is an intestinal nematode first reported in 1964 from Luzon, the Philippines. It has also been reported from Thailand. Over 1,000 cases with 100 deaths were reported in an epidemic in the late 1960s in the Philippines. The female worm measures 2.5 to 4.3 mm in length by 20 to 50 μm in diameter. The male is smaller. The adult worms live burrowed in the small intestine, predominantly the jejunum. Eggs measure 36 to 45 μm by 21 μm, are bioperculate, and diagnostic of infection when found in the feces. Transmission occurs, it is believed, by the ingestion of larvae in three species of mainly marine fish. Soil seeded with eggs in a rural community maintains human transmission. The ability of the worms to reproduce in the intestine (autoinfection) results in a heavy build-up (200,000 recovered from 1 liter of intestinal content) of adult worms and larvae.

Symptomatology and pathology. The disease is characterized at the onset by generalized or epigastric abdominal pain, chronic diarrhea, and loud gurgling sounds (borborygmi). Malaise, anorexia, nausea, and vomiting follow and severe diarrhea leads to ascites, weight loss, cachexia, and death. Infections run a course of 6 to 12 months. Stools are numerous, very watery, and contain increased amounts of fat. Decrease in subcutaneous fat and muscular wasting reveals the outline of muscles and tendons through the skin and also peristalsis. Protein loss in the stool is about 15 times higher than normal. IgM and IgG may be decreased and bacterial enteritis or septicemia may develop as a consequence. Malabsorption of fats and sugar, loss of protein, low levels of carotene, potassium, and calcium, and decreased protein in the plasma occur. The small intestine is thickened, indurated, congested, and distended with fluid. Crypts of the jejunal mucosa, upper ileum and, at times, the duodenum reveal worms. Villi are flattened and show atrophy. The liver reveals fatty metamorphosis, congestion, atrophy, and hemosiderin.

Diagnosis and treatment. Eggs bear a close resemblance to those of *Trichuris trichiura* but are diagnostic of capillariasis when found in the feces. Treatment centers around restoration of fluid and electrolytes, particu-

larly potassium. A high protein diet is recommended. The drug of choice is given in Table 8-1.

Anisakidae

Anisakiasis or herring worm disease is an infection of the gastrointestinal tract caused by the larvae of ascarioid nematodes, *Anisakis*, *Phocanema*, and *Contracecum* of the family Anisakidae.

Geographical distribution and life cycle. The ascarioid nematodes are common parasites of herring, cod, Alaskan pollack, and other fishes of the North Sea and the Atlantic and North Pacific Oceans. The habit of eating raw or insufficiently cooked, salted or slightly pickled fish in areas of Japan, Holland, Brittany, Scandinavia, and the Pacific coastal area of South America accounts for the wide distribution among humans. Such dishes as suski and sashimi in Japan, green herring in Holland, and ceviche in South America serve as excellent vehicles for infection. Various marine mammals such as seals, porpoises, and whales harbor the adult worms in their intestinal tract. Details of the life cycles of these worms have not been worked out but eggs are passed in the feces and hatching of second-stage larvae occurs. It is believed that small crustaceans ingest the larvae and development to the next larval stage takes place. Fish or squid feeding on the crustaceans acquire the larvae which penetrate the gut wall and reach the body cavity or somatic muscles. The fish or squid serve as transport hosts to other fish or squid tending to concentrate within a few commonly eaten species by man.

Symptomatology and pathology. Third-stage larvae ingested by man are at a dead end and do not develop into adult worms as they do in marine mammals. They attach to the stomach or bowel mucosa, causing local ulceration. Patients have nausea and epigastric pain and vomit within 12 hours after exposure. Sometimes hematemesis occurs. In Japan, half of the patients have hypo-

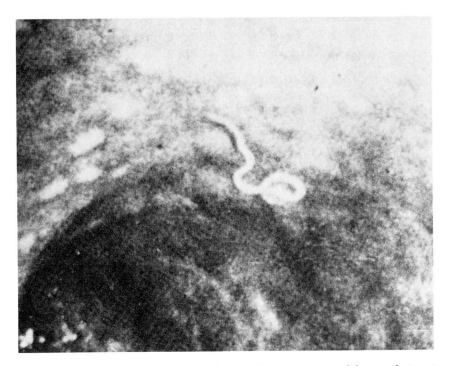

Fig. 8-26. Visualization of the worm causing anisakiasis in the gastric mucosa of the prepyloric region is shown here by gastroscopy. (AFIP 76-2118.)

chlorhydria or achlorhydria, which probably predisposes them to infection. X ray reveals single or multiple ulcers. Gastroscopy often reveals motile larvae penetrating the gastric wall (Fig. 8-26), and they sometimes can be removed under direct vision. Chronic infections mimic peptic ulcer, chronic gastritis, and carcinoma, making diagnosis difficult. There may be leukocytosis with a mild to moderate eosinophilia. Chronic infection in the small intestine often mimics appendicitis or regional enteritis, with nonspecific radiologic changes compatible with either diagnosis. Laporotomy, sometimes as an emergency measure, reveals the intestine diffusely thickened and edematous with inflammation of the peri-intestinal fat. Mesenteric lymph nodes are hyperplastic. Perforation of the bowel with larvae escaping into the peritoneal cavity may lead to localization of larvae in the mesentery, omentum, and pancreas. Preoperative diagnosis of anisakiasis is impossible unless visualization of larvae has been done through gastroscopy or radiographic techniques. Microscopically the lesions range from diffuse interstitial edema, accompanied by a filtrate of numerous eosinophils along with neutrophils, lymphocytes, monocytes, and plasma cells, to abscesses of eosinophils. Advanced lesions may show granulomas.

Diagnosis and treatment. Larvae expelled from the mouth or recovered from intestinal biopsy specimens are definitive. Radiographic and gastroscopic studies are helpful. Cure is obtained by removing the larvae by gastroscopy. Surgery may be necessary at times. The gastronomic tastes of the foreign traveler as well as the featuring of foreign dishes in this country are a cause of concern by the U.S. Food and Drug Administration. Outbreaks in Europe and Asia have stimulated research into this disease in the United States.

REVIEW QUESTIONS

1. Describe the basic life pattern of a nematode.
2. Why are pinworms the most common helminth infection in the temperate regions of the United States?
3. What is the significance of whipworm infection in the United States?
4. Contrast the life cycle of *Ascaris lumbricoides* with that of *Trichuris trichiura*.
5. What are the outstanding pathologic features of an ascarid infection that a physician should know?
6. Why is *T. spiralis*, an intestinal nematode, such a potentially dangerous parasite? How can infection be prevented?
7. Discuss the significance of hookworm infection and hookworm disease.
8. Why is eradication, rather than just reduction in worm burden, important in strongyloidiasis and ascariasis?
9. Discuss the differential diagnosis of hookworm infection and *Strongyloides* infection.
10. Discuss the treatment of trichinosis, hookworm infection, and strongyloidiasis.
11. What is oesophagostomiasis? Discuss.
12. What is the significance of anisakiasis in the United States?
13. What are the symptoms and pathologic findings of *Capillaria philippinensis* infections?
14. Identify the geographical distribution of and the symptoms and pathologic findings of the diseases caused by *Physaloptera caucasica*, *Diploscapter coronata*, and *Ternidens deminutus*.

REFERENCES

Adam, M., and others. 1973. Hyperinfection syndrome with *Strongyloides stercoralis* in malignant lymphoma. Br. Med. J. **1:**264-266.

Banzon, T. C., R. W. Lewert, and M. G. Yogore. 1975. Serology of *Capillaria philippinensis* infection: reactivity of human sera to antigens prepared from *Capillaria obsignata* and other helminths. Am. J. Trop. Med. Hyg. **24:**256-263.

Beaver, P. C. 1966. Zoonoses with particular reference to parasites of veterinary importance. In Biology of parasites. Academic Press, New York.

Beaver, P. C., J. J. Kriz, and T. J. Lau. 1973. Pulmonary nodule caused by *Enterobius vermicularis*. Am. J. Trop. Med. Hyg. **22:**711-713.

Beck, J. W., and others. 1959. The treatment of pinworm infections in humans (enterobiasis) with pyrvinium chloride and pyrvinium pamoate. Am. J. Trop. Med. **8:**329-352.

Beck, J. W., and M. Beverly-Burton. 1968. The pathology of *Trichuris*, *Capillaria*, and *Trichinella* infections. Helminthol. Abstr. **37:**1-26.

Bezjak, B. 1975. Immunoglobulin studies in stron-

gyloidiasis with special reference to raised serum IgE levels: preliminary communication. Am. J. Trop. Med. Hyg. **24:**945-948.

Binford, C. H., and D. H. Connor, Editors. 1976. Pathology of tropical and extraordinary diseases: an atlas. Vol. II. Armed Forces Institute of Pathology, Washington, D.C.

Boyd, W. P., Jr., F. W. Campbell, and W. L. Trudeau. 1978. *Strongyloides stercoralis:* hyperinfection. Am. J. Trop. Med. Hyg. **27:**39-41.

Bradley, S. L., D. E. Dines, and N. S. Brewer. 1978. Disseminated *Strongyloides stercoralis* in an immunosuppressed host. Mayo Clin. Proc. **53:**332-335.

Brashear, R. E., R. R. Martin, and J. L. Glover. 1971. Trichinosis and respiratory failure. Am. Rev. Respir. Dis. **104:**245-248.

Chandler, A. C. 1948. *Diploscapter coronata* as a facultative parasite of man, with a general review of vertebrate parasitism by rhabtoid worms. Parasitology **30:**44-55.

Chavn, H. 1967. The treatment of chronic strongyloidiasis with thiabendazole. Trans. R. Soc. Trop. Med. Hyg. **61:**812-816.

Chitwood, M. B., and C. Valesquez, and N. G. Salazar. 1972. *Capillaria philippinensis* sp. n. (Nematoda: Trichinellidae) from the intestine of a man in the Philippines. J. Parasitol. **54:**368-371.

Chowdhury, A. B., and G. A. Schad. 1972. *Ancylostoma ceylanicum:* a parasite of man in Calcutta and environs. Am. J. Trop. Med. Hyg. **21:**300-301.

Clark, P. S., and others. 1972. Bear meat trichinosis: epidemiologic, serologic, and clinical observations from two Alaskan outbreaks. Ann. Intern. Med. **76:**951-956.

Cruz, T., G. Reboucas, and H. Rocha. 1966. Fatal strongyloidiasis in patients receiving corticosteroids. N. Engl. J. Med. **275:**1093-1096.

Despommier, D., M. Muller, B. Jenks, and M. Fruitstone. 1974. Immunodiagnosis of human trichinosis using counterelectrophoresis and agar gel diffusion techniques. Am. J. Trop. Med. Hyg. **23:**41-44.

Eng-Lam, L., and others. 1976. Therapeutic evaluation of oxantel pamoate (1, 4, 5, 6-tetrahydro-1-methyl-2 [trans-3-hydroxystyryl] pyrimidine pamoate) in severe *Trichuris trichiura* infection. Am. J. Trop. Med. Hyg. **25:**563-567.

Eveland, L. K., M. Kenney, and V. Yermakov. 1975. Laboratory diagnosis of autoinfection in strongyloidiasis. Am. J. Clin. Pathol. **63:**421-425.

Foy, H., and G. S. Nelson. 1963. Helminths in the etiology of anemia in the tropics, with special reference to hookworms and schistosomes. Exp. Parasitol. **14:**240-262.

Fozard, G. 1978. Major helminthic diseases of North America: a review. J. Fam. Pract. **6:**1195-1203.

Gould, S. E. 1970. Trichinosis in man and animals. Charles C Thomas, Publisher, Springfield, Ill.

Graham, C. F. 1941. A device for the diagnosis of *Enterobius* infection. Am. J. Trop. Med. **21**:159-161.

Harada, Y., and O. Mori. 1955. A new method for culturing hookworm. Yonago Acta Med. **1**:177-179.

Higenbottam, T. W., and B. E. Heard. 1976. Opportunistic pulmonary strongyloidiasis complicating asthma with steroids. Thorax **31**:226-233.

Jaramillo, D., W. León, V. Cárdenas, and A. Cortes. 1978. Reiter's syndrome, immunodepression, and strongyloidiasis: report of a fatal case. J. Gut Pathol. **5**:200-208.

Jung, R. C., and P. C. Beaver, 1951. Clinical observations of *Trichocephalus trichiurus* (whipworm) infestation in children. Pediatrics **8**:548-557.

Kojima, S., M. Yokogawa, and T. Tada. 1972. Raised levels of serum IgE in human helminthiases. Am. J. Trop. Med. Hyg. **21**:913-918.

Little, M. D., G. J. Cuello, and A. D'Alessandro. 1973. Granuloma of the liver due to *Enterobius vermicularis:* report of a case. Am. J. Trop. Med. Hyg. **22**:567-569.

Louw, J. H. 1966. Abdominal complications of *Ascaris lumbricoides* infestation in children. Br. J. Surg. **53**:510-521.

Mansour, T. E. 1979. Chemotherapy of parasitic worms: new biochemical strategies. Science **205**:462-469.

Martin, L. K., and P. C. Beaver, 1968. Evaluation of Kato thick smear technique for quantitative diagnosis of helminthic infection. Am. J. Trop. Med. Hyg. **17**:382-391.

Meltzer, R. S., and others. 1979. Case report: antemortem diagnosis of central nervous sytem strongyloidiasis. Am. J. Med. Sci. **277**:91-98.

Miller, T. A. 1968. Pathogenesis and immunity in hookworm infection. Trans. R. Soc. Trop. Med. Hyg. **62**:473-485.

Moens, M., and others. 1978. Levamisole in ascariasis. Am. J. Trop. Med. Hyg. **27**:897-904.

Most, H. 1975. The epidemiology of common intestinal helminths. J. Sch. Health **45**(6):343-345.

Most, H. 1978. Current concepts in parasitology. Trichinosis: preventable yet still with us. N. Engl. J. Med. **298**:1178-1180.

Nawalinski, T., G. A. Schad, and A. B. Chowdhury. 1978. Population biology of hookworms in children in rural West Bengal: II. Acquisition and loss of hookworms. Am. J. Trop. Med. Hyg. **27**:1162-1173.

Neefe, L. L., and others. 1973. Disseminated strongyloidiasis with cerebral involvement. Am. J. Med. **55**:832-838.

Oshima, T. 1972. *Anisakis* and anisakiasis in Japan and adjacent areas. Prog. Med. Parasitol. Japan **4**:301-393.

Osturu, M. 1962. *Trichostrongylus brevis* sp. nov. from man (Nematoda: Trichostrongylidae). Acta. Med. Biol. **9**:273-278.

Paulino, G. B., Jr., and J. Wittenberg. 1973. Intestinal capillariasis: a new cause of a malabsorption pattern. Am. J. Roentgenol. Rad. Therapy, Nuclear Med. **117**:340-345.

Peña-Chavarría, A., J. C. Swartzwelder, V. M. Villarejas, and R. Zeledón. 1973. Mebendazole, an effective broad-spectrum anthelminthic. Am. J. Trop. Med. Hyg. **22**:592-595.

Pradatsundarasar, A., K. Pecharanond, C. Chintanawongs, and P. Ungthavorn. 1973. The first case of intestinal capillariasis in Thailand. Southeast Asian J. Trop. Med. Public Health **4**:131-134.

Purtillo, D. T., W. M. Meyers, D. H. Connor. 1974. Fatal strongyloidiasis in immunosuppressed patients. Am. J. Med. **56**:488-493.

Rivera, E., and others. 1970. Hyperinfection syndrome with *Strongyloides stercoralis*. Ann. Intern. Med. **72**:199-204.

Sandground, J. H. 1931. Studies on the life history of *Ternidens deminutus*, with observations on its incidence in certain regions of southern Africa. Ann. Trop. Med. Parasitol. **25**:147.

Singston, C. N., T. C. Banson, and J. H. Cross. 1975. Mebendazole in the treatment of intestinal capillariasis. Am. J. Trop. Med. Hyg. **24**:932-934.

Stone, O. J., G. B. Newell, and J. F. Mullins. 1972. Cutaneous strongyloidiasis: larva currens. Arch. Dermatol. **106**:734-736.

Suzuki, H., and others. 1972. *Terranova* (Nematoda: Anisakidae) infection in man: I. Clinical features of five cases of *Terranova* larva infection. Jap. J. Parasitol. **21**:252-256.

Swartzwelder, J. C. 1939. Clinical *Trichocephalus trichiurus* infection: an analysis of 81 cases. Am. J. Trop. Med. **19**:473-481.

Swartzwelder, J. C. 1946. Clinical ascariasis: an analysis of 202 cases in New Orleans. Am. J. Dis. Child. **72**:172-180.

Swartzwelder, J. C., J. H. Miller, and R. W. Sappenfield. 1955. The treatment of cases of ascariasis with piperazine citrate, with observations on the efficacy of the drug on other helminthiases. Am. J. Trop. Med. **4**:326-331.

Tripathy, K., F. González, H. Lotero, and O. Bolaños. 1971. Effects of *Ascaris* infection on human nutrition. Am. J. Trop. Med. Hyg. **22**:212-218.

Turner, K. J., L. Feddema, and E. H. Quinn. 1979. Nonspecific potentiation of IgE by parasitic infections in man. Int. Arch. Allergy Appl. Immunol. **58**:232-236.

Van Thiel, P. H. 1966. The final host of the Perringworm *Anisakis marina*. Trop. Geogr. Med. **18**:310-328.

Villarejos, V. M., J. A. Arguedas, G. Vargas, and A. Peña-Chavarría. 1975. Evaluation of the skin test for hookworm as an epidemiological tool. Am. J. Trop. Med. Hyg. **24**:250-255.

Wallace, L., R. Kenkin, and A. Mathies. 1956. *Trichostrongylus* infestation with profound eosinophilia. Ann. Intern. Med. **45:**146-150.

Wang, C. C., and G. A. Galli. 1975. Strongyloidiasis treated with pyrvinium pamoate. J.A.M.A. **193:**847-848.

Wassom, D. L., and G. J. Gleich. 1979. Damage to *Trichinella spiralis* newborn larvae by eosinophil major basic protein. Am. J. Trop. Med. Hyg. **28:**860-863.

Whalen, G. E., and others. 1971. Treatment of intestinal capillariasis with thiabendazole, bithionol, and bephenium. Am. J. Trop. Med. Hyg. **20:**95-100.

World Health Organization. 1967. The control of ascariasis. WHO Technical Report Series no. 379. Geneva, Switzerland, pp. 1-47.

CHAPTER 9

The tissue roundworms

The tissue roundworms of medical importance occur chiefly in the superfamilies Filarioidea and Dracunculoidea. These are worms for which humans are the definitive host. A variety of nematodes of lower animals, which invade human tissue in their larval stages, is included in this chapter.

Filarioidea

The filarial worms parasitic in humans are as follows:

Wuchereria bancrofti
Brugia malayi
Loa loa
Onchocerca volvulus
Dipetalonema streptocerca
Dipetalonema perstans
Mansonella ozzardi

The adults of each species inhabit preferentially certain human tissues. The adults are long and slender and vary in length within a given species. Male worms usually are smaller than females. Females give birth to living embryos, called microfilariae, that reach the circulation or the skin. Bloodsucking arthropods pick up this stage while taking a blood meal. Within the body of the arthropod the larvae develop to the infective larval stage. From the thoracic muscles they move forward and invade the labium or sheath surrounding the mouth parts. At time of feeding, the labium comes in contact with the host, and infective larvae, attracted by the warmth of the host, migrate onto the skin surface. They quickly enter the puncture wound and move through the lymphatics, circulation, or tissue migration to the habitat in the host where they are destined to become adults. Maturation requires 6 months to 1 year. Adult worms in general are noted for their longevity, averaging about 15 years (Fig. 9-1).

Diagnosis is chiefly dependent on recovery and identification of the microfilariae (Fig. 9-2) from the blood or skin. *Dipetalonema streptocerca*, confined to tropical Africa and less common than *Onchocerca volvulus*, also has microfilariae in the skin. Differentiation can be made morphologically. Confusion with the blood microfilariae presents no problem. Recovery of adults may be feasible also in some instances. Differential characteristics of the blood microfilariae are present in Table 9-1. (See also Fig. 9-3.)

Both the indirect hemagglutination (IHA) test and the bentonite-flocculation test (BFT) using the dog heart worm *Dirofilaria immitis* as the source of antigen show good sensitivity but lack specificity (see Tables 15-1 and 15-2). Many reactions with low titers make interpretation difficult. Titers of 1:128 (IHA test) and 1:5 (BFT) when obtained simultaneously are considered significant by the Center for Disease Control diagnostic laboratory.

There is no satisfactory chemotherapeutic agent effective against the adult filarial worms. Diethylcarbamazine (Hetrazan) will kill the microfilariae and, at times, some adults (Table 9-2). Larvicidal treatment of stagnant waters with temephos (Abate) is a good preventive step in endemic areas.

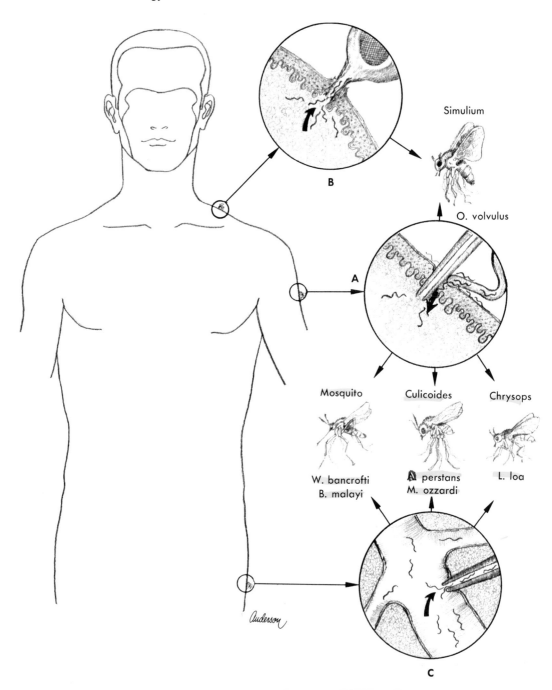

Fig. 9-1. Life cycle of the filarial worms. Infective larvae enter the skin from the labium of the intermediate host at time of feeding, **A,** and pass on to the appropriate tissues of the body where they become adults worms. Microfilariae, in turn, are picked up by the appropriate host at time of feeding, either from the skin, **B,** or the bloodstream, **C.**

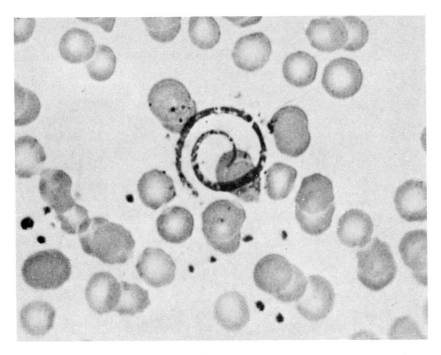

Fig. 9-2. Germinated spore of fungus in a blood film. Artifact mistaken for microfilaria. (AFIP 67-10245.)

Wuchereria bancrofti

Geographic distribution. The filarial worm *Wuchereria bancrofti*, causing Bancroft's filariasis (elephantiasis) in humans, has a spotty worldwide distribution throughout the tropics and subtropics, Africa, the Near East, and the Far East. It occurs predominately in coastal areas and islands with sustained high humidity and heat for long periods. At one time it was prevalent in Charleston, South Carolina, but is no longer present in the United States. In the western hemisphere it is found in the West Indies and along the coast of South America from Brazil to Colombia. A small focus along the Atlantic Coast of Costa Rica is gradually diminishing. Isolated foci are found along the Mediterranean coast of North Africa and southern Europe. Filariasis, for the most part, is endemic across Central Africa, from coast to coast, as well as along the coastal areas of Asia from India through China, Japan, the Philippines, Taiwan, the East Indies, the northern part of Australia, and the Pacific Islands in the southwest. The nonperiodic strain in the South Pacific is considered by some as a different species, *W. pacifica*, or a strain variation, *W. bancrofti* var *pacifica*.

Morphology and life cycle. The third-stage, or infective, larvae, after entering the skin, migrate to the lymphatics where the developing and adult worms spend their entire life, up to 12 years or more, not, as is generally believed, in the lymph nodes but in the main afferent lymphatics. The adult female varies in size from 60 to 100 mm in length by 150 to 250 μm in diameter, while the male averages 40 mm by 100 to 150 μm. Maturation is slow and microfilariae (Fig. 9-4) may not appear in the circulation for a year or more after infection. Except for the South Pacific strain that shows no periodicity, the microfilariae show a nocturnal periodicity, appearing most abundantly at night. Mosquitoes of the genera *Anopheles*, *Culex*, *Aedes*, and *Mansonia* are the inter-

Table 9-1. Differential characteristics of microfilariae

	Wuchereria bancrofti	Brugia malayi	Loa loa	Dipetalonema streptocerca	Dipetalonema perstans	Mansonella ozzardi	Onchocerca volvulus
Location	Blood	Blood	Blood	Skin and subcutaneous tissues	Blood	Blood	Skin and subcutaneous tissues
Periodicity	Nocturnal; South Pacific strain, nonperiodic	Nocturnal, less absolute than W. bancrofti	Diurnal	Nonperiodic	Nonperiodic	Nonperiodic	Nonperiodic
Sheath	Present	Present	Present	Absent	Absent	Absent	Absent
Nuclei	Not terminal	Terminal; tip of tail swollen with two nuclei	Terminal	Terminal	Terminal	Not terminal	Not terminal
Appearance	Graceful, sweeping curves; cephalic space, length equals width	Irregular, kinky curves; varying girth; cephalic space, length twice width	Irregular, kinky curves; varying girth	Taper at both ends; body relatively straight but posterior end bent in a shepherd's crook angle	Slender, delicate curves	Slender, delicate curves	Graceful, sweeping curves

mediate hosts. When ingested in a blood meal, the sheaths of the microfilariae are lost and the organisms penetrate the stomach wall, migrating to the thoracic muscles where first-stage larvae develop. After the filariform stage develops, migration continues to the tip of the sheath covering the proboscis. Contact with the warm skin of the human host at time of feeding stimulates the larvae to leave the proboscis and penetrate the skin of the host. The complete cycle in the mosquito takes about 2 weeks.

Epidemiology. The incidence of Bancroft's filariasis is determined chiefly by the presence and distribution of the moquito vectors. Dense populations living in unsanitary environments in tropical climates where mosquitoes breed unhampered offer ideal conditions for the spread of filariasis. In the vast area of India, as well as in many other parts of the world, *Culex fatigans*, the vector, which has acquired resistance to almost all of the residual insecticides, is a problem of man's own doing. This mosquito is a "messmate" of man, breeding in pit latrines and polluted water around homes and feeding at night on humans in houses not equipped to keep the mosquitoes out. Badly needed is community effort to clean up the environment and provide better housing. Reduction of mosquitoes will lead to the eventual elimination of *W. bancrofti*. Unlike schistosomiasis, which is increasing in the world both in prevalence and distribution, chiefly because of the development of water resources, filariasis is increasing because of the population explosion. It is estimated that at least 400 million persons are at risk of contracting filariasis in these endemic areas. Fortunately, however, only a small proportion of the infected community will develop elephantiasis, but other serious complications will occur. It is estimated that at least 80 species and subspecies of mosquitoes, including the genera *Anopheles*, *Culex*, *Aedes*, and *Mansonia*, are known intermediate hosts for *Wuchereria*. Since no known reservoir hosts

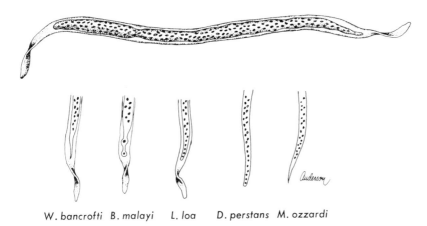

W. bancrofti   B. malayi   L. loa   D. perstans   M. ozzardi

Fig. 9-3. Differential characteristics of the blood microfilariae. On the top, a typical microfilaria with sheath is shown, and on the bottom, the differential characteristics of the terminal ends can be seen. (Compare with Table 9-1.)

exist, transmission depends on the presence of microfilariae in the bloodstream of humans at the time of the biting of the mosquito. Night-biting mosquitoes transmit the nocturnal periodic strains, whereas day-biting mosquitoes account for most of the transmission of the nonperiodic strains. Experimental evidence has shown that even when microfilariae cannot be detected in the blood, mosquito infection can still occur. Fortunately, the worldwide malaria eradication program of mosquito control has served effectively as a two-edged sword.

Symptomatology and pathology. From the time of exposure until microfilariae appear in the circulation, the developing worms produce minimal symptoms—mild fever, malaise, and a transient lymphatic inflammation. Preceding the local inflammation, the filaroid fever may last a week with temperatures up to 104° F, followed by several febrile attacks. Following maturation of the worms, lymphatic inflammation becomes severe. Common complaints are headache, nausea, fatigue, malaise, backache, anorexia, insomnia, and muscle pain. An urticarial rash may appear. This acute phase is characterized by fever, lymphadenitis, lymphangitis, orchitis, and hydrocele. Most

lesions eventually appear in the lower lymphatics, being concentrated in the scrotum in the male.

The chronic stage is characterized by lymph varices, chyluria, hydrocele, and elephantiasis. Repeated episodes of lymphangitis lead to blockage of vessels. Experimental studies indicate that the obstructive lymphangitis is preceded by the immune complexes in the dilated varicose lymphatics leading to lymphedema. Prior to obstruction, chemotherapy can reverse this pathologic process with complete return of the lymphatics to normal. Blockage of the lymphatics of the urinary bladder causes chyluria while blockage of peritoneal lymphatics leads to ascites. Lymphedema predisposes the tissues to secondary bacterial invasion. Elephantiasis rarely follows short exposure in an endemic area. Repeated bites of infective mosquitoes over many years lead to a buildup of many worms. Eventual destruction of the worms, caseation, granulomas, and fibrosis lead to vessel breakdown, and pools of lymph collect in the tissues, resulting in elephantiasis (Fig. 9-5).

Microfilariae in the bloodstream produce no significant symptoms or pathologic changes. They appear in the circulation most

Table 9-2. Treatment for tissue roundworms

Infection	Drug	Adult dose*	Pediatric dose*
Filariasis			
Wuchereria bancrofti, Brugia (W.) malayi, Dipetalonema perstans. Loa loa, Dipetalonema streptocerca			
Drug of choice	Diethylcarbamazine[1]	Day 1: 50 mg Day 2: 50 mg tid Day 3: 100 mg tid Day 4 through 21: 2 mg/kg tid	Day 1: 25-50 mg Day 2: 25-50 mg tid Day 3: 50-100 mg tid Day 4 through 21: 2 mg/kg tid
Alternative	None		
Tropical eosinophilia			
Drug of choice	Diethylcarbamazine[1]	2 mg/kg tid × 7-10d	2 mg/kg tid × 7-10d
Alternative	None		
Onchocerca volvulus			
Drug of choice	Diethylcarbamazine[1]	25 mg/d × 3d, then 50 mg/d × 5d, then 100 mg/d × 3d, then 150 mg/d × 12d	0.5 mg/kg tid × 3d (max. 25 mg/d), 1.0 mg/kg tid × 3-4d (max. 50 mg/d), 1.5 mg/kg tid × 3-4d (max. 100 mg/d), 2.0 mg/kg tid × 2-3 wk (max. 150 mg/d)
	followed by suramin[2]	100-200 mg (test dose) IV, 1 gm IV at weekly intervals × 5 wk	10-20 mg (test dose) IV, then 20 mg/kg IV at weekly intervals × 5 wk
Infections with animal filariae (Dirofilaria)			
Drug of choice	None	Surgical excision of subcutaneous and pulmonary nodules	
Dracunculus medinensis (guinea worm)			
Drug of choice	Niridazole[2]	25 mg/kg (max. 1.5 gm)/d × 15d	12.5 mg/kg bid × 15d (max. 1.5 gm/d)
Alternative	Metronidazole[3,4,5]	250 mg tid × 10d	25 mg/kg/d (max. 750 mg/d) in 3 doses × 10d
Visceral larva migrans[6]			
Drug of choice	Thiabendazole[4]	25 mg/kg bid × 5d	25 mg/kg bid × 5d
Alternative	Diethylcarbamazine	2 mg/kg tid × 30d	2-4 mg/kg tid × 3 wk

From The Medical Letter, Inc., 56 Harrison Street, New Rochelle, N.Y.
*The letter d indicates day.

1. Diethylcarbamazine should be administered with special caution in heavy infections with *Loa loa* because it can provoke an encephalopathy. Antihistamines or corticosteroids may be required to reduce allergic reactions due to disintegration of microfilaria in the treatment of all filarial infection, especially those caused by *Onchocerca* and *Loa loa*. Surgical excision of subcutaneous *Onchocerca* nodules is recommended by some authorities before starting drug therapy in order to diminish allergic manifestations.
2. In the U.S.A. this drug is available from the Parasitic Diseases Division, Center for Disease Control, Atlanta, Georgia 30333; telephone 404-329-3311.
3. Metronidazole is carcinogenic in rodents and mutagenic in bacteria; it should generally not be used in pregnant women, particularly in the first trimester.
4. Considered an investigational drug for this condition by the U.S. Food and Drug Administration.
5. Metronidazole is not believed to be vermicidal and does not prevent new lesions from appearing.
6. Visceral larvae migrans is usually a self-limited disease. Treatment should be restricted to severe cases. For severe symptoms or eye involvement, corticosteroids can be used in addition.

Table 9-2. Treatment for tissue roundworms—cont'd

Adverse effects of antiparasitic drugs

Diethylcarbamazine citrate USP (Hetrazan)
    Frequent: severe allergic or febrile reactions, due to the filarial infection; GI disturbances
    Rare: encephalopathy
Suramin sodium (Germanin)
    Frequent: vomiting; pruritus; urticaria; paresthesia; hyperesthesia of hands and feet; photophobia; peripheral
      neuropathy
    Occasional: kidney damage; blood dyscrasias; shock
Niridazole (Ambilhar)
    Frequent: immunosuppression; vomiting; cramps; dizziness; headache
    Occasional: diarrhea; slight ECG changes; rash; insomnia; paresthesia
    Rare: psychosis; hemolytic anemia in G6PD deficiency; convulsions
Metronidazole (Flagyl)
    Frequent: nausea; headache; metallic taste
    Occasional: vomiting; diarrhea; insomnia; weakness; stomatitis; vertigo; paresthesia; rash; dark urine; dry mouth
    Rare: ataxia; depression; irritability; confusion; mild Antabuse-like reaction with alcohol
Thiabendazole USP (Mintezol)
    Frequent: nausea; vomiting; vertigo
    Occasional: leukopenia; crystalluria; rash; hallucinations; olfactory disturbance
    Rare: shock, tinnitus; Stevens-Johnson syndrome

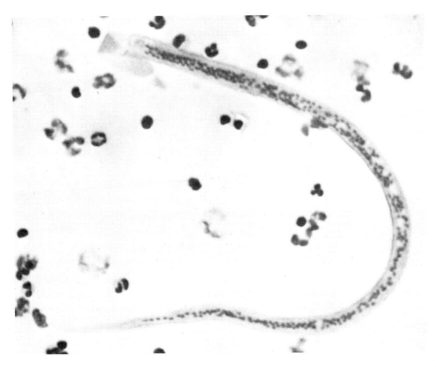

Fig. 9-4. Microfilaria of *Wuchereria bancrofti* showing sheath and nuclei not extending to the tip of the tail. (AFIP 70-10516.)

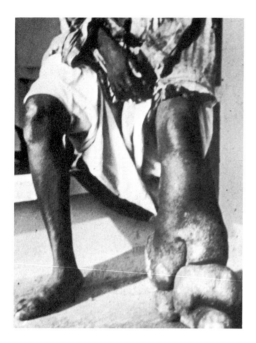

Fig. 9-5. Elephantiasis of the leg. (From a nonprofit cooperative endeavor by numerous colleagues under the editorship of Dr. Herman Zaiman, Valley City, N.D.)

commonly in infections which begin in childhood and persist for some years before major pathologic changes develop. Here they serve as a source of infection for mosquitoes. Microfilariae are seldom seen in chronic cases of elephantiasis.

Evidence suggests that filarial infections are one of the underlying causes of tropical eosinophilia (eosinophilic lung), a syndrome characterized by coughing, asthmatic-like dyspnea, fatigue, and malaise. Tubercle-like nodules, suggestive of miliary tuberculosis, are seen in chest films. In the eosinophilic infiltrate, degenerate microfilariae have been observed at autopsy or in biopsy specimens, but microfilaremia is absent and no evidence of adult worms is found. Filariasis, with or without pulmonary manifestations, was common among the American servicemen in the South Pacific during World War II. Out of more than 12,000 who had infections in a one-year period, only 20 persons developed

a demonstrable microfilaremia. Many continued to have recurrent attacks of lymphangitis and scrotal swelling 15 years after leaving the area. Enemy propaganda, including pictures of natives with massive elephantoid limbs and scrotums, induced severe mental anguish requiring psychiatric therapy. No servicemen, however, ever developed elephantiasis.

Diagnosis. In endemic areas chronic filariasis may be diagnosed by the lymphangitis, lymphadenitis, and elephantiasis present. However, sometimes it is too readily assumed that lymphedema and elephantiasis are caused by filarial worms. Of the many causes of dependent lymphedema and consequent elephantiasis, tuberculosis, for example, is very important in the tropics. In the highlands of Ethiopia and Kenya, where the low temperature does not permit transmission of *W. bancrofti* or *Brugia malayi*, elephantiasis is common. It has been suggested that the damage to the lymphatics is caused by the absorption of chemicals from the soil through abrasions in the skin. Microfilariae may be present early in the infection, but blood smears rarely show microfilariae during the chronic stage. Lymph node biopsy specimens may reveal live or dead adult worms but biopsy is not generally approved as a diagnostic technique because surgery may further compromise lymphatic drainage. Detection of microfilariae in the blood is conclusive. Thick blood films are best made between the hours of 10:00 P.M. and 2:00 A.M. for the nocturnal strains. Relatively aperiodic strains are best detected in the early afternoon. Failure to find microfilariae, however, does not rule out infection. An advance in diagnostic methods is the membrane filtration technique in which blood is passed directly from the syringe through a membrane filter (commercially available) of 5-μm pore size. Blood cells are removed and the microfilariae are left on the filter where they can be washed, stained, and identified (Appendix B). This technique has disclosed high infection rates in communities where thick blood films revealed no infections. In American Samoa, where mass infections were thought to be practically eliminated, the membrane filtration technique revealed continuing infections. Complement-fixation, precipitin, and skin tests, employing other filarial worms as antigen, give a group reaction and are not conclusive when positive. False reactions also occur.

Details of techniques for the laboratory diagnosis of filariasis are given in Appendix B.

Treatment. The administration of diethylcarbamazine serves as an important public health measure in breaking the cycle of infection. This drug kills the microfilariae, and, at times, the adult worms (more slowly). Side effects of diethylcarbamazine include vertigo, malaise, fever, headache, nausea, vomiting, and inflammatory reactions in the lymph nodes. The drug is nontoxic and the side effects are probably allergic reactions to toxic products from the worms under treatment. Bullous reactions and abscess formation sometimes occur. The former can be arrested quickly with cortisone and prednisone, but it must be remembered that corticosteroids must be used with extreme care when secondary bacterial infections are present. Injections of sclerosing agents such as sodium psylliate and sodium morrhuate are effective in treating hydrocele. Chyluria requires complete bed rest with elevation of the lower extremities. Antihistamines are helpful for symptomatic relief of lymphangitis, but acetylsalicylic acid is better for pain and fever. Pressure bandages, along with elevation of the limbs, aid in reducing swollen extremities. Surgical intervention is sometimes indicated for definitive treatment of elephantiasis. In acute illness of recent onset, rest during the attacks, moving to a cool climate, and, occasionally, psychotherapy are all that is usually required for someone traveling into an endemic area. Supportive therapy for lymph node swelling may be indicated.

Brugia malayi

Brugia malayi, formerly known as *Wuchereria malayi*, is common in areas of India, Malaysia, Thailand, Burma, Vietnam, coastal areas of China, Taiwan, South Korea, Japan, Borneo, and Indonesia. Natural infections occurs in the Kra monkey, *Macaca irus*. The genus *Brugia* was created for this species on the basis of studies in these animals. *B. pahangi* was designated as the name for species in cats, dogs, and monkeys in Malaysia, and *B. patei* for the species in dogs and cats in East Africa. Human infections with *Brugia* sp from animals have been reported in the New England area.

The adult worms morphologically resemble those of *W. bancrofti* but are somewhat smaller. Sheathed microfilariae are described in Table 9-1 and Figs. 9-2 and 9-6. Most strains show nocturnal periodicity, but in Malaysia and Indonesia, where the reservoir population is numerous in monkeys and a variety of carnivores, little periodicity exists. Two peaks often occur, one around 8:00 P.M., the other around 4:00 A.M. Much of the transmission in these areas is by day-biting mosquitoes that are chiefly zoophilic in the forest areas. Malaysian filariasis is an occupational disease among those working on rubber plantations. Filariasis control is difficult in such areas in spite of mass therapy. Where *Mansonia* mosquitoes are the chief vectors, larvicidal measures such as the use of Paris Green, DDT spray, and oil are ineffective because the moquitoes attach themselves to green plants for oxygen.

The pattern of infection and disease produced is similar to that seen in Bancroft's filariasis. Lymphadenopathy and lymphadenitis precede the eventual elephantiasis in severe chronic cases. Scrotal involvement and elephantiasis of the upper limbs are uncommon. Chyluria and chylous hydrocele have not been observed. In some cases, pulmonary changes, an increase in local eosinophils, and adenopathy suggestive of tropical eosinophilia are reported. Elephantiasis,

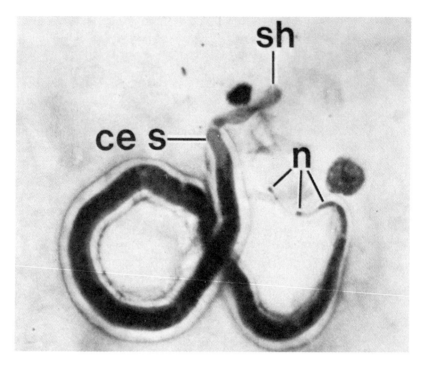

Fig. 9-6. Microfilaria of *Brugia malayi*. Sheath *(sh)*, cephalic space *(ces)*, nuclei *(n)*. (AFIP 74-9264.)

when present, occurs chiefly in the legs. Diagnosis is essentially the same as for *W. bancrofti*, with consideration for the nature of the periodicity factor. The ready availability of animal models (not accessible for *W. bancrofti*) affords opportunity for research in the development of vaccines and new chemotherapeutic agents and basic information about the pathogenesis of disease. At present, therapy follows the same pattern as for Bancroft's filariasis.

Loa loa

Loa loa, the eye worm, is restricted to western and central Africa, occurring chiefly in the rain forest areas. It is endemic along the Congo River watershed and extends southward to Angola, eastward to the Rift valley, and westward to Sierra Leone. The adult worms live in the subcutaneous tissues, wandering about freely. Attracted by warmth, they come to the skin surface when the person sits before a fire. They are most spectacular and therefore most often noticed

when they move across the cornea (Fig. 9-7). The female worms vary in size from 50 to 70 mm and move about one-half inch per minute. The males are about half the size of the female. Microfilariae are sheathed (Fig. 9-8) and show a diurnal periodicity in the bloodstream, retreating to the lungs primarily at night. Diagnostic features are given in Table 9-1 and Fig. 9-3. A variety of tabanid flies *(Chrysops)*, commonly known as mango or deer flies, are the intermediate hosts. Experimentally, *Chrysops atlanticus*, the American deer fly has been infected with larvae infective for monkeys. Only the females bite. Development of the third-stage larvae takes place in the thoracic muscles and migration to the fleshy parts of the proboscis follows, with transmission to humans at time of biting. The pattern is similar to that of other filarial worms. Larvae migrate to the subcutaneous tissues where development to adults occurs very slowly. The life span of the adults is 15 years or more.

Symptoms usually are mild and temporary,

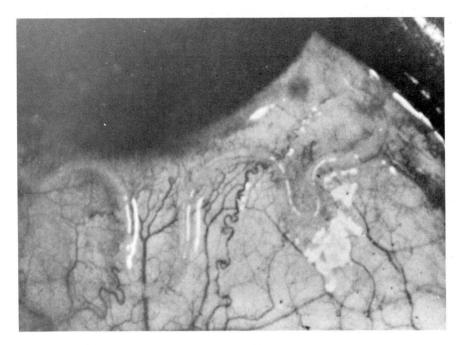

Fig. 9-7. Adult *Loa loa* moving across the eye of a patient. (AFIP 73-6554.)

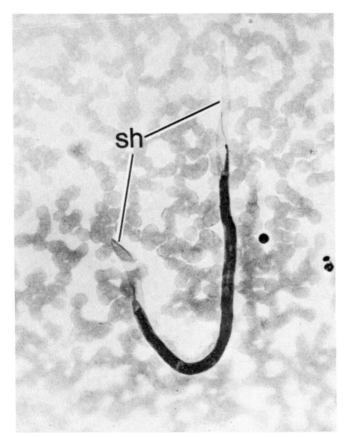

Fig. 9-8. Microfilaria of *Loa loa* showing sheath *(sh)*. Note that nuclei extend to the tip of the tail. (AFIP 75-6618.)

provoking inflammatory responses as they go. Calabar and fugitive swellings, sometimes the size of a hen's egg, appear at various sites throughout the body and are believed to be associated with local sensitization as the worms remain stationary for a while, but these swellings disappear as the worms move on. Neurologic symptoms related to worm migration occur rarely. The pattern of host response varies, some patients being essentially symptomless while others manifest allergic responses such as edema, pruritus, and eosinophilia with or without demonstrable worms and microfilariae. Diagnosis is based on a history of exposure to an endemic area, seeing migrating subcutaneous or corneal worms, the presence of eosinophilia, and the demonstration of microfilariae by thick blood film or, preferably, the membrane filter technique described in Appendix B and in the section on diagnosis of *W. bancrofti*.

Diethylcarbamazine (Table 9-2) has been used successfully, but indications for therapy must be weighed against the risk of encephalopathy associated with treatment. Initially, a low dose of 0.7 mg/kg body weight three times a day for 10 days is given to avoid severe allergic reactions. Mild symptoms may appear. An increase of 2.0 mg/kg daily for 14 days is followed by a respite from treatment for at least 2 weeks before repeating treatment. Both adult and microfilariae are killed. For chemoprophylaxis, 2.0 mg/kg twice daily for 3 consecutive days each month is recommended.

Surgical removal may lead to breakage of the worm and severe allergic reaction. A young surgeon in Africa related that upon seeing his first case, with great care and precision using complete sterile techniques and new surgical instruments, he deftly removed a worm from the cornea of a patient. Turning to his native assistant, he pointed with pride to his accomplishment, only to learn that the natives did it frequently with two pine needles.

Onchocerca volvulus

Geographic distribution. Onchocerciasis, a filarial infection in humans, occurs endemically in two regions of the world—the tropical zone of Africa and Central and South America. A small focus has been found in the Yemen Arab Republic. Endemic foci are found most commonly near rivers or streams in hilly or mountainous regions where the black flies, *Simulium*, breed in fast-running streams. The disease is found throughout most of the tropical rain forest areas of Africa and the savanna belt extending from the Atlantic coast of Senegal to the Indian Ocean coast of Tanzania. Onchocerciasis has emerged as a great world health problem, afflicting an estimated 40 million persons in the world, approximately 2 million of whom are blind. The disease has aptly been named "river blindness" by the natives. *Simulium damnosum* and *S. naevei* are the chief vectors in Africa, while in Central America it is *S.*

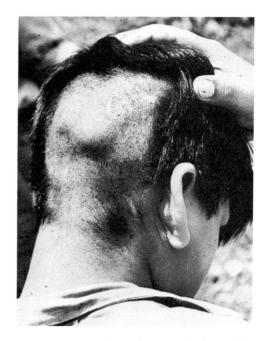

Fig. 9-9. Patient with *Onchocerca volvulus* nodules. (Courtesy Department of Pathology, University of Miami, School of Medicine.)

ochraceum. Foci discovered in Venezuela, Colombia, and Brazil are found in the lowland hilly areas. The major endemic areas in the western hemisphere are in southern Mexico and Guatemala.

Epidemiology. Onchocerciasis is associated with an environment containing fast-running streams where the larvae and pupae of the black fly or buffalo gnat develop. Although the wind may carry flies great distances from their breeding places, infections usually occur close by since the flies have a limited flight range dependent on their degree of infection. Heavily parasitized thoracic muscles may prevent some flies from reaching their hosts. Thus transmission is usually limited to areas around the rivers and streams in which the flies breed, where washing, wading, fishing, and water collection take place. Repeated trips to the rivers and streams result in repeated exposure and

a buildup of worms in the people. As in regions of Africa where larviciding is practical, this means of control is highly recommended. Long stretches of streams and rivers in Africa are readily accessible and lend themselves well to larviciding. In Guatemala, however, the topography prevents elimination of the fly by attacking its breeding place and the control method is the extirpation of detectable nodules to reduce the microfilariae population and thus the severity of eye infection.

Morphology and life cycle. Adult worms live in a tangled mass in the subcutaneous tissues of the human host. They become encapsulated under the skin in fibrous connective tissue nodules. Female worms vary from 33 to 50 cm in length by 270 to 400 μm in diameter. Male worms are smaller, averaging 19 to 42 cm by 130 to 210 μm. Nodules over bony prominences become quite con-

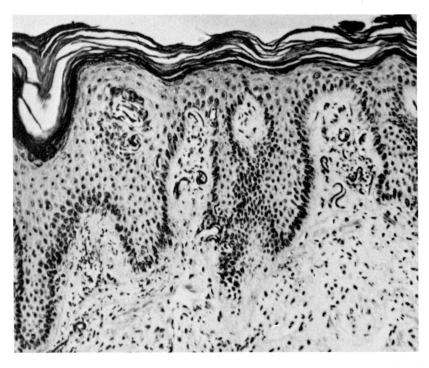

Fig. 9-10. Microfilariae of *Onchocerca volvulus* within the dermis. Note the inflammatory cells, edema, and fibrosis. (AFIP 68-9448.)

spicuous as on the head or over the ribs and hips. In Africa about 95% of the nodules appear on the chest, lower trunk, or near joints, while in Mexico and Guatemala the majority appear in the head and neck regions (Fig. 9-9). Since microfilariae produced are most abundant in the skin (Fig. 9-10) in the vicinity of the nodules it has been postulated that the African species of black flies prefer the trunk and lower areas of the body while biting; those in Mexico and Central America prefer the head and neck areas. The microfilariae are two sizes—one is 285 to 368 μm in length by 6 to 9 μm in diameter, the other is 150 to 287 μm by 5 to 7 μm. Development of microfilariae to the third-stage larvae takes place in the thoracic muscles of the black fly or buffalo gnat. A number of species of *Simulium*, as previously indicated, are involved. Infective larvae in the labium of the proboscis migrate onto the skin of the host and penetrate to the subcutaneous tissues where development into adults takes place. In the early stage of infection the worms live free or are simply enclosed in loose fatty tissue. In later stages, chronic inflammation develops, cellular infiltration and eventual fibrous encapsulation follows, and the worms become surrounded by a fibrous connective tissue wall. Micro-

filariae migrate through this wall into the skin. Flies become infected by rasping the skin of the infected host and ingesting the microfilariae in their blood meal. Although previously thought to occur only in the skin and eyes, microfilariae have now been recovered from the lungs, liver, spleen, and kidneys.

Symptomatology and pathology. Onchocerciasis in the western hemisphere characteristically shows milder skin lesions than elsewhere with the exception of the rare "erysipela de la costa" in Guatemala. The subcutaneous nodules containing adult worms cause very few pathologic changes and rarely any symptoms (Fig. 9-11). The disease is associated chiefly with the microfilariae. In Guatemala and Mexico the nodules and thus the skin microfilariae, as indicated, are found mainly on the head, neck, and upper parts of the body. This is probably linked with the biting habits of *S. ochraceum*, an organism that attacks these areas of the body. Thus eye lesions from microfilariae become a serious problem. In Venezuela and the remainder of South America *S. metallicum* and *S. exiguum* bite and produce lesions lower on the body and thus diminish the chances of eye lesions. In Africa more blindness occurs in the savanna than in the

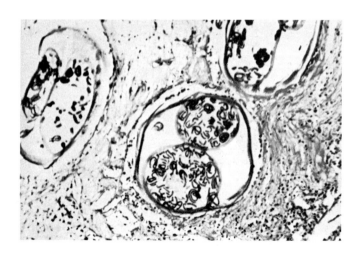

Fig. 9-11. Onchocercoma. Section of adult worm embedded in an inflammatory nodule showing microfilariae. (From Anderson, W. A. D., and Scotti, T. M.: Synopsis of pathology, ed. 9, St. Louis, 1976, The C. V. Mosby Co.)

forest area. In the Yemen Arab Republic pruritus, swelling, darkening papules, and unusual enlargement of regional lymph nodes are frequently limited to one limb. This severe dermatitis is known as "swoda," meaning black.

Onchocerca nodules, called onchocercomas, tend to lie over bony prominences and are usually flattened or bean shaped, movable, and nontender. Nodules may be discrete or bound together as conglomerates (Fig. 9-11). In patients with heavy infections of long duration lymphedema and especially hanging groin may be present. In some areas elephantiasis may occur. Yemenites with swoda have nodules suggestive of lymphosarcomas. Early changes in the dermis caused by microfilariae are minimal, with edema and a few proliferating fibroblasts and cells. More advanced stages show hyperkeratosis, focal parakeratosis, dilated lymphatics, and inflammatory mucin between dermal collagen fibers. Fibrosis continues leading to replacement of dermal collagen with hyalinized scar tissue. This is the most serious skin change. Degenerating microfilariae elicit a granulomatous reaction or eosinophilic infiltration. Lymph nodes in African patients become fibrotic while those in Yemenites with swoda become large, soft, tumorlike, and hyperplastic. Microfilariae and their inflammatory reaction, as previously indicated, have been found in various organs of the body, including the lungs, liver, spleen, and kidneys. Damage to the eyes is caused by living or dead microfilariae. An early sign of infection is photophobia and lacrimation, although many victims may have no symptoms and visual impairment will be minimal. Punctate keratitis is an early sign and each opacity is the result of the inflammatory reaction around the degenerating microfilariae. Often called "snowflake" or "fluffy" opacities, they develop in all parts of the cornea and disappear usually in a few weeks. Sclerosing keratitis, a stromal inflammation, is a common cause of blindness in Central America and in the savanna in Africa. Numerous microfilariae invade the cornea, the lesions developing peripherally and moving centrally. The process may stop before total opacity occurs (Fig. 9-12). Early treatment will reverse the process. Persons with many parasites may develop a severe iridocyclitis. Numerous microfilariae may be seen in the anterior chamber as wriggling silver threads. The pupil is frequently distorted slightly and a fibrinous exudate covers the lower margin. Posterior synechiae and occlusion of the pupil are common after bouts of plastic iritis. Lesions in the choroid and retina reveal focal depigmented areas of mottling, with mild atrophy of the retinal pigment epithelium. In severe lesions atrophy of the choriocapillaris also occurs. Optic atrophy is believed to result from inflammation of the optic nerve. Microfilariae have been found in essentially all tissues of the eye.

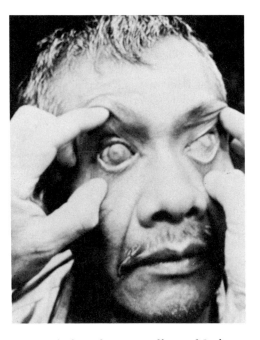

Fig. 9-12. Blindness due to microfilariae of *Onchocerca volvulus*. (Courtesy Department of Pathology, University of Miami, School of Medicine.)

Diagnosis. In endemic areas the diagnosis is readily suggested by skin nodules or corneal opacities, but not all patients show these findings. Eosinophilia is frequent but nonspecific. Diagnosis is best made by superficial skin snips. Tissue obtained without bleeding and examined in saline solution under a coverslip will reveal microfilariae leaving the skin. Biopsies are best performed near a nodule. In Africa, skin snips from the lower trunk and legs give the best yield, while in Central America the shoulders and head give the best results. At times, examination of urine and sputum may reveal microfilariae. In persons infected with *O. volvulus*, itching and a rash will develop within a few hours after taking 2 mg/kg of diethylcarbamazine. This is known as the Mazzotti test for onchocerciasis.

Treatment. Diethylcarbamazine is useful in onchocerciasis because it destroys the microfilariae. The drug is given cautiously in increasing doses, usually starting with 25 mg daily for 3 days, then 50 mg daily for 5 days, 100 mg daily for 3 days, and finally 150 mg daily for 12 days. In addition a test dose of 100 to 200 mg of suramin (Germanin) given intravenously followed by 1 gm intravenously at weekly intervals for 5 weeks is recommended (Table 9-2). Vomiting, pruritus, urticaria, paresthesia, hyperesthesia of the hands and feet, photophobia, and peripheral neuropathy are frequent with the use of suramin. Occasionally, kidney damage, blood dyscrasia, and shock may occur. Suramin is available from the Parasitic Disease Drug Service of the Center for Disease Control, Atlanta, Georgia. When the eyes are involved, treatment may be started with even lower doses, and antihistamines or corticosteroids may be required to reduce allergic reactions to the disintegration of microfilariae. In endemic areas, where prolonged drug therapy under close observation is not feasible, extirpation of the nodules offers a partial solution by reduction in the worm burden.

Dipetalonema streptocerca

The filarial worm *Dipetalonema streptocerca* is found in the tropical rain forest areas of western and central Africa with a high prevalence in central Zaire. Adults and microfilariae occur in the dermis, the latter being more superficial in location. The microfilariae are unsheathed and taper at both ends, with the tail being strongly bent like a fishhook or shepherd's crook. Nuclei extend to the tip of the tail. The average size is 180 to 240 μm $\times$ 3 μm and they can readily be distinguished from *O. volvulus*, which also occurs in the skin. Species of *Culicoides* are the intermediate hosts and vector. Infections are essentially symptomless, although in some a dermatitis characterized by an itchy rash, somewhat suggestive of *O. volvulus*, may appear. Hypopigmented macules and papules are aggravated by diethylcarbamazine, the reaction of the Mazzotti test for *O. volvulus*. The drug apparently kills both microfilariae and adults.

Dipetalonema perstans and Mansonella ozzardi

The two filarial worms *Dipetalonema perstans* and *Mansonella ozzardi* are considered by most as being nonpathogenic although some attribute a mild allergic reaction to *D. perstans*. Unexplained eosinophilia is usually the first clue to diagnosis. *D. perstans* is found in western and central Africa and from Panama to Argentina in the western hemisphere, whereas *M. ozzardi* occurs in Yucatan, Panama, the islands of St. Vincent and Dominica, as well as in several countries in South America. Species of tiny biting midges or gnats of the genus *Culicoides* are the intermediate hosts for both worms. Microfilariae in the blood show no periodicity. Characteristics are given in Table 9-1. *D. perstans* adults are found in various body cavities, such as the pleural, peritoneal, and pericardial cavities, whereas *M. ozzardi*, in addition to the body cavities, occurs also in the mesentery and visceral fat. Treatment is rarely indicated.

Dracunculoidea
Dracunculus medinensis

Geographic distribution. Guinea worms (worm of Medina, *Dracunculus medinensis*) date back to biblical times and are believed to have been the "fiery serpents" that afflicted the Israelites while in the Sinai Peninsula. In the eastern hemisphere they are found in central and northern Africa, as well as in vast areas of Asia. In the western hemisphere they occur in the West Indies, the Guianas, and parts of Brazil. In the United States, as well as elsewhere, the same or similar species occurs in fur-bearing animals, particularly the raccoon, but human infection is not seen.

Morphology and life cycle. The gravid females, living in the subcutaneous tissue, may reach lengths of 2½ to 4 feet (Fig. 9-13) with a diameter of 1 mm. The males average 20 to 30 mm in length and apparently are short lived. The female, when gravid, comes to the skin surface and produces a blister into which the anterior end of the worm protrudes. A break in the cuticle of the worm results in a prolapse of the uterus into the blister. Breaking of the blister leaves an ulcer, with the protruding uterus and worm in the center. Then immersion in water causes rupture of the uterine loop and discharge of numerous larvae. After removal of the skin surface from the water, healing takes place until the next immersion, which again causes a release of more larvae.

Copepods, of the genus *Cyclops*, living in the water, ingest the larvae, and develop-

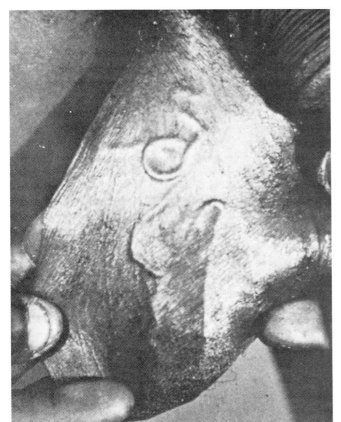

Fig. 9-13. Female *Dracunculus medinensis* in the subcutaneous tissue of the scrotum. (AFIP 74-9011.)

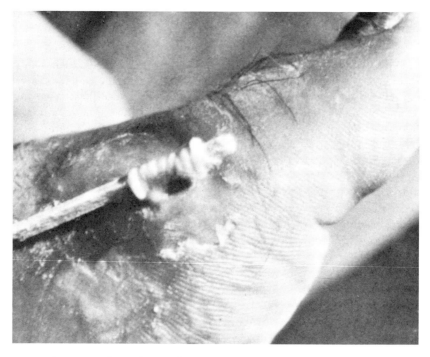

Fig. 9-14. Female *Dracunculus medinensis* being removed from the foot by winding on a stick. (AFIP 67-1563-6.)

ment to the infective larval stage takes place in their body cavity. When the copepods are accidentally ingested by humans, digestion releases the larvae and they penetrate the intestinal wall, migrating to the deep subcutaneous tissues. Probably much of the migration takes place through the lymphatics. By the third or fourth month mature worms of both sexes appear. Gravid females appear beneath the skin surface about 1 year after infection.

Epidemiology. In the Orient, step-in wells are the chief source of drinking water. Instead of the conventional bucket and rope, natives walk down steps into the well with their vessels to obtain water; sometimes they walk knee deep into the water. Blisters on the lower extremities break, and larvae are released into the well where *Cyclops* can ingest them. The natives drinking this water unknowingly ingest infected copepods, thus

ensuring completion of the life cycle. In Africa, ponds are used in a similar manner.

Immunity develops over the years, but complete resistance is not evident.

Symptoms and pathology. The major pathologic condition is probably related to secondary infection of the blister, with resulting infections of deep structures including tendons, joints, and bones. In some parts of India over 20% of the population have joint involvement with later fixation and deformity as a result of secondarily infected dracontiasis. A few hours before the gravid female appears beneath the skin, erythema, generalized urticaria, severe itching, dyspnea, giddiness, and asthma-like symptoms appear, believed to be caused by toxic secretions of the worm. Sometimes nausea and vomiting occur. As the female nears the surface a reddish papule with a vesicular center appears. Tenderness and erythema are noted at the site of the forming ulcer. Symptoms usually disappear with the formation of the ulcer.

Diagnosis and treatment. The worms can often be seen beneath the surface of the skin. The examination of ulcers for larvae and the protruding female ensure diagnosis.

The age-old treatment of catching hold of the worm and carefully and slowly winding it on a stick is, with few modifications, still the best treatment widely available (Fig. 9-14). Its danger lies in rupture of the worm, which then retracts and later causes secondary infection. Niridazole is the drug of choice (Table 9-2). With niridazole, vomiting, diarrhea, cramps, dizziness, and headache are frequent, and slight electrocardiographic changes, rash, insomnia, and paresthesia are occasional. Convulsions, psychosis, and anemia (in a glucose-6-phosphate dehydrogenase deficient person) are rare.

NEMATODES AS ACCIDENTAL PARASITES OF HUMANS
Spiruroidea

Some members of the superfamily Spiruroidea are occasionally accidental parasites of humans. For the most part, the eggs of this group are voided in the feces of the normal definitive host. The embryonated eggs, ingested by arthropods, develop into larvae within the body cavity. Infections in humans occur chiefly by the accidental ingestion of the arthropod.

Gongylonema pulchrum is a slender, filaria-like worm living in the walls of the esophagus or mouth cavity of pigs and various ruminants. The female reaches a length of 15 cm with a diameter of 0.2 to 0.5 mm. Males are much smaller. Rows of wartlike bosses on the anterior end are characteristic of this parasite. Dung beetles and roaches are the intermediate hosts; thus human infections are uncommon since our appetite veers in other directions. Cases in humans, however, have been reported from around

the world including the United States. Patients are aware of the migrating worms under the lips and cheek and find them very annoying. Nervousness is common. Removal of worms solves the problem.

Thelazia californiensis is a slender, little worm that inhabits the conjunctival sac and lacrimal ducts of various wild cats, dogs, rabbits, sheep, black bear, and other animals in California, New Mexico, Oregon, and Nevada. The adult female is about 7 to 19 mm long, the males being smaller in size. Eggs containing a larva are laid by the female. Intermediate hosts are flies (*Fannia* sp) in California. Roaches have been shown to be intermediate hosts for species in chickens. About a half dozen cases have been recorded in humans. Common symptoms are considerable infection of the eye, causing tearing and infection of blood vessels, pain, and nervousness. Over time scratching of the eyeball by the cuticle of the worm causes scar tissue formation and gradual cloudiness of vision. The worms may be removed with forceps after desensitizing the eye with a few drops of novocaine. *Thelazia callipaeda* is found in the Orient. Human infections have been reported in China, Korea, Thailand, and India.

Gnathostomiasis, known indigenously as Yangtze edema in China, Choko-Fushu in Japan, and tua chid in Thailand, is caused by the larval stage of the nematode *Gnathostoma spinigerum*. In natural hosts, the adult worms, measuring 2 to 3 cm in length, are found in the stomach walls of dogs and various felines such as leopards, tigers, domestic cats, wild cats, and lions. Human infections are most common in southeast Asia and India, with major foci in Thailand and Japan. A variety of different species occur in a variety of animals in both North and South America as well as in the Middle East and Africa. The source of human infections in the southern United States is unknown. Eggs passed in the feces of the natural host hatch and the larvae, eaten by crustaceans, develop to the next larval stage. Crustaceans, in turn, are eaten by fish and snakes wherein further larval development occurs. These third-stage larvae eaten by the definitive (natural) hosts migrate through the stomach wall, into the peritoneal cavity, through the liver, and eventually into skeletal muscle and connective tissue. They return to the stomach in about 3 months, penetrate and become embedded in the mucosa, and in about 6 months become adults. The entire cycle takes about 1 year. In abnormal hosts, such as humans, larvae from infected fish migrate through the stomach wall and into the body tissues producing symptoms of "larva migrans." Snake poultices applied to the skin effect transfer of larvae to skin lesions. Within 24 to 48 hours after exposure, nausea, salivation, vomiting, pruritus, urticaria, and upper abdominal pain or discomfort appear. An eo-

sinophilia reaching 90% has been recorded. Larvae migrating through the body mimic cholecystitis, appendicitis, cystitis, and salpingitis. Pulmonary infiltration resulting in hemoptysis or pneumothorax may occur. In 3 to 4 weeks larvae reach the subcutaneous tissues and systemic symptoms are reduced. In the chronic phase, migrating larvae (Fig. 9-15) in the subcutaneous tissues produce intermittent swellings, which recur every 2 to 6 weeks and last, at times, as long as 10 days, but become milder and shorter in time. Penetration of the central nervous system is rare. Treatment involves removal of the worms when found. The intradermal skin test has been used in diagnosis in some areas. Proper cooking of infected fish is necessary for prevention of infection. When domestic animals for human consumption have eaten infected fish adequate cooking procedures must also be employed.

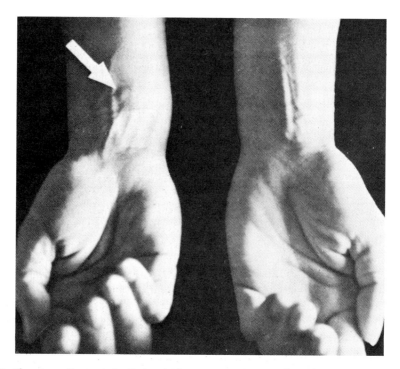

Fig. 9-15. Chronic gnathostomiasis. Patient had recurrent migrating edema (*arrow*) of forearm, wrist, and hand for 12 years. Carpal tunnel syndrome required surgical release of median nerve compression. (AFIP 75-10880.)

Reported in the literature is the finding of a nematode, *Cheilospirura* sp, in a nodule on the conjunctiva of a Filipino. Since these worms normally live under the lung or gizzard of birds, this is an example of abnormal behavior in an abnormal host.

Filarioidea

Species of *Dirofilaria* occur commonly in many lower animals. Mosquitoes are their arthropod host. Numerous cases in humans have been reported from the southern United States. There appear to be two types, both associated with adult worms in humans, an unnatural host. In one type, worms are found in the heart or lungs, and this worm is identical with the dog parasite, *D. immitus*, so prevalent in the coastal states of the southeastern United States. Lesions are usually identified as "coin lesions" in routine chest x rays. Most often they are spherical and about 1 to 3 cm in diameter. The common symptoms noted are chest pain, cough, fever, chills, malaise, and hemoptysis. Many patients are asymptomatic. Usually only one worm is found in the necrotic tissue, often fragmented and sometimes focally calcified. Diagnosis is made at surgery or autopsy. The second type, found in a subcutaneous tumor, is called *D. conjunctivae*. It is identical with the *D. tenui* of raccoons. Subcutaneous nodules on the face, arms, breast, and conjunctiva may be tender, painful, and erythematous. At times, the worms may migrate. Lesions usually contain a single, dead or degenerating worm, but live worms have also been removed. Diagnosis is made at surgery. *D. repens* is probably the species involved in Europe, Africa, and Asia. In either case, infection is acquired from a mosquito bite and usually only one adult parasite is found. Systemic symptoms and peripheral eosinophilia are rare. As indicated previously for filarial worms in general, the serologic indirect hemagglutination and bentonite-flocculation tests are quite sensitive but lack specificity. Treatment is surgical removal of the worms.

Dog and cat hookworms

Ancyclostoma braziliense, a common hookworm in dogs and cats along the southeastern coast and gulf coast of the United States, as well as in many tropical and subtropical parts of the world, is the causative agent of "creeping eruption" or cutaneous larva migrans. The filariform larvae penetrate human skin and wander aimlessly above the germinative layer for periods of up to 3 months or longer, producing serpiginous tunnels in their wake. Indurated, itchy papules develop at the point of invasion with linear, serpiginous tunnels 1 to 2 mm in diameter, produced by the migrating larvae (Fig. 9-16). Allergic response varies with the host. Intense itching leads to scratching and frequently secondary infection. Plumbers, electricians, carpenters, and others who must crawl on their backs under buildings frequented by cats and dogs are highly susceptible to infection. Children playing in sandboxes frequented by cats may fall victim to creeping eruption. Freezing the skin area with ethyl chloride or carbon dioxide snow, by producing a vesicle, causes sloughing of the skin containing the larvae and thus effects a cure, although the larvae themselves are

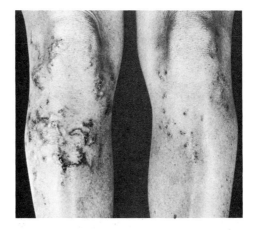

Fig. 9-16. Creeping eruption, or cutaneous larva migrans. (From Katz, R., and Hood, R. W.: J. Invest. Derm. 46[3]:309, 1966.)

unaffected by repeated freezing and thawing. The drug of choice is thiabendazole, applied topically or given orally at the dosage of 25 mg/kg twice daily for 2 days (maximum 3 gm/day) and repeated in 2 days, if necessary. Topical application is very effective.

Ascarids

Embryonated eggs of the ascarid worms of the dog and cat, chiefly *Toxocara canis* but also *T. cati*, when ingested, usually by children playing in contaminated soil, hatch larvae that penetrate the intestinal mucosa, wander aimlessly in the visceral and pleural cavities, and produce granulomas in their wake. Protean manifestations are produced. Patients typically exhibit fever, hepatomegaly, and eosinophilia. Not all patients have

hepatomegaly, and pulmonary infiltrates, which appear early, are probably missed in many cases. Symptoms may last for months or even years.

Clinically, an eosinophilia together with a history of pica for dirt or playing in a contaminated environment will be suggestive of visceral larva migrans. A definitive diagnosis is made only by identification of the larva in tissue biopsy specimens. The liver is the best source of tissue for diagnosis, but the number of worms is small and biopsy findings are diagnostic in less than half the cases. Infection of the brain, heart, eyes, and other organs of the body have been recorded from around the world (Fig. 9-17). Ocular lesions are fairly numerous, frequently resulting in the loss of vision and the eye itself

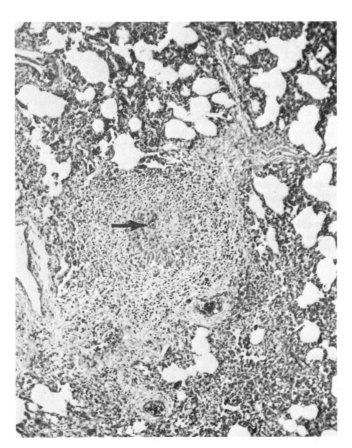

Fig. 9-17. *Toxocara canis (arrow)* within a granuloma in the lung. (AFIP 69-4369.)

as well. In young children strabismus is observed or the infection is noticed accidentally by routine examination of the fundus. Eye lesions are usually painless, unilateral, and without signs or symptoms. They usually lead, however, to total retinal detachment. Lesions in the liver become necrotic and are surrounded by many inflammatory cells including many eosinophils but fewer giant cells, lymphocytes, and plasma cells. Fibrosis eventually occurs, with mineralization often following.

The serologic diagnosis of visceral larva migrans (VLM) is far from satisfactory. Using two antigens, one an extract from *Ascaris lumbricoides* and the other from *Toxocara canis*, gives considerable cross-reactions, but occasionally the difference in titers using the two may give a specific diagnosis. Both the indirect hemagglutination (IHA) test and the bentonite-flocculation test (BFT) should be positive. These tests are being replaced by the enzyme-linked immuno-specific assay (ELISA), which is superior in both sensitivity and specificity (see Tables 15-1 and 15-2). History and clinical evaluation are relevant to making a diagnosis. Very high titers of anti-A or anti-B blood group antibodies are also suggestive. No satisfactory treatment is available at the present time. Visceral larva migrans is usually a self-limiting disease, and treatment should be instituted only in severe cases. Administration of 20 to 40 mg of prednisone daily, reduced after 3 to 5 days, is recommended by some. As an alternative, 2 mg/kg three times daily of diethylcarbamazine (Hetrazan) for 30 days may be used or 25 mg/kg twice daily of thiabendazole is also recommended until the symptoms subside or toxicity is manifested (Table 9-2).

Lagochilascaris minor is an ascarid found normally in the cloudy leopard. Sexually mature specimens have been found in the subcutaneous or tonsillar abscesses about the heads of several patients in Trinidad. Other reports also of similar infections about the neck, ear, and jaw area in patients from Tobago, Costa Rica, and Brazil are recorded. The life history of this parasite is unknown. The adults are about the size of hookworms and are identifiable by their lips and keel-like expansion of the cuticle extending the length of the worm.

Angiostrongylus

Angiostrongylus cantonensis, the rat lungworm, first reported in rats in Canton, China, has since been observed in various parts of the world. It has been found from Madagascar to Hawaii. Infections in humans have been recorded in the Philippines, Taiwan, Vietnam, Thailand, Indonesia, New Caledonia, Tahiti, Hawaii, and some of the smaller islands of Oceania. The adult female worm measures 22 to 34 mm by 340 to 560 μm in diameter. Males are smaller. The adults live in the branches of the pulmonary artery where eggs are produced. Hatching occurs in the capillary bed and the larvae pass over into the alveoli, up the bronchial tree, and down the esophagus. First-stage larvae are excreted in the feces where survival, up to 2 weeks under optimum conditions, enhances opportunity for invasion of terrestrial slugs and various aquatic or land-snails by ingestion or penetration of the integument. In the tissues of these intermediate hosts, development to the third-stage larva takes place. Land crabs, freshwater prawns, and frogs have been found naturally infected, and oysters have been infected experimentally. Rats become infected usually by eating the intermediate host. Larvae penetrate the gastrointestinal tract and, via the lymphatics and venules, enter the circulation from whence they travel to the pulmonary circuit and on to the viscera. Within 4 days they leave the vascular system and can be found in the interstitial spaces of the cord and brain. After two molts, young adults enter cerebral veins and are carried to the pulmo-

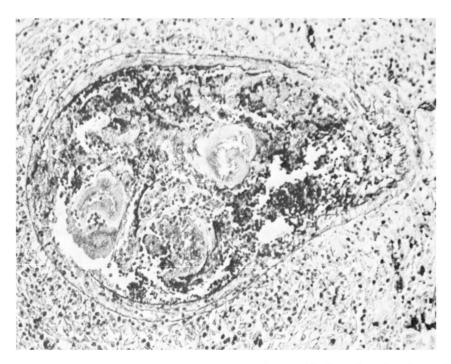

Fig. 9-18. Granulomatous reaction within the lumen of a pulmonary blood vessel resulting from a degenerating *Angiostrongylus cantonensis.* (AFIP 74-11640.)

nary system where development is completed (Fig. 9-18). The total cycle in the rat takes about 6 weeks.

Humans become infected by ingesting third-stage larvae in raw or insufficiently cooked invertebrates. Various transport hosts such as freshwater prawns and land crabs may be eaten. Eating raw fruits and vegetables contaminated by the mucus of intermediate or transfer hosts may cause infections in humans. European settlers in French Oceania, for example, are sometimes infected by eating the fresh salad greens they relish. Larvae migrate into the brain and die, causing an encephalitis. The incubation period in humans is about 2 weeks but may vary from 12 to 28 days. The most common complaint is headache, usually associated with stiff neck, photophobia, vertigo, nausea, vomiting, and low-grade fever. Usually a slight leukocytosis develops, with eosinophilia sometimes very high. Cerebrospinal fluid cell counts are highest in the first 2 weeks and range from 200 to 5,000 per cu mm, with eosinophils being about 25%. Convalescence usually takes several weeks to months. Patients with isolated ocular invasion do not have symptoms and the cerebrospinal fluid is normal. The chief complaint is painless loss of vision. Very few autopsies have been performed, inflammation and necrosis being associated chiefly only with dead worms. Patients in endemic areas with brain dyscrasia and eosinophilia both peripherally and in the spinal fluid should be prime suspects. There is no known therapy at present. Surgical removal of the worms from the eye is ineffective. Infection may be prevented by proper dietary habits.

Angiostrongylus costaricensis, a related species, is a parasite of wild rodents in Central America. It is found in rats (*Sigmodon hispidus, Rattus rattus,* and others). The cotton rat *S. hispidus* is the major reservoir host in Panama. Cotton rats in Texas have also been found to be infected. The life cycle differs from that of *A. cantonensis* in that adult worms live in the mesenteric arteries near the cecum. Eggs are laid in either the tissues or capillaries of the intestinal wall. Hatched larvae migrate into the intestinal lumen and pass out in the feces. Slugs *(Vaginulus plebeius)* eat rat feces, and larvae develop to the third stage. Rats in turn eat the slugs to continue the life cycle, with the larvae developing in lymph nodes and lymphatics. Young adults migrate to the arterioles of the ileocecal area. Humans who eat unwashed vegetables contaminated with the mucus secretions of infected slugs become infected. The same migration pattern occurs in humans as in rats. However, eggs produced do not hatch but degenerate, producing granulomas. Abdominal infection has been reported in Venezuela, Honduras, southern Mexico, and El Salvador. Approximately 10 to 30 cases, mostly in children, are diagnosed in Costa Rica every year. The inflammation is usually centered in the wall of the appendix but may extend into the ileum, cecum, and ascending colon. Thickening may cause partial obstruction of the intestinal lumen. Local thrombosis is caused by adult worms in the mesenteric arteries. Diagnosis is based on clinical findings, and surgical intervention may sometimes be indicated. Treatment with thiabendazole is successful. This drug is also used postoperatively to kill residual worms. Radiologic examination reveals a filling defect over the cecum with spasticity and bowel irritability. The white blood cell count varies between 10,000 and 50,000 with eosinophilia from 10% to 80%.

MORE TISSUE ROUNDWORMS

Capillaria hepatica is a fairly common parasite in the liver of rodents and other animals. The adult worms are closely related to *Trichuris trichiura* but are more delicate in appearance. Eggs produced resemble those of *T. trichiura* and are retained in the liver parenchyma. Such infected liver eaten by other animals results in the eggs being disseminated in the feces. Development in the soil produces infective larvae, which, when ingested by the definitive host, enter the intestinal wall and reach the liver, becoming adults. Infective larvae in humans, likewise, penetrate the intestinal wall and produce a clinical picture similar to that of visceral larva migrans. Maturation of adult worms takes about 1 month. No therapy is known. Over 20 cases in humans have been reported. Eosinophilia with an acute or subacute hepatitis, substantiated by liver biopsy findings, characterizes human infection.

Micronema deletrix, a free-living nematode found in soil, manure, and decaying humus, has been reported once—in a five-year-old farm boy in Canada who fell into a manure spreader and passed through its mechanism. He suffered severe lacerations, fractures, a penetrating sucking chest wound, and a penetrating wound of the abdomen. He died 24 days after the accident. Autopsy revealed an extensive and unusual meningoencephalomyelitis. Various stages of the worm, including gravid females, juveniles, larvae, and eggs, were found throughout the leptomeninges, cerebral hemispheres, pons, medulla, midbrain, cerebellum, and spinal cord. The concentration of worms indicated that reproduction took place until time of death.

Dioctophyma renale, the giant kidney worm, is a huge, blood-red nematode. The female reaches a length of 3 feet at times, with a diameter the size of a little finger. The males are insignificant in size. *D. renale* is found in the pelvis of the kidney of a variety of fish-eating mammals such as the dog, wolf, various wildcats, raccoon, skunk, and mink. Eggs passed in the urine develop in water, and freshwater fishes apparently harbor the larval stage. About a dozen human infections are recorded. The worms gradually destroy the kidney, leaving only the capsule. At times they migrate into the ureters. Diagnosis is based on finding typical eggs in the urine or finding a worm passed through the urethra. There is no known chemotherapy.

Species of *Syngamus* are normally parasitic in the trachea and bronchi of birds and mammals. They are commonly called gapeworms, or forked worms, so called because the male is permanently attached to the vulva of the female by its bursa, giving the pair a forked appearance. The female, the larger of the sexes, is about 15 to 20 mm long. Eggs are about 85 × 50 μm in size and in an early stage of segmentation when oviposited. Infections in humans occur from eating uncooked food or drinking unboiled or unfiltered contaminated water. Reports of human infections in Puerto Rico, Martinique, St. Lucia, Trinidad, British Guiana, Brazil, and the Philippines are recorded. All are believed to be accidental infections with *S. laryngeus* of cattle, water buffaloes, and goats, although *S. nasicola* from goats is also involved. Worms in the trachea are irritating; hemoptysis and sometimes asthma occur. Violent attacks of coughing will frequently discharge the worms and eggs in the sputum. Diagnosis is made by recovering the characteristic eggs in sputum or feces.

REVIEW QUESTIONS

1. Describe the characteristics common to the filarial worms of humans.
2. What is the significance of infection with *Wuchereria bancrofti* to the tourist in Samoa?
3. Of what importance are filarial infections to physicians in the United States?
4. Discuss larva migrans.
5. How does onchocerciasis differ mainly from the other filariases?
6. Discuss the epidemiology of dracontiasis (dracunculiasis).
7. What is the significance of *Angiostrongylus cantonensis*? Of *A. costaricensis*?
8. What is the significance of free-living nematodes in the soil with regard to human infection? Discuss.
9. Discuss the significance and ramifications of improperly cooked food and unboiled or unfiltered water to the itinerant traveler in an underdeveloped country.

REFERENCES

Alicata, J. E., and K. Jindrak. 1970. *Angiostrongylus* in the Pacific and Southeast Asia. Charles C Thomas, Publisher, Springfield, Ill.

Aljeboori, T. I., and M. H. Ivey. 1970. An improved hemagglutination technique for detecting antibody against *Toxocara canis*. Am. J. Trop. Med. Hyg. **19**:244-248.

Anderson, J., and H. Fuglsang. 1973. Topical diethylcarbamazine in ocular onchocerciasis. Trans. R. Soc. Trop. Med. Hyg. **67**:710-717.

Anderson, R. I., L. E. Fazen, and A. A. Buck. 1975. Onchocerciasis in Guatemala. II. Microfilariae in urine, blood, and sputum after diethylcarbamazine. Am. J. Trop. Med. Hyg. **24**:58-61.

Anderson, R. I., L. E. Fazen, and A. A. Buck. 1975. Onchocerciasis in Guatemala. III. Daytime periodicity of microfilariae in skin. Am. J. Trop. Med. Hyg. **24**:62-65.

Bartlett, A., and others. 1978. Variation in delayed hypersensitivity in onchocerciasis. Trans. R. Soc. Trop. Med. Hyg. **72**:372-377.

Beaver, P. C. 1964. Cutaneous larva migrans. Industr. Med. Surg. **33**:319-321.

Beaver, P. C. 1969. The nature of visceral larva migrans. J. Parasitol. **53**:3-12.

Beaver, P. C., and I. R. Carn. 1974. *Wuchereria*-like Filaria in an artery, associated with pulmonary infarction. Am. J. Trop. Med. Hyg. **23**:869-876.

Beaver, P. C., G. S. Horner, and J. Z. Bilos. 1974. Zoonotic onchocercosis in a resident of Illinois and observations on the identification of *Onchocerca* species. Am. J. Trop. Med. Hyg. **23**:595-607.

Beaver, P. C., and T. C. Orihel. 1965. Human Infection with filariae of animals in the United States. Am. J. Trop. Med. **14**:1010-1029.

Beverley-Burton, M., and V. F. Crichton. 1973. Identification of guinea-worm species. Trans. R. Soc. Trop. Med. Hyg. **67**:152.

Binford, C. H., and D. H. Connors. 1976. Pathology of tropical and extraordinary diseases: an atlas. Vol. II. Armed Forces Institute of Pathology. Washington, D.C.

Buck, A. A., Editor. 1974. Onchocerciasis; symptomatology, pathology, diagnosis. WHO, Geneva, Switzerland.

Chandra, R., and others. 1978. *Brugia malayi* infective larval whole worm antigen in the diagnosis of filariasis by skin test. Indian J. Med. Res. **68**:61-66.

Chitanondh, H., and L. Rosen. 1967. Fatal eosinophilic encephalitis caused by the nematode *Gnathostoma spinigerum*. Am. J. Trop. Med. Hyg. **16**:638-645.

Choyce, D. P. 1966. Onchocerciasis: ophthalmic aspects. Trans. R. Soc. Trop. Med. Hyg. **60**:707-719.

Collins, R. F., and M. H. Ivey. 1975. Specificity and sensitivity of skin test reactions to extracts of *Toxocara canis* and *Ascaris suum.* I. Skin tests done in infected guinea pigs. Am. J. Trop. Med. Hyg. **24:**455-459.

Connor, D. H. 1978. Current concepts in parasitology: onchocerciasis. N. Engl. J. Med. **298:**379-381.

Connor, D. H., and others. 1970. Onchocerciasis: onchocercal dermatitis, lymphadenitis, and elephantitis in the Ubangi territory. Hum. Pathol. **1:**553-579.

Coolidge, C., and others. 1979. Zoonotic *Brugia* filariasis in New England. Ann. Intern. Med. **90:**341-343.

DeSavigny, D. H., and I. R. Tizard. 1977. Toxocaral larva migrans: the use of larval secretory antigens in haemagglutination and soluble antigen fluorescent antibody tests. Trans. R. Soc. Trop. Med. Hyg. **71:**501-507.

Desowitz, R. S., and J. C. Hitchcock. 1974. Hyperendemic Bancroftian filariasis in the Kingdom of Tonga: the application of the membrane filter concentration technique to an age-stratified blood survey. Am. J. Trop. Med. Hyg. **23:**877-879.

Dutta, S. N., and H. J. Diesfeld. 1978. Indirect immunofluorescence test against *Dipetalonema vitae* in detection of filariasis in Dhanbad coal mines area. Indian J. Med. Res. **67:**553-561.

Eberhard, M. L. 1979. Studies on the *Onchocerca* (Nematoda: Filariodea) found in cattle in the United States. I. Systematics of *O. gutturosa* and *O. lienalis* with a description of *O. stilesi* sp. N. J. Parasitol. **65:**379-388.

Edeson, J. F. B. 1972. Filariasis. Br. Med. Bull. **28:**60-65.

Fuglsang, H., and J. Anderson. 1974. Collapse during treatment of onchocerciasis with diethylcarbamazine. Trans. R. Soc. Trop. Med. Hyg. **68:**72-73.

Glickman, L., P. Schantz, R. Dombroske, and R. Cypress. 1978. Evaluation of serodiagnostic tests for visceral larva migrans. Am. J. Trop. Med. Hyg. **27:**492-498.

Glickman, L. T., and others. 1979. *Toxocara* infection and epilepsy in children. J. Pediatr. **94:**75-78.

Grove, D. I., and others. 1977. Sensitivity and specificity of skin reactivity to *Brugia malayi* and *Dirofilaria immitis* antigens in Bancroftian and Malayan filariasis in the Philippines. Am. J. Trop. Med. Hyg. **26:**220-229.

Grove, D. I., and R. S. Davis. 1978. Serological diagnosis of Bancroftian and Malayan filariasis. Am. J. Trop. Med. Hyg. **27:**508-513.

Grove, D. I., F. S. Valeza, and B. D. Cabrera. 1978. Bancroftian filariasis in a Philippine village: clinical, parasitological, immunological, and social aspects. Bull. WHO **56:**975-984.

Hawking, F., and D. A. Denham. 1976. The distribution of human filariasis throughout the world. Part I. The Pacific region including New Guinea. Trop. Dis. Bull. **73:**348-373.

Heather, C. J., and E. W. Price. 1972. Non-filarial elephantiasis in Ethiopia: analytical study of inorganic material in lymph nodes. Trans. R. Soc. Trop. Med. Hyg. **66:**450-458.

Kagam, I. G., and L. Norman. 1976. Serodiagnosis of parasitic diseases. Manual of clinical immunology. Chapter 51. American Society of Microbiology.

Kale, O. O. 1975. Mebendazole in the treatment of dracontiasis. Am. J. Trop. Med. Hyg. **24:**600-605.

Kazacos, K. R., and L. E. Smith, Jr. 1979. Loiasis *(Loa loa)* in an African student in Indiana. Am. J. Trop. Med. Hyg. **28:**213-215.

King, L. A. 1974. The identification of anti-parasitic antibodies in bloodstains using an indirect fluorescent antibody technique. J. Forensic Sci. **14:**117-121.

Krupp, I. M. 1974. Hemagglutination test for the detection of antibodies specific for *Ascaris* and *Toxocara* antigens in patients with suspected visceral migrans. Am. J. Trop. Med. Hyg. **23:**378-384.

Laing, A. B. G., J. F. B. Edeson, and R. H. Wharton. 1960. Studies on filariasis in Malaya: the vertebrate hosts of *Brugia malayi* and *B. pahangi*. Am. Trop. Med. Parasitol. **54:**92-99.

Meyers, W. M., and others. 1972. Human streptocerciasis: a clinico-pathologic study of 40 Africans (Zairians) including identification of the adult filaria. Am. J. Trop. Med. Hyg. **21:**528-545.

Mitra, A. K., and D. R. W. Haddock. 1970. Paraplegia due to Guineaworm infection. Trans. R. Soc. Trop. Med. Hyg. **64:**102-106.

Miyazaki, J. 1966. *Gnathostoma* and gnathostomiasis in Japan. Progress of medical parasitology in Japan. Meguro Parasitological Museum **3:**531-586.

Morera, P. 1973. Life history and redescription of *Angiostrongylus costaricensis* Morera and Céspedes. 1971. Am. J. Trop. Med. Hyg. **22:**613-621.

Morera, P. and R. Céspedes. 1971. *Angiostrongylus costaricensis* n. sp. (Nematoda: Metastrongyloidea), a new lung worm occurring in man in Costa Rica. Rev. Biol. Trop. **18:**173-185.

Morgan, H. C., G. F. Fotto, R. F. Jackson, and C. H. Courtney, Editors. 1978. Proceedings of the Heartworm Symposium 1977. Veterinary Medicine Publishing Co., Bonner Springs, Ks.

Muller, R. 1971. Dracunculus and dracunculiasis. Pages 73-151. In B. Dawes, Editor. Advances in parasitology. Academic Press, Inc., New York.

Muller, R. 1972. Maintenance of *Dracunculus medinensis* (L.) in the laboratory and observations on experimental infections. Parasitol. **64:**107-116.

Murthy, P. K., and others. 1978. Inhibition of filarial skin test reactions by diethylcarbamazine therapy. Indian J. Med. Res. **68:**428-434.

Neafie, R. C., D. H. Connor, and W. H. Meyers. 1975. *Dipetalonema streptocerca* (Macfie and Corson, 1922): description of the adult female. Am. J. Trop. Med. Hyg. **24:**264-267.

Neilson, J. T. M. 1979. Kinetics of *Dipetalonema vitae:* infections established by surgical implantation of adult worms into hamsters. Am. J. Trop. Med. Hyg. **28:** 216-219.

Nelson, G. S. 1966. The pathology of filarial infections. Helminthol. Abstr. **35:**311-336.

Nelson, G. S. 1970. Onchocerciasis. Adv. Parasitol. **8:** 173-223.

Nelson, G. S. 1979. Current concepts in parasitology: filariasis. N. Engl. J. Med. **300:**1136-1139.

Neppert, J. 1979. Immunologic response in onchocerciasis: relations to microfilaria density in the skin biopsy and to some frequent symptoms. Dermatologica **158:**137-141.

Neva, F. A., and E. A. Ottesen. 1978. Current concepts in parasitology: tropical (filarial) eosinophilia. N. Engl. J. Med. **298:**1129-1131.

Ngu, J. L. 1978. Immunological studies on onchocerciasis. Acta Trop. **35:**269-279.

Nitidandhaprabhas, P., S. Hanchansin, and Y. Vongsloesvidhya. 1975. A case of expectoration of *Gnathostoma spinigerum* in Thailand. Am. J. Trop. Med. Hyg. **24:**547-548.

Nitidandhaprabhas, P. and others. 1975. Human urinary gnathostomiasis: a case report from Thailand. Am. J. Trop. Med. Hyg. **24:**49-51.

Orihel, T. C., and P. C. Beaver. 1975. Morphology and relationship of *Dirofilaria tenuis* and *Dirofilaria conjunctivae.* Am. J. Trop. Med. Hyg. **14:**1030-1043.

Orihel, T. C., and R. C. Lowrie. 1975. *Loa loa:* development to the infective stage in an American deerfly, *Chrysops atlanticus.* Am. J. Trop. Med. Hyg. **24:**610-615.

Padonu, K. O. 1973. A controlled trial of metronidazole in the treatment of dracontiasis in Nigeria. Am. J. Trop. Med. Hyg. **22:**42-44.

Patterson, R., C. C. Huntley, M. Roberts, and J. S. Irons. 1975. Visceral larva migrans: immunoglobulins, precipitating antibodies and detection of IgG and IgM antibodies against *Ascaris* antigen. Am. J. Trop. Med. Hyg. **24:**465-470.

Peña Periero, A., and others. 1978. Larva migrans visceral. Rev. Cubana Med. Trop. **30:**60-67.

Polley, L. 1978. Visceral larva migrans and alveolar hydatid disease: dangers real and imagined. Vet. Clin. North Am. **8:**353-378.

Price, E. W. 1974. Endemic elephantiasis of lower legs: natural history and clinical study. Trans. R. Soc. Trop. Med. Hyg. **68:**44-52.

Samuel, A. M., and others. 1978. Cell mediated and humoral immune response in tropical eosinophilia. Indian J. Med. Res. **68:**444-449.

Sasa, M. 1976. Human filariasis. University Park Press, Baltimore, Md.

Saverbrey, M. 1977. A precipitin test for the diagnosis of human abdominal angiostrongyliasis. Am. J. Trop. Med. Hyg. **26:**1156-1158.

Sodeman, T. M., and N. Dock. 1976. Laboratory diagnosis of parasitic and fungal diseases of the central nervous system. Ann. Clin. Lab. Sci. **6:**47-55.

Somorin, A. O., D. C. Heines, and R. E. Ajugwo. 1970. Immunoglobulin E in Nigerian onchocerciasis. Am. J. Trop. Med. Hyg. **26:**872-876.

Sondergaard, J. 1971. Filariasis caused by *Acanthochielonema perstans.* Arch. Dermatol. **106:**547-548.

Subrahmanyam, D., and others. 1978. Immune reactions in human filariasis. J. Clin. Microbiol. **8:**228-232.

Tannehill, A. W., Jr., and H. B. Hatch, Jr. 1968. Coin lesions of the lung due to *Dirofilaria immitis:* report of a case. Dis. Chest **53:**369-371.

Taylor, A. E. R., and J. R. Baker, Editors. 1978. Methods of cultivating parasites in vitro. Academic Press, Inc. New York.

Thomas, D. B., R. I. Anderson, and A. A. MacRae. 1973. Microfilariae of *Onchocerca volvulus* in a vaginal irrigation specimen. J. Parasitol. **59:**941-942.

Trent, S. C. 1963. Reevaluation of World War II: veterans with filariasis acquired in the South Pacific. J. Trop. Med. Hyg. **12:**877-887.

Tungkanak, R., S. Sirisinha, and S. Punyagupta. 1972. Serum and cerebrospinal fluid in eosinophilic meningoencephalitis: immunoglobulins and antibody to *Angiostrongylus cantonensis.* Am. J. Trop. Med. Hyg. **21:**415-420.

Ubelaker, J. E., and N. M. Hall. 1979. First report of *Angiostrongylus costaricensis* Morera and Céspedes 1971 in the United States. J. Parasitol. **65:**307.

Walls, K. W. 1979. Immunoserology of parasitic diseases. In Friedman, H., T. J. Linna, and J. E. Prier, Editors. Immunoserology in the diagnosis of infectious diseases. University Park Press, Baltimore, Md.

Wiseman, R. A., and A. W. Woodruff. 1970. Evaluation of a skin sensitivity test for the diagnosis of toxocariasis. Trans. R. Soc. Trop. Med. Hyg. **64:** 239-245.

Woodruff, A. W. 1970. Toxocariasis. Br. Med. J. **3:** 663-669.

Woodruff, A. W., and D. DeSavigny. 1978. Study of toxocaral infection in dog breeders. Br. Med. J. **2:** 1747-1748.

Wright, K. A. 1979. *Trichinella spiralis:* an intracellular parasite in the intestinal phase. J. Parasitol. **65:**441-445.

Yoshimura, H., and M. Yokogawa. 1970. *Dirofilaria* causing infarct in human lung. Am. J. Trop. Med. Hyg. **19:**63-67.

Zaman, V., and W. P. Fung. 1973. Treatment of eosinophilic lung with levamisole. Trans. R. Soc. Trop. Med. Hyg. **67:**144-145.

Zaman, V., and H. Lal. 1973. Treatment of *Wuchereria bancrofti* with levamisole. Trans. R. Soc. Trop. Med. Hyg. **67:**610.

THE FLATWORMS (Platyhelminthes) AND SPINY-HEADED WORMS (Acanthocephala)

■ The flatworms, unlike the nematodes, have no body cavity. They are flattened dorsoventrally, with the internal organs embedded in a spongy parenchyma. An alimentary tract, when present, is usually a blind sac with no anal pore. The nervous system consists of a primitive ganglion in the anterior part of the worm, with nerve cords or fibers extending into the body. The excretory or osmoregulatory system consists of a series of tubes conducting fluid to the outside through the excretory pore. Nearly all are hermaphroditic and many have asexual as well as sexual means of reproduction. Life cycles often are complicated with both an alternation of generations and an alternation of hosts. Humans may be either definitive or intermediate hosts, or both in some instances.

Those of medical importance occur in two classes—Cestoidea, the tapeworms or cestodes, and Trematoda, the flukes or trematodes.

THE TAPEWORMS (CESTOIDEA)

The tapeworms are so called because they resemble a measuring tape. The habitat of the adult worm is the intestinal tract of the definitive host. Most of those parasitic in humans are intestinal parasites, although a few invade the tissues of the body in the larval stages and are known as somatic tapeworms.

The adult worm is considered by many not to be a single individual, but a family consisting sometimes of thousands of individuals, one behind the other like links in a chain. For practical reasons it is convenient, however, to refer to this family as a single tapeworm.

The chain or strobila can be divided into regions. At one end is a hold-fast organ, called the scolex, which is round to oval in shape and contains either four suction cups (suckers) or two elongated sucking grooves. The scolex tapers into a neck region from which are proliferated proglottids or "segments" as they are commonly called. The series of segments adjacent to the neck region comprises the region of immature proglottids. As more are formed, the existing ones are pushed posteriorly, grow, and develop male and female sex organs within. They comprise the region of mature proglottids. After fertilization they develop eggs and are gravid proglottids. Thus, the fully grown strobila consists of a scolex, neck region, and regions of immature, mature, and gravid proglottids.

The tapeworm, with no digestive tract, is dependent on the absorption of simple food

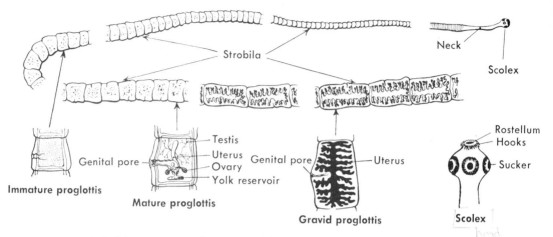

Fig. 1. Cyclophyllidean tapeworm showing morphologic features. Rostellum may be "armed" or "unarmed" depending on species. (From Medical protozoology and helminthology. 1955. Bethesda, Md., United States Naval Medical School, National Naval Medical Center.)

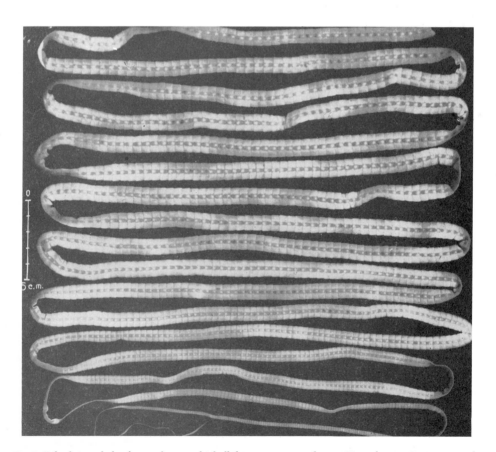

Fig. 2. *Dibothriocephalus latus,* the pseudophyllidean tapeworm of man. Note the persistent terminal proglottid. Shedding of proglottids does not occur normally as in the cyclophyllidean tapeworms. (From Kourí, P., and Basnuevo, J. G. Lecciones de parasitología y medicina tropical, Editorial Profilaxis S.A., Havana.)

elements. Studies show that tapeworms can utilize only monosaccharides, not disaccharides, ingested by the host, and that essential nutriments such as vitamins and amino acids are supplied by both active and passive transfer across the mucosal epithelium. Radioactive thiamine, for example, when given parenterally to the host is absorbed by the tapeworm. Analysis of the intestinal mucosa reveals a high concentration of this vitamin.

Even though the size of some tapeworms is considerable, they are in general tolerated rather well by the host. The old notion that a person with no weight gain despite a voracious appetite has a tapeworm is a fallacy. In most instances major complaints are absent until the patient observes proglottids; then alarm, intestinal cramps, and discomfort may ensue. Intestinal obstruction is possible but rare. Tapeworms may trigger nutritional deficiency in borderline cases. The general reaction to most tapeworm infections is usually one either of undue alarm or of indifference; both points of view are to be avoided. Any patient with an intestinal tapeworm certainly should be treated.

Two orders of tapeworms have representative parasites in humans. All these parasites with the exception of one species are found in one order, the Cyclophyllidea. The remaining parasite is in the order Pseudophyllidea.

Two divergent types of reproductive systems, which are useful in diagnosis, are found in these orders. The gravid proglottids of the Cyclophyllidea are little more than uterine sacs full of eggs, surrounded by protective tissue or parenchyma (Fig. 1). The distended uterus may assume various shapes of diagnostic value, depending on the species. Rupture of the uterus and the surrounding parenchyma is necessary to effect liberation of the eggs. Gravid proglottids either rupture within the host or pass out intact in the feces. The pseudophyllidean tapeworm is characterized by having gravid proglottids that contain a very small uterus, often described as a rosette, and a uterine pore through which eggs are passed directly into the intestinal lumen of the host. Thus, rather than store a large quantity of eggs as in the Cyclophyllidea, this tapeworm gets rid of them as soon as they are formed and are ready for liberation. The gravid proglottid with the rosette uterus is readily identifiable (Fig. 2).

FLUKES (TREMATODA)

The flukes, or trematodes, represent a primitive class of worms. Those parasitic in humans have rather complicated life cycles involving an alternation of generations and alternation of hosts. Aside from one aberrant group, the schistosomes, all are hermaphroditic. The hermaphroditic adult is flat and leaflike and contains an oral and a ventral sucker as hold-fast organs, a primitive digestive tract, a nervous and excretory system, and genital organs of both sexes. Eggs produced are operculated and either unsegmented or embryonated when passed. The embryo within is designated as a miracidium, resembling in many ways a ciliate. The miracidium, within the appropriate species of snail, undergoes asexual multiplication through several generations. Eventually cercariae are produced. Cercariae are shed by the snail and pass to the next appropriate intermediate host where they encyst, becoming metacercariae. This intermediate host may be a plant, or an appropriate freshwater fish, crab, or crayfish. When the raw or improperly cooked intermediate host is eaten by humans, the metacercariae excyst, migrate to their destination, and become adults.

The schistosomes differ in that the sexes are separate and, in gross appearance, somewhat resemble roundworms more than typical flukes. The eggs are not operculated, and hatching occurs by breaking of the shell membrane. The cercariae shed by the appropriate snails penetrate directly into the skin of the definitive host and enter the circulation to reach their final abode and become adults. Thus no second intermediate hosts are involved.

The typical life pattern for the trematodes may be represented as follows:

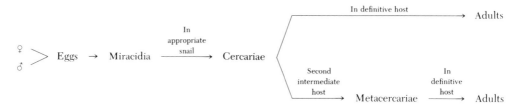

The flukes parasitizing humans may be conveniently grouped according to their location in the host, as follows:

Intestinal flukes
Lung flukes
Liver flukes
Blood flukes

THE SPINY-HEADED WORMS (ACANTHOCEPHALA)

The Acanthocephala, or spiny-headed worms, were previously considered with the nematodes but are now believed to be closer to the tapeworms. They have received recognition of their own, being given phylum status.

Sexes are separate and no free-living phase is noted in the life cycle. Eggs are passed in the feces of a variety of definitive vertebrate hosts. When ingested by the appropriate arthropod (insect, crustacean, myriapod) they hatch, develop to maturity, and mate in the intestinal tract. Humans are an occasional accidental host. *Macracanthorhynchus hirudinaceus*, a common parasite of pigs, is reported to occur in peasants of the Volga valley in southern Russia where the white grubs of beetles are eaten. *Acanthocephalus rauschi* has been reported in the peritoneum of an Eskimo, the true definitive host undoubtedly being a fish. *Corynosoma stromosum*, a seal parasite, has been found in humans. Rather interesting is the report of a toad worm, *Acanthocephalus bufonis*, in an Indonesian. One patient reputedly vomited an adult male *Moniliformis moniliformis*, the rat spiny-headed worm, which was recovered from a soiled towel.

Worms vary in size, according to species and sex, from 4 to 5 cm in length for males and up to 60 cm or more for females. The spiny proboscis burrows into the mucosal wall, is firmly attached, and, in some instances, perforates the gut wall of animals, causing a fatal peritonitis.

CHAPTER 10

The cyclophyllidean tapeworms (Cyclophyllidea)

The members of the order Cyclophyllidea have a life pattern consistent throughout the species. The hermaphroditic adult produces eggs composed of shell membranes surrounding a six-hooked embryo or onchosphere. The latter is often referred to as a hexacanth embryo. The hexacanth embryos differ from one another in the nature of their shell membranes. This embryonated egg is passed in the feces of the definitive host, either free or within the gravid proglottid, and is ingested by the appropriate intermediate host. The liberated onchosphere burrows through the gut wall and develops into the next larval stage in the body tissues of the intermediate host. This larval stage may be one of several types. It may be a cysticercus, cysticercoid, cenurus, or hydatid cyst (Fig. 10-1). When the infected intermediate host is ingested by the definitive host, the larvae grow into adult worms in the small intestine. This life pattern may be represented in the diagram below.

The cysticercus larva, commonly referred to as a bladder worm, is a small bladder 6 mm to 18 mm in diameter, filled with fluid and containing one invaginated scolex attached to the inner wall. The cysticercoid is quite similar to the cysticercus except that the invaginated scolex lies within solid tissue instead of fluid. The body often tapers into a taillike projection. The cenurus larva is almost identical to the cysticercus except that it is much larger (30 mm or more) and contains up to 20 or more invaginated scolices in the fluid-filled bladder. The hydatid cyst represents the most advanced type of tapeworm larva from the standpoint of budding; it likewise is a bladder filled with fluid, sometimes reaching the size of a large grapefruit. The outer wall is laminated and the inner or germinative layer gives rise to numerous secondary or daughter cysts known as brood capsules. Within each brood capsule numerous invaginated scolices may also develop. Secondary or granddaughter cysts with more scolices may also develop. The possibilities for scolex formation seem endless; a fertile cyst can harbor up to 2 million scolices. Liberated scolices and bits of germinative tissue in the cyst are known collectively as hydatid sand.

The cyclophyllidean tapeworms parasitizing the intestinal tract of humans are as follows:

Taenia saginata   Hymenolepis nana
Taenia solium   Dipylidium caninum
Hymenolepis diminuta

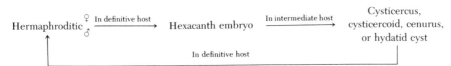

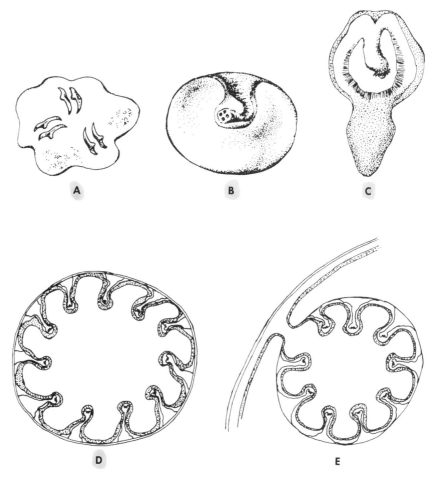

Fig. 10-1. Larval stages of cyclophyllidean tapeworms. The liberated onchosphere, **A,** ingested by the appropriate intermediate host may develop into a cysticercus, **B,** cysticercoid, **C,** cenurus, **D,** or hydatid cyst, **E,** depending on the species involved.

Taenia saginata

Geographic distribution. Wherever beef is eaten raw or insufficiently cooked, *Taenia saginata* may be found. It is cosmopolitan in distribution, particularly in Islamic countries. In Ethiopia, where raw beef is a delicacy, a man boasts of the number of tapeworms he harbors. In some parts of the world, sewage systems are periodically plugged by the large number of worms. Infections occur in the United States.

Morphology and life cycle. Humans are the only known definitive host. The life span is estimated to be up to 25 years. The strobila, creamy white in color, averages 25 feet in length, although specimens as long as 50 feet have been recovered. The scolex is piriform with four well-developed suckers and a rostellum without hooks (unarmed) (Fig. 10-2). Attachment to the mucosal wall of the upper jejunum occurs; the remainder of the strobila lies free in the lumen and folded on itself. Arising posteriorly from the constricted neck region are a series of 1,000 to 2,000 segments, or proglottids, ranging from immature to gravid. As growth continues from

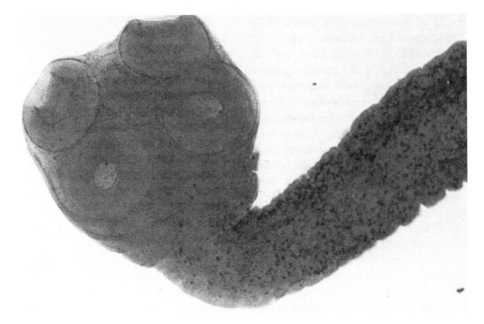

Fig. 10-2. Scolex of *Taenia saginata*. Note the absence of hooks. (From a nonprofit cooperative endeavor by numerous colleagues under the editorship of Dr. Herman Zaiman, Valley City, N.D.)

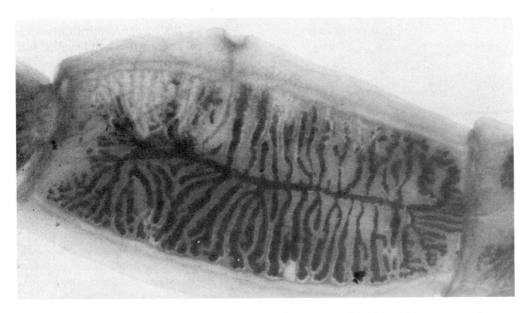

Fig. 10-3. Gravid proglottid of *Taenia saginata*. Note the numerous lateral branches emanating from the median stem—more than thirteen on a side. (From a nonprofit cooperative endeavor by numerous colleagues under the editorship of Dr. Herman Zaiman, Valley City, N.D.)

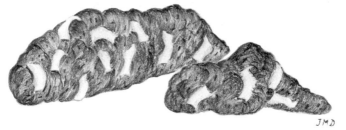

Fig. 10-4. Stool specimen showing numerous motile gravid proglottids of *Taenia saginata*.

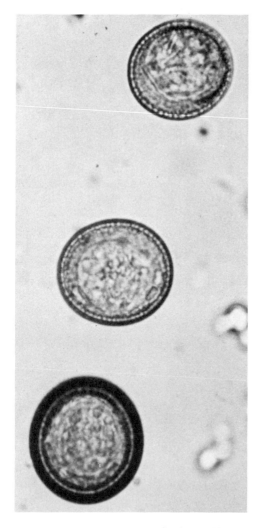

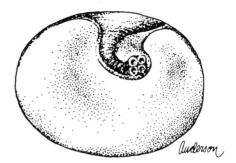

Fig. 10-6. Cysticercus larva of *Taenia saginata*. Note the unarmed scolex.

Fig. 10-5. Eggs of *Taenia* sp. Note the discernible hooks in the young egg at the top of the photo. Eggs of *Taenia solium* and *Taenia saginata* are identical in appearance. (From a nonprofit cooperative endeavor by numerous colleagues under the editorship of Dr. Herman Zaiman, Valley City, N.D.)

the neck region, gravid proglottids, measuring approximately 20 mm in length by 6 mm in width, are shed and passed out in the feces intact (Fig. 10-3). They usually occur singly and, because of the well-developed musculature, often show great activity, moving across the fecal mass with a typical "wormlike" motion (Fig. 10-4). Many times they are mistaken, by untrained observers, as other adult worms. The officer in charge of the clinical laboratory in an Air Corps Hospital during World War II, much to the consternation of the more experienced technicians of lower rank, identified a gravid proglottid moving across a fecal specimen as the adult of *Echinococcus granulosus*, a tapeworm ironically enough never occurring in humans in the adult stage. Eggs may also occur in the feces as a result of partial rupturing of the uterine branches in the region of the separation of proglottids (Fig. 10-5).

Gravid proglottids passed in the feces onto the soil and vegetation are eaten by cattle and allied animals, such as water buffalo, camels, llamas, antelopes, and other herbivores, while grazing. Each proglottid is packed full of eggs containing six-hooked, or hexacanth, embryos within. When ingested, these embryos, liberated from their shells, penetrate the mucosal wall, enter lymphatics and blood vessels, and are carried by the circulation over the entire body. They come to rest and develop into cysticerci in the various muscles of the host. To a lesser degree various organs may also be invaded. The intermediate host apparently tolerates the cysticerci rather well. Development of this larval stage takes place in approximately 12 to 15 weeks after ingestion of the eggs. The cysticerci average about 5 mm × 9 mm and are readily discernible to the naked eye when heavily infected measly beef is examined (Fig. 10-6). When humans eat infected beef or other meat, the scolex liberated from the "bladder worm" evaginates in the intestine, attaches itself to the mucosa, and from the neck region develops the strobila. Development of the mature tapeworm takes about 2 to 3 months. Although three cases of cysticercosis in humans have been reported in the literature, humans are *not* considered to be suitable intermediate hosts (Fig. 10-7).

Epidemiology. Infections occur in humans chiefly by the eating of raw or insufficiently cooked beef. In areas where night soil is used for fertilizer, or sewage is allowed to drain into a meadow, cattle become infected from grazing on the contaminated soil. Eggs, under ideal conditions, may remain viable for as long as 6 months. Chemical treatment of the soil does not kill the ova, well protected in the muscular proglottids. The most effective prophylaxis is the prevention of soil contamination where cattle are grazing. The thorough cooking of beef before eating will also break the cycle, as will adequate deep-freeze refrigeration before human consumption. Pickling in 25% salt solution for 5 days will also destroy the cysticerci.

Symptomatology and pathology. Many

people harbor this parasite with no noticeable disturbances of any kind. Anemia and eosinophilia are uncommon but sometimes occur. Because of their size, the worms may conceivably cause intestinal obstruction, though this is very rare. The majority of patients are asymptomatic. The most prevalent symptoms, when present, are epigastric pain, weight loss, and anorexia. Many believe some of these symptoms to be psychosomatic. In areas where malnutrition is widespread, the presence of *Taenia saginata* in the intestinal tract may play a role in nutritional deficiency.

Tolerance to this tapeworm is well illustrated by the professor who harbored a beef tapeworm, much to his pleasure, because it furnished teaching material for his class. In time he became quite attached to the parasite. Much to his dismay, however, one day the tapeworm lost its grip on things and passed on, thus severing a mutual friendship of long standing.

Diagnosis. Eggs in the feces cannot be differentiated from those of *Taenia solium*. The gravid proglottids, when pressed between two slides and examined over a strong light, reveal the characteristic uterine branching. Injecting india ink into the central uterine system using a 25 gauge needle and syringe will dye the branches. The number of lateral branches on one side of the median stem averages 15 to 35. For the sake of convenience, the number 13 is easier to remember, and more than 13 branches on a side means *T. saginata* versus the proglottid of *T. solium*, which averages 7 to 10 (less than 13) branches. Cellophane tape impressions of the perianal region may reveal ova when stool specimens are negative. If the scolex is recovered, identification can be further verified. Proglottids not infrequently migrate out of the anus, even when defecation is not involved.

Treatment. Many preparations have been used in the treatment of tapeworm infections in humans. A crude extract of pumpkin seeds

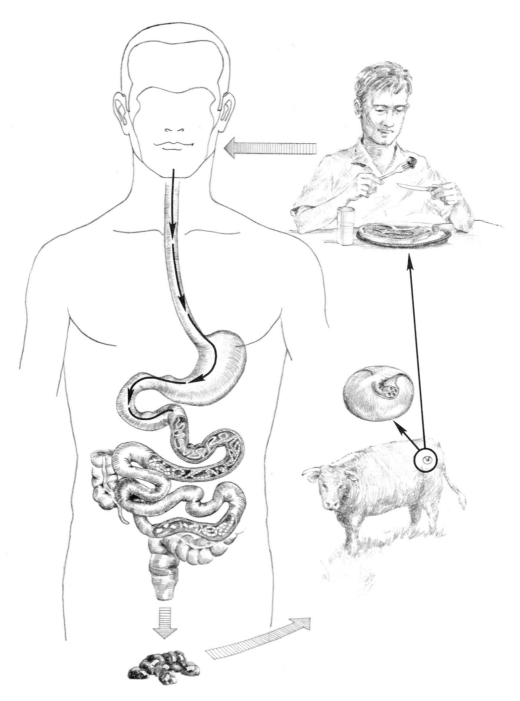

Fig. 10-7. Life cycle of *Taenia saginata*. Gravid proglottids passed in the feces of the host are ingested by cattle grazing in the meadow. Cysticerci develop in the skeletal muscle. The ingestion of raw or insufficiently cooked beef by man results in the establishment of the strobila in the small intestine.

Table 10-1. Treatment for tapeworms

Infection	Drug	Adult dose*	Pediatric dose*
Adult or intestinal stage			
Dibothriocephalus (Diphyllobothrium) latus (fish tapeworm), *Taenia saginata* (beef tapeworm), *Taenia solium* (pork tapeworm),[1] *Dipylidium caninum* (dog tapeworm), *Hymenolepis diminuta* (rat tapeworm)			
Drug of choice	Niclosamide[2]	A single dose of 4 tablets (2 gm) chewed thoroughly	*11-34 kg:* a single dose of 2 tablets (1 gm); *>34 kg:* a single dose of 3 tablets (1.5 gm)
Alternative	Paromomycin[3]	1 gm q15min × 4 doses	11 mg/kg q15min × 4 doses
Hymenolepis nana (dwarf tapeworm)			
Drug of choice	Niclosamide[2]	A single daily dose of 4 tablets (2 gm) chewed thoroughly × 5d	*11-34 kg:* a single daily dose of 2 tablets (1 gm) × 5d; *>34 kg:* a single daily dose of 3 tablets (1.5 gm) × 5d
Alternative	Paromomycin[3]	45 mg/kg once/d × 5-7d	45 mg/kg once/d × 5-7d
Larval or tissue stage			
Echinococcus granulosus (sheep, cattle, human, deer hydatid cysts)			
Drug of choice	See footnote 4		
Cysticercus cellulosae (T. solium)			
Drug of choice	None (surgical)		

Adverse effects of antiparasitic drugs

Niclosamide (Yomesan)
  Occasional: nausea; abdominal pain
Paromomycin (Humatin)
  Frequent: GI disturbance
  Rare: eighth-nerve damage (mainly auditory); renal damage

From The Medical Letter, Inc., 56 Harrison Street, New Rochelle, N.Y.
*The letter d indicates day.
1. Niclosamide and paromomycin are effective for the treatment of *T. solium* but since they disintegrate segments and release viable eggs their use creates a theoretical risk of causing cysticercosis.
2. In the U.S.A., this drug is available from the Parasitic Diseases Division, Center for Disease Control, Atlanta, Georgia 30333; telephone 404-329-3311.
3. Considered an investigational drug for this condition by the U.S. Food and Drug Administration.
4. Surgical resection of cysts is the treatment of choice. When surgery is contraindicated, or cysts rupture spontaneously during surgery, mebendazole (experimental for this purpose) can be tried (Bekhti, A., et al., Br. Med. J. **2:**1047, 1977; Beard, T. C., et al., Med. J. Austr. **1:**633, 1978). For details, call the Parasitic Diseases Division, Center for Disease Control (404-329-3311).

has been shown to be effective for both beef and pork tapeworms. For many years oleoresin of aspidium (filixmas, or the male fern of *Dryopteris*) was the drug of choice, and in some areas it is still used. Quinacrine hydrochloride (Atabrine) has been widely used also, but the drug of choice for *T. saginata* is niclosamide (Yomesan) in the dosage of 4 tablets (2 gm) chewed thoroughly in a single dose after a light meal (Table 10-1). Occasional nausea and abdominal pain may occur. The drug is available from the Para-sitic Disease Drug Service of the Center for Disease Control, Atlanta, Georgia. As an alternative, four doses of paromomycin (Humatin), given as 1 gm once every 15 minutes, is recommended. Gastrointestinal disturbances and renal damage are frequent. Occasionally eighth-nerve damage (mainly auditory) may occur. This drug is considered investigational only for this infection by the U.S. Food and Drug Administration.

Beef tapeworms are normally few; only one or two are usually present. The value of searching for the scolex in the feces to determine the efficacy of treatment seems rather dubious. It is akin to searching for a needle in a haystack, and the reward is questionable since another scolex may still be present in the patient. If the scolex still remains, a wait of 2 to 3 months will reveal another strobila and treatment will have to be reinstituted.

Taenia solium

Geographic distribution. The pork tapeworm, *Taenia solium*, is cosmopolitan in distribution and most common in countries where raw or insufficiently cooked pork is eaten. It is common throughout Mexico and South America as well as in the Balkan states and the Slavic countries. Among the Jews and Muslims it is noticeably absent because of the religious taboo against eating pork. One of the enigmas of parasitology is the fact that in the United States cysticerci in pork is quite common in some areas, whereas adult tapeworms in humans are practically nonexistent. Humans are the only known definitive host.

Morphology and life cycle. Many similarities exist between *T. solium* and *T. saginata*. The essential differences are that the chief intermediate host for *T. solium* is the pig and, most important medically, is the fact that humans may also be the intermediate host. The adult tapeworm averages 6 to 10 feet in length and has less than 1,000 proglottids in the strobila. The scolex is small, about 1 mm in diameter (Fig. 10-8). In addition to the four typical suckers, the rostellum is armed with two rows of hooks, an addi-

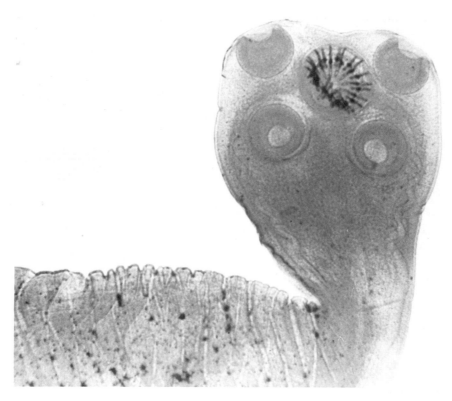

Fig. 10-8. Scolex of *Taenia solium*. Note the presence of hooks. (From a nonprofit cooperative endeavor by numerous colleagues under the editorship of Dr. Herman Zaiman, Valley City, N.D.)

tional aid for holding on to the mucosa. Like *T. saginata*, this tapeworm is found in the upper regions of the small intestine, and gravid proglottids are passed in the feces singly or in short chains. (Unlike those of *T. saginata*, they are flabby and inactive) (Fig. 10-9). To the experienced observer this difference will readily identify the tapeworm. The coprophagic habit of pigs leads to heavy infections that apparently are tolerated well by this animal. When measly pork is eaten by a human, the scolex is liberated from the cysticercus, evaginates, attaches itself to the mucosal wall, and develops a mature strobila in 2 to 3 months. The gravid proglottids contain eggs morphologically similar to those of *T. saginata*. Eggs average around 35 μm in diameter and contain hexacanth embryos within (Fig. 10-5). They are seen less frequently in the stool than those of *T. saginata*, undoubtedly because the uterine branches are less frequently ruptured in the separation of gravid proglottids from the strobila. In the intermediate host, which, in addition to the pig, may also be humans, camels, dogs, monkeys, sheep, deer, and other animals, each liberated onchosphere claws its way through the mucosal wall and penetrates lymphatics and blood vessels. After traveling around the body, the majority come to rest and undergo development to the cysticercus stage in the musculature (Fig. 10-10).

Epidemiology. Although humans are the only definitive host for *T. solium*, the incidence of human infection is relatively rare in some areas, compared with the prevalence of cysticercosis in hogs, the chief source of infection for humans. The acceptance by hogs of fecally contaminated slop and their habit of foraging in polluted areas results in a high incidence, which in some regions runs as high as 25%. The thorough cooking of pork and pork products is, obviously, essential in the prevention of infection and is more economically feasible in many areas than is changing the diet of pigs, though the latter approach is certainly to be desired. As indicated, the presence of *T. solium* in the intestinal tract of humans requires treatment, to prevent not only autoinfection but also dissemination of eggs to humans and other animals, chiefly the hog.

Symptomatology and pathology. Like *T. saginata*, the pork tapeworm in the intestinal tract of humans will frequently produce few if any symptoms. However, the fact that humans may be an intermediate host as well, with major tissue pathologic changes, signs, and symptoms, places a different significance on this tapeworm. This manifestation of infection, cysticercosis, is discussed on p. 214.

Diagnosis. Usually only one adult is pres-

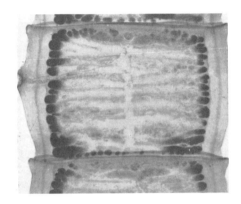

Fig. 10-9. Gravid proglottid of *Taenia solium*. Note the smaller number of lateral branches (less than thirteen) emanating from the median stem on each side, as compared with *T. saginata*. (Courtesy Dr. Michael Ivey, Department of Preventive Medicine and Public Health, University of Oklahoma School of Medicine.)

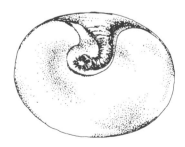

Fig. 10-10. Cysticercus larva of *Taenia solium*. Note the armed scolex.

ent. Gravid proglottids in the feces can readily be identified by counting the 7 to 10 uterine branches on one side of the median stem, less than 13 being easily remembered as diagnostic. Eggs, not common in the feces, are morphologically similar to those of *T. saginata*. When the scolex is recovered, specific identification can easily be made by the presence of the armed rostellum not seen with *T. saginata*.

Treatment. Treatment for the adult tapeworm is the same as for *T. saginata*. The drug of choice is niclosamide administered as 4 tablets (2 gm) chewed thoroughly in a single dose after a light meal. Paromomycin is likewise its alternative in the same dosage (1 gm every 15 minutes for 4 doses) as for *T. saginata* (Table 10-1). It is particularly important to avoid nausea and vomiting because of the danger of gravid proglottids and eggs being brought into the stomach by reverse peristalsis, with the resultant risk of cysticercosis. Purgation should follow 1 to 2 hours after treatment. The efficacy of treatment can be determined in 2 to 3 months by the presence or absence of proglottids in the stool.

Hymenolepis diminuta

The parasite *Hymenolepis diminuta*, a rat tapeworm, is an accidental, sporadic tapeworm in the small intestine of humans throughout the world. It is most prevalent where sanitation is poor, occurring most commonly in the tropics and subtropics. Infections have been reported in numerous states in the United States. The adult tapeworm may reach lengths of 90 cm with gravid proglottids about 5 mm in diameter. The scolex with four suckers is unarmed. Gravid proglottids disintegrate in the lumen of the intestine, liberating the embryonated eggs, which average 60 to 80 μm in diameter and become bile stained before passage from the intestinal tract (Fig. 10-11). The chief intermediate hosts are the larvae of rat and mice fleas and adult grain beetles. In the body cavity of the intermediate host the oncho-

sphere develops into a cysticercoid type of larva. When the adult intermediate host is accidentally eaten by humans, the liberated scolex evaginates, holds on to the intestinal mucosa, and develops a strobila. Human infections are associated chiefly with the contamination of cereals, grains, and other foodstuffs by infected grain beetles. Symptoms in humans are usually mild and, since humans are an abnormal host, the tapeworms are frequently lost spontaneously. Diagnosis is

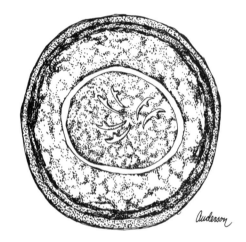

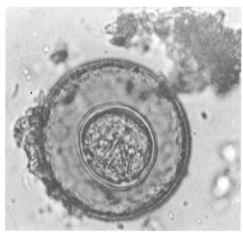

Fig. 10-11. Egg of *Hymenolepis diminuta*, with drawing. Note the characteristic shell membranes with the absence of polar knobs and filaments. (Photomicrograph courtesy Department of Pathology, University of Miami, School of Medicine.)

made by recovery and identification of the typical bile-stained ova in the feces. The onchosphere within is surrounded by an inner shell membrane without knobs. Surrounding this is the outer bile-stained shell layer. Treatment, when necessary, is the same as for the taenias. Many times a strong cathartic is sufficient.

Hymenolepis nana

Geographic distribution. The dwarf tapeworm, *Hymenolepis nana*, was first described in rats and mice, but subsequently humans have been added to the list of com-

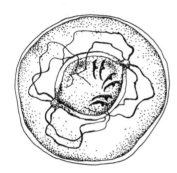

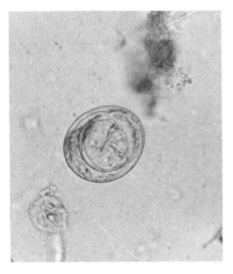

Fig. 10-12. Egg of *Hymenolepis nana*, with drawing. Note the characteristic shell membranes with the presence of polar knobs and filaments. (Photomicrograph courtesy Department of Pathology, University of Miami, School of Medicine.)

monly infected hosts. It is cosmopolitan in distribution, occurring most frequently in children in the tropics and subtropics. It is the most common human tapeworm in the southeastern United States.

Morphology and life cycle. The size of the adult worm is inversely proportional to the number present in the intestinal tract. In a moderate infection the average size varies from 20 to 30 mm, with a maximum width of about 500 μm. The scolex, with the usual tetrad of cuplike suckers, is armed. The entire strobila presents the appearance of a mucus thread. The gravid proglottids disintegrate in the bowel, liberating embryonated eggs that pass out of the feces. The eggs average about 40 μm $\times$ 50 μm in size and are composed of a hexacanth embryo surrounded by an inner shell (Fig. 10-12). This embryophore is oval and contains knobs on either end, from which emanate delicate filaments extending into the gelatinlike matrix. It is surrounded by a thin, colorless, round to oval shell membrane. When ingested by the larvae of rat and mice fleas or the adults of grain beetles, the eggs develop in the body cavity into cysticercoid larvae (cercocystis larvae). When the adult intermediate hosts are eaten by humans or other appropriate definitive hosts, the adult tapeworm develops in the small intestine. Like *T. solium*, humans may also serve as an intermediate host. When eggs are swallowed, the six-hooked embryos claw their way into the villi of the intestinal wall and there undergo development to the cysticercoid stage. This takes about 4 days. No invasion of the deeper tissues or circulation occurs. The cysticercoid attaches itself to the mucosal wall and a strobila is developed, egg production appearing in about 15 to 20 days. Experimental evidence in mice shows that these eggs in turn may hatch while still in the intestinal tract, invade the villi, and thus establish new infections. In this manner an initially light infection in a person may become a very heavy one.

Epidemiology. Infections with *Hymenolepis nana* are confined chiefly to children. The incidence declines after 8 years of age. In the southern United States approximately 3% of the population is infected. Infections are transmitted chiefly by hand-to-mouth contact, the children soiling their hands in contaminated areas of play. Though humans themselves are the chief source of human infection, rodents (rats and mice) may also be involved. The murine strains show varying degrees of susceptibility to humans. The accidental ingestion of mouse "pills" (feces) is believed by some to account chiefly for human infections in some areas of the southern United States. The incidence of infection is similar in cities with sewer systems and in rural areas without sewer systems. The role of infection by the ingestion of infected intermediate hosts apparently is overshadowed by murine and human fecal transmission.

Symptomatology and pathology. In light infections, symptoms may be absent or be limited to vague abdominal discomfort. In heavy infections, particularly in children, abdominal pain, nausea, vomiting, weight loss, nervousness, headaches, diarrhea, and other toxic manifestations may be present. Since the cysticercoid larvae develop in the villi, extensive erosion may be caused by overwhelming infections. Fortunately, however, no bloodstream invasion occurs and extraintestinal cysticercosis does not ensue.

Diagnosis. Recovery and identification of the eggs in the feces establish the diagnosis. Adults, when recovered, can be identified by their size and morphology.

Treatment. The drug of choice currently is niclosamide (Yomesan), available from the

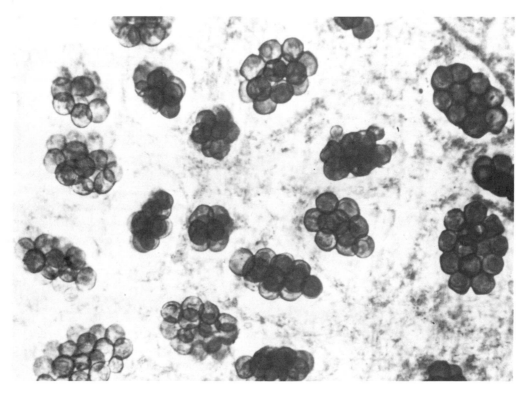

Fig. 10-13. Gravid proglottid of *Dipylidium caninum* showing area of uterine packets containing eggs. (From a nonprofit cooperative endeavor by numerous colleagues under the editorship of Dr. Herman Zaiman, Valley City, N.D.)

Parasitic Disease Drug Service, Center for Disease Control, Atlanta, Georgia, given in four tablets (2 gm), single dose, and chewed thoroughly. This is repeated daily for 5 days. The problem of autoinfection makes successful therapy difficult. Paromomycin is the alternative drug in the dosage of 45 mg/kg daily for 5 to 7 days (Table 10-1). As indicated for the taenias, this is considered an investigational drug for this infection by the U.S. Food and Drug Administration.

Dipylidium caninum

Dipylidium caninum is a common tapeworm of dogs and cats around the world. Humans are only an accidental host for the adult worm, and infections are rare. The adult tapeworm averages up to 70 cm in length. The gravid proglottids, averaging 12 mm × 2 to 5 mm, are passed in the feces and show remarkable activity, squirming about on the fecal mass. When pressed between two glass slides and examined microscopically, the barrel-shaped proglottids show typical uterine balls containing about 15 eggs per packet (Fig. 10-13). Infections occur predominantly in infants and very young children closely associated with dogs and cats. Accidental ingestion of the intermediate host, the flea, harboring the cysticercoid larva results from the licking of the child's face and mouth by the animal nurturing some fleas it has recently nipped. Abdominal discomfort, diarrhea, and pruritus may be present. Infections are often spontaneously lost. A purge may be sufficient to dislodge the worms. If treatment becomes necessary, it should be as for the taenias.

REVIEW QUESTIONS

1. Contrast the flatworms with the roundworms.
2. Describe the strobila of a tapeworm.
3. What is the source of nutrients for the tapeworm?
4. Describe the life pattern of a cyclophyllidean tapeworm.
5. Describe each of the following: cysticercus, cysticercoid, cenurus, hydatid cyst.
6. Why is an intestinal infection with *Taenia solium* more serious than one with *T. saginata?*
7. What is the treatment for tapeworm infections?
8. How can a differential diagnosis be made between *T. saginata* and *T. solium?*
9. Why are infections with *Hymenolepis nana* more common than with other tapeworms?
10. How are infections with *Hymenolepis diminuta* contracted? *Dipylidium caninum?*

REFERENCES

Beck, J. W. 1951. Effect of diet upon singly established *Hymenolepis diminuta* in rats. Exp. Parasitol. **1:**46-59.

Daugherty, J. W., and W. B. Foster. 1958. Comparative studies on amino acid absorption by cestodes. Exp. Parasitol. **7:**99-107.

Fetterman, L. E. 1965. Radiographic demonstration of *Taenia saginata:* an unsuspected cause of abdominal pain. N. Engl. J. Med. **272:**364-365.

Gleason, N. N. 1962. Records of *Dipylidium caninum,* the double-pored tapeworm. J. Parasitol. **48:**812.

Heyneman, D. 1962. Studies on helminth immunity. IV. Rapid onset of resistance by the white mouse against a challenging infection with eggs of *Hymenolepis nana* (Cestoda: Hymenolepididae). J. Immunol. **88:**217-220.

Keeling, J. E. D. 1968. The chemotherapy of cestode infections. Pages 109-152. In Advances in chemotherapy. Academic Press, Inc., New York.

Most, H., M. Yoeli, J. Hammond, and G. P. Scheinesson. 1971. Yomesan (Niclosamide) therapy of *Hymenolepis nana* infections. Am. J. Trop. Med. Hyg. **20:**206-208.

Pawlowski, Z., and M. G. Schultz. 1972. Taeniasis and cysticercosis *(Taenia saginata).* Adv. Parasitol. **10:**269-343.

Proctor, E. M. 1972. Identification of tapeworms. S. Afr. Med. J. **46:**234-338.

Read, C. P. 1959. The role of carbohydrates in the biology of cestodes. VIII. Some conclusions and hypotheses. Exp. Parasitol. **8:**365-382.

Slais, J. 1970. The morphology and pathogenicity of the bladder worm *Cysticercus cellulose* and *Cysticercus bovis.* The Hague, Netherlands.

Ulivelli, A. 1968. Paromomycin and taeniasis. Lancet **1:**696.

Upton, A. C. 1950. Taenial proglottids in the appendix: possible association with appendicitis. Am. J. Clin. Pathol. **20:**1117-1120.

Wardle, R. A., J. A. McLeod, and S. Radinovsky. 1974. Advances in the zoology of tapeworms, 1950-1970. University of Minnesota Press, Minneapolis.

Wittner, M., and H. Tanowitz. 1971. Paromomycin therapy of human cestodiasis with special reference to hymenolepiasis. Am. J. Trop. Med. Hyg. **20:**433-435.

CHAPTER 11

The pseudophyllidean tapeworms (Pseudophyllidea)

Only one pseudophyllidean tapeworm is of medical importance because it parasitizes the intestinal tract of humans—*Dibothrioceph-alus latus (Diphyllobothrium latum)*. References occur in the literature to sporadic infections in humans, with closely related species of lower animals, such as *Diphyllobothrium cordatum* in the seal, walrus, and dog in Greenland and Iceland, *D. houghtoni* in the dog and cat in China, *D. ursi* in bears in North America. Those invading human tissues are discussed under somatic tapeworms on p. 221.

Dibothriocephalus latus

Geographic distribution. The tapeworm *Dibothriocephalus latus* is most frequently found in the temperate regions where the eating of freshwater fish is quite common. In the western hemisphere this is around the Great Lakes in both Canada and the United States. *D. latus* occurs also in Alaska and other parts of western and central Canada and the United States. In South America it is prevalent in Chile and Argentina. It is common in many parts of Europe, approximately 20% of the Finnish people being infected. In some areas in the Baltic region, infection runs as high as 100%. Endemic areas are also reported in central Africa and parts of Asia.

Morphology and life cycle. In addition to humans, the definitive host may be the dog, cat, or, less frequently, a variety of other fish-eating mammals. The adult tapeworm lives predominately in the ileum and attaches itself to the mucosal wall by the almond-shaped scolex, which contains two slitlike grooves or suckers running longitudinally almost the length of the scolex (Fig. 11-1). From the neck region is elaborated a long chain of segments or proglottids numbering 3,000 to 4,000 per strobila and reaching lengths of 30 feet or more. Usually only one tapeworm is found per host; when more than one is present, the size of each is proportionately smaller. The segments are broader than they are long, measuring approximately 3 mm × 11 mm. Because of this feature, the parasite is commonly known as the "broad tapeworm" of humans. Since the definitive host acquires the infection from eating fish, the worm is also referred to as the "fish tapeworm" of humans. The majority of the proglottids mature simultaneously and produce eggs that are deposited through a uterine pore (Fig. 11-2). The eggs that pass out in the feces are oval in shape, with a shell membrane, and average 60 μm × 40 μm in size. They are characterized by an operculum or lid at one end that opens at hatching to allow exit of the embryo. At the opposite end of the egg is a knoblike structure that helps in identification. The shell membrane is filled with yolk material surrounding the small fertilized ovum. When egg laying is complete, the spent proglottid atrophies but usually remains attached to the strobila. The life span of the tapeworm may be 30 years or more (Fig. 11-3).

Two intermediate hosts are necessary to complete the life cycle. The eggs, in fresh water, undergo development, and in 1 to 2 weeks a ciliated embryo called a coracidium hatches through the operculum. The coracidium consists of a typical hexacanth embryo surrounded by a ciliated membrane. It swims about in the fresh water until ingested by the appropriate species of copepods (a type of crustacean) within 24 hours. Otherwise death occurs. Within the copepod the liberated onchosphere burrows its way through the gut wall into the body cavity. In approximately 2 weeks the onchosphere develops into an elongated wormlike organism with a large knoblike structure (cercomer) on the posterior end, which contains the embryonic hooks. The cercomer is eventually discarded. At the anterior end of the larva, a slight depression is formed, in which lytic glands develop (Fig. 11-4). This larval form is now known as the procercoid and averages about 500 μm in length. When the copepod is eaten by the appropriate freshwater fish, the liberated procercoid larva burrows through the gut wall into the body cavity, eventually reaches the flesh of the fish, and within a month develops into the next larval stage, the plerocercoid, or sparganum. The plerocercoid larva lies unencysted in the flesh of the fish. It averages 4 to 5 mm or longer, with great variation in size. The anterior end is characterized by the development of an inverted scolex. The remainder of the larva is an elongated, wrinkly, flattened, white mass of tissue. When humans or other suitable definitive hosts eat raw fish containing the plerocercoid larva, the body of the larva degenerates, the scolex everts itself, attaches to the mucosa, and develops a strobila. A fully developed worm results in about 3 weeks (Fig. 11-5).

Epidemiology. Credit for the presence of this parasite in humans in the western hemisphere has been given to the Scandinavians

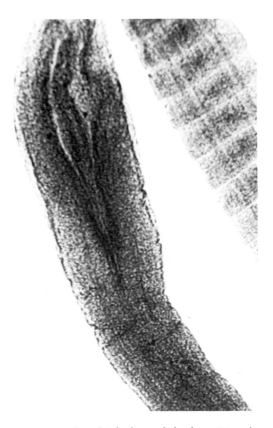

Fig. 11-1. Scolex of *Dibothriocephalus latus*. Note the longitudinal groove or bothrium and the portion of immature segments to the side. (From a nonprofit cooperative endeavor by numerous colleagues under the editorship of Dr. Herman Zaiman, Valley City, N.D.)

who migrated to the northern woods in the early colonizing period, but the possibilities of the infection being carried across the Bering Straits or the presence of a native species in wild carnivores (brown bear) of the western hemisphere also exist.

The role of first intermediate host in the United States and Canada is restricted to certain species of the copepod, *Diaptomus*. These copepods are quite commonly eaten by small fish, such as minnows, in which the procercoid larvae do not undergo further development but merely lie dormant. When these small fish are in turn eaten by larger fish, the same dormancy occurs again. Only

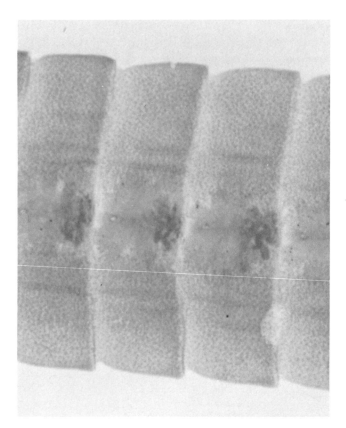

Fig. 11-2. Gravid proglottid of *Dibothrio-cephalus latus.* Note the rosette uterus. (From a nonprofit cooperative endeavor by numerous colleagues under the editorship of Dr. Herman Zaiman, Valley City, N.D.)

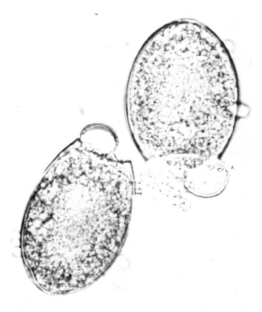

Fig. 11-3. Eggs of *Dibothriocephalus latus* showing open opercula. Note the slight thickening of the shell membrane at the opposite end of each egg. (From a nonprofit cooperative endeavor by numerous colleagues under the editorship of Dr. Herman Zaiman, Valley City, N.D.)

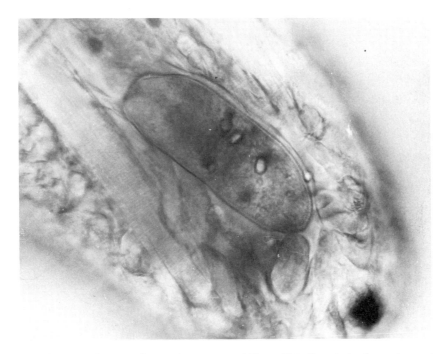

Fig. 11-4. Body cavity of a copepod containing a procercoid larva. Note the anterior depression, posterior cercomer, and internal calcareous granules. (Photograph by Justus F. Mueller. From Schmidt, G. D. and Roberts, L. S.: Foundations of parasitology, St. Louis, 1977, The C. V. Mosby Co.)

when the proper second intermediate hosts, such as the larger game fish, eat the smaller infected fish do the procercoid larvae continue their development. In the northern United States and Canada, predominately in the lake regions, a large percentage of pike and walleyed pike had been infected with the plerocercoid larvae of *D. latus*. The high incidence was attributable to the pollution of the lakes and streams by sewage pumped directly into these waters from small towns bordering them. However, recent surveys of fish for plerocercoid larvae suggest that the incidence has dropped. Dogs and cats, given the fish refuse from camp cookouts, hotels, and the like, help to sustain the tapeworm life cycle. Pike and walleyed pike are considered choice fish in the preparation of gelfilte fish by Jewish housewives; tasting for seasoning before cooking is a gastronomic necessity, and thus the housewives become infected. In other countries, a taste for raw fish dishes contributes to the prevalence of infection. Obviously the pollution of streams and lakes is a major factor in the continuance of this disease, and the prevention of this pollution along with adequate cooking of all freshwater fish would break the life cycle and eliminate the parasite from the human domain.

Symptomatology and pathology. Single-worm infections are most common and most infected persons apparently are asymptomatic. As with the other large tapeworms, intestinal obstruction is possible. Some catarrhal inflammation of the mucosa may occur. A modest eosinophilia and the various complaints of nausea, abdominal discomfort, nervousness, weakness, loss of appetite, or hunger pains have been attributed to the parasite. This tapeworm, however, is unique in that in 1% of infected persons its presence is associated with a megaloblastic anemia, which may be associated with combined sys-

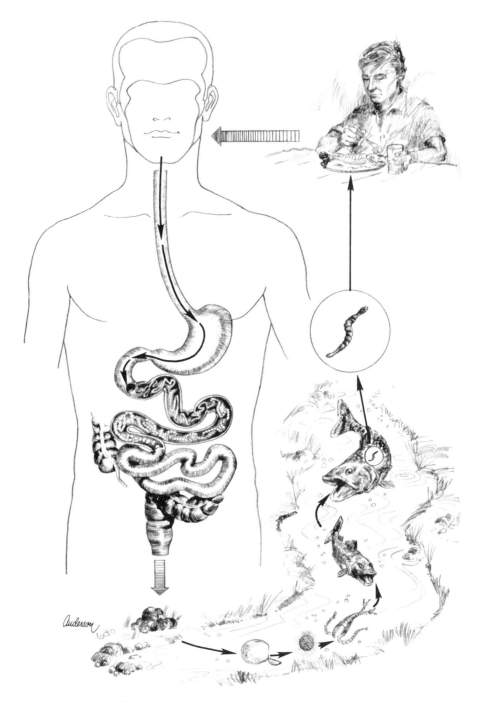

Fig. 11-5. Life cycle of *Dibothriocephalus latus*. The plerocercoid larva in raw or insufficiently cooked freshwater fish, when ingested, develops into the strobila of *D. latus* in the small intestine of humans. Immature eggs passed in the feces of humans into freshwater develop a ciliated embryo within, called a coracidium. Hatching occurs and appropriate species of copepods, commonly *Diaptomus* and *Cyclops*, ingest the coracidia, which develop into procercoid larvae in the body cavity. Small game fish ingest infected copepods and, in turn, are eaten by large game fish. In the flesh of the appropriate freshwater fish the procercoid larvae develop into plerocercoid larvae, which serve as the source of infection for humans.

temic degeneration. Unlike true pernicious anemia, it occurs in all age groups regardless of gastric acidity. The location of the worms in the intestinal tract seems to be important; in anemic patients they are always high up in the jejunum, whereas nonanemic patients seem to harbor them in the ileum. It is postulated that the tapeworms near the duodenum compete for vitamin B_{12}. Analyses of the worms show a very high absorption of vitamin B_{12}, over 50 times greater than that of *Taenia saginata*. (Several workers have demonstrated that the administration of powdered worms along with gastric juice will cure pernicious anemia as effectively as vitamin B_{12} alone.) The absorption of folic acid by the tapeworm contributes to the megaloblastic anemia. This anemia is prevalent among the Finnish people where one third of all pernicious anemias are associated with *D. latus* infection. It is commonly referred to as "bothriocephalus anemia," or "dibothriocephalus anemia."

Diagnosis. The diagnosis of infection can readily be made by recovery and identification of the typical operculated eggs in the feces of the host. Spent proglottids when found in the feces, though atrophied, will reveal the diagnostic rosette uterus.

Treatment. Treatment is the same as for the taenias with niclosamide 4 tablets (2 gm) chewed thoroughly in a single dose and paromomycin as the alternative (1 gm every 15 minutes for 4 doses) (Table 10-1). Temporary remission of the anemia may be effected with

the administration of vitamin B_{12}, with the worm in place. Removal of the worms is necessary for permanent cure.

REVIEW QUESTIONS

1. What are the essential differences in the morphology of *Dibothriocephalus latus* as compared with a cyclophyllidean tapeworm?
2. What is the epidemiology of the broad fish tapeworm infections in the United States?
3. What is "bothriocephalus anemia"? Discuss.
4. What is the treatment for the broad fish tapeworm in humans?

REFERENCES

Baer, J. G. 1969. *Diphyllobothrium pacificum*, a tapeworm from seal lions endemic in man along the coastal area of Peru. J. Fish Res. Bd. (Canada) **26**:717-723.
Baer, J. G., C. H. Miranda, R. W. Fernandez, and T. J. Medina. 1967. Human diphyllobothriasis in Peru. Z. Parasitenkd. **28**:277-289.
Birkeland, I. W. 1932. Bothriocephalus anemia. Medicine **11**:1-139.
Faust, E. C. 1952. Some morphologic characters of *Diphyllobothrium latum*. An. Inst. Med. Trop. (Lisboa) **9**:1277-1300.
Margolis, L., R. L. Rausch, and E. Robertson. 1973. *Diphyllobothrium ursi* from man in British Colombia: first report of this tapeworm in Canada. Can. J. Public Health. **64**:588-589.
Tanowitz, H. B., and M. Wittner. 1973. Paromomycin in the treatment of *Diphyllobothrium latum* infection. J. Trop. Med. Hyg. **76**:151-152.
Von Bonsdorff, B. 1956. *Diphyllobothrium latum* as a cause of pernicious anemia. Exp. Parasitol. **5**:207-230.
Von Bonsdorff, B. 1977. Diphyllobothriasis in man. Academic Press, Inc., New York.
Wardle, R. A., J. A. McLeod, and S. Radinovsky. 1974. Advances in the zoology of tapeworms, 1950-1970. University of Minnesota Press, Minneapolis.
Wolfgang, R. W. 1954. Indian and Eskimo diphyllobothriasis. Canad. Med. Assoc. J. **70**:536-539.

CHAPTER 12

The somatic tapeworms

The larval stages of several species of tapeworms develop in the extraintestinal tissues of humans. The cysticercus, cenurus, hydatid cyst, and plerocercoid larva are represented in this group.

CYSTICERCOSIS

Humans may serve as the intermediate host for *Taenia solium*. Hexacanth embryos, when ingested by mouth in contaminated food or drink, or by hand-to-mouth contact, hatch in the small intestine, where the liberated onchospheres burrow into the mucosal circulation and are carried throughout the body. Systemic infection may also occur with the displacement of eggs into the stomach through reverse peristalsis; for this reason, vomiting may be dangerous for persons with intestinal *T. solium* infection.

Cysticerci may develop in any organ or tissue of the body (Fig. 12-1). The fully developed cysticercus is a small bladder filled with fluid and measuring approximately 5 mm × 10 mm in size. Developed from the inner wall is an invaginated scolex on a small stalk. This white spot within the cysticercus is readily discernible with the naked eye. Cysticerci survive for 3 to 5 years (Fig. 12-2).

The clinical picture depends on their location and number. Light infections are probably common and asymptomatic. Symptoms usually result from the death of the larvae in the visceral organs, secondary to swelling or to the release of foreign proteins. Cysticerci in the musculature and subcutaneous tissues are well tolerated. Palpable lesions or radiographic calcifications in muscles may be noted. Invasion of the eye (Fig. 12-3), spinal cord, and brain may present serious complications, even death. Epilepsy is a common sequel of central nervous system invasion; large numbers of British soldiers stationed only briefly in endemic areas during World War II were later afflicted. Unencapsulated larvae (racemose type), with numerous branches and reaching lengths of 15 cm, may be found in the subarachnoid spaces at the base of the brain. Both this form, which clinically presents as intermittent hydrocephalus, and epilepsy have a poor prognosis. The death of increasing numbers of cysticerci over a period of years produces cumulative effects.

Diagnosis can be made by biopsy, occasionally by visualization of the motile larvae in the eye, or by the characteristic appearance of calcified larvae on x-ray film of muscles; cysticerci in the brain rarely calcify. A history of present infection with the adult tapeworm is highly suggestive but frequently absent.

Treatment is unsatisfactory. Antiepileptic drugs can be used for epilepsy. Surgery is sometimes useful in treating cerebral cysticercosis.

CENUROSIS

Multiceps multiceps is a common cyclophyllidean tapeworm of dogs, particularly in sheep-raising countries of the world. The intermediate host is a herbivore, usually a goat or sheep, in which the cenurus larva develops. Invasion of the central nervous system results in a condition referred to as

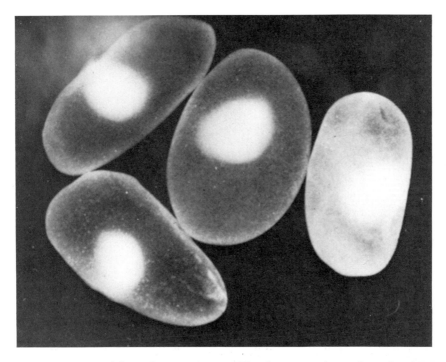

Fig. 12-1. Cysticerci excised from subcutaneous tissue. Note the opaque white scolex within. (AFIP 69-9754.)

"gid," or "vertigo." The cenurus is a bladder worm similar to the cysticercus but larger, at times containing up to 75 scolices on the inner wall. A limited number of larval infections in humans have been reported around the world, including the United States. Other species of *Multiceps* have also been incriminated. The prognosis is grave. There is no specific treatment, and diagnosis is rarely made during life. Obviously, prevention of contamination of food and drink is essential.

HYDATID DISEASE (HYDATIDOSIS)

The larval stage of species of the cyclophyllidean tapeworm *Echinococcus* is known as the hydatid cyst. Several species occur in humans.

Echinococcus granulosus

Geographic distribution. The tapeworm *Echinococcus granulosus*, parasitic in the dog

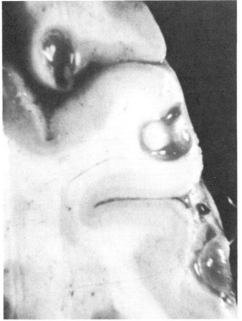

Fig. 12-2. Cysticercosis of the brain. (From a nonprofit cooperative endeavor by numerous colleagues under the editorship of Dr. Herman Zaiman, Valley City, N.D.)

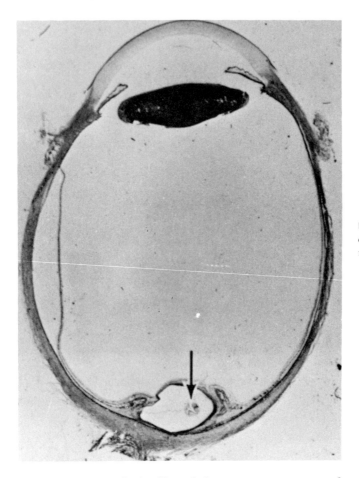

Fig. 12-3. Cysticercus *(arrow)* in the eye between the retina and vitreous, near the macula. (AFIP 74-12712.)

and similar animals (wolf, jackal, coyote, wildcat, and fox), is cosmopolitan in distribution but particularly common in sheep- and cattle-raising countries of the world. Human infections are found in Uruguay, Chile, Argentina, areas of Africa, eastern and southern Europe, the Middle East, Australia, New Zealand, extensive areas of central Asia, north China, southwestern United States, Canada, the Central Valley in California, and Utah.

Morphology and life cycle. The adult tapeworm is small, measuring only 2 to 9 mm in length, and consists of an armed scolex and one immature, one or two mature, and one gravid proglottid (Fig. 12-4). It lives in the small intestine of the dog and related animals and has a life span of about 5 months.

Heavy infections produce no apparent harm to their hosts. The eggs, passed in the feces, are similar to *Taenia* eggs. When ingested by the appropriate intermediate herbivorous host, such as sheep, cattle, horses, pigs, rabbits, moose, elk, and also humans, the liberated onchosphere claws its way into the intestinal wall and passes through the portal system to the liver. Most of the eggs are trapped in the liver and develop into hydatid cysts. Initially a hollow bladder is formed and, growing slowly, reaches a size of about 10 mm in 5 months. A cross-section of the cyst wall reveals a white laminated membrane about 1 mm thick without nuclei and an inner germinal layer about 10 to 15 μm in thickness with nuclei (Fig. 12-5). As the cyst grows, host reaction results in the formation

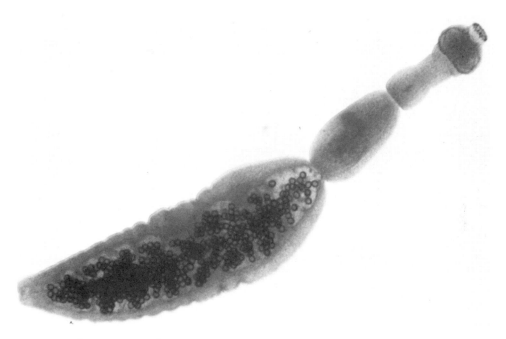

Fig. 12-4. *Echinococcus granulosus*, adult tapeworm of dogs and similar animals. Note the eggs in the gravid proglottid. (From a nonprofit cooperative endeavor by numerous colleagues under the editorship of Dr. Herman Zaiman, Valley City, N.D.)

of a fibrous connective-tissue cyst wall. From the inner germinative wall of the parasite itself, hollow secondary cysts develop. They are known as brood capsules and, as they grow, invaginated scolices develop from their inner wall. Each scolex is ovoid and contains the typical four suckers, a double crown of hooklets, and calcareous bodies or granules. Escaped scolices from brood capsules, free-floating brood capsules, and bits of the germinative wall broken off from the parent wall, floating free within the nearly colorless fluid, are known as "hydatid sand." At times, buds from the germinative wall of the mother cyst, perhaps by herniation or broken bits of germinative tissue, give rise to daughter cysts and, in turn, to granddaughter cysts, which grow independently within the cyst fluid. Over the years the mother cyst may reach the size of a grapefruit or larger, containing 15 quarts or more of fluid. Over 2 million scolices may be produced in one such cyst. Because this type of hydatid

is single, it is also referred to as a unilocular cyst. Some cysts fail to develop brood capsules; they then become "sterile" cysts. Multiple cysts in the liver may be the result of multiple egg infections or the formation of exogenous daughter cysts as a result of herniation of the germinative layer before the host response has resulted in a fibrous connective tissue wall. Hydatid cysts in bone do not become spherical but fill the narrow cavities and cause erosion.

The life cycle is completed when the infected intermediate host is eaten by the definitive host, each scolex ingested being capable of developing into an adult worm in the intestinal tract in about 7 weeks.

Epidemiology. Infections are heaviest in cattle- and sheep-raising countries where domestic dogs are used. Infections are also sylvatic when dogs, foxes, wolves, jackals, or other animals supply infective eggs for pigs, rabbits, moose, elk, and the like. The dogs and related animals ingest numerous scolices

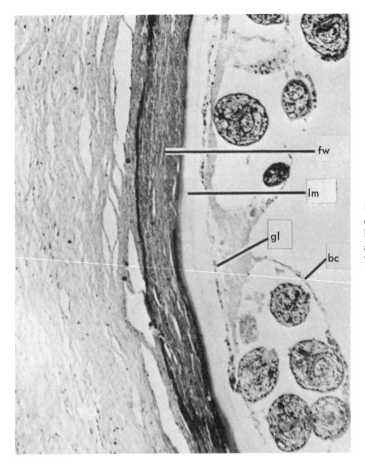

Fig. 12-5. Section of unilocular hydatid cyst. Brood capsule *(bc)*, germinal layer *(gl)*, laminated membrane *(lm)*, and fibrous wall of host *(fw)*. (AFIP N-74378.)

while eating the entrails of animals with hydatid cysts and develop very heavy infections. They, in turn, sow the tapeworm eggs over extensive land areas. Cattle and sheep grazing on contaminated pastures thus become infected. Cattle, however, do not play a significant role as a reservoir source of infection for dogs and related animals since the majority of hydatid cysts are sterile in those animals. Humans become an accidental host chiefly by intimate association with dogs. In circumpolar areas, wolves, moose, and elks maintain the cycle. In slaughterhouses in the United States, it is not uncommon to find pig livers with hydatid cysts, either dogs, foxes, or wild furbearing animals serving as the source of infection. Hydatid disease in the United States

is reported in the southwest, chiefly among Navaho Indians. In Utah, more surgical cases have occurred than in any other state except Alaska. More than 40 cases requiring surgical removal from the liver or lungs have been recorded since 1944, labeling Utah an endemic area for hydatid disease. In the central part of the state it is estimated that about 1% of the population in some of the smaller communities has had or will have surgical removal of a cyst some time in the future. In a survey during the period from 1971 to 1976 around 11% of more than 800 dogs examined were positive for *E. granulosus*, while 9.8% of around 9,000 sheep examined were positive. Over the 6-year period a definitive decline in infection rates was noted, suggesting that preventive and con-

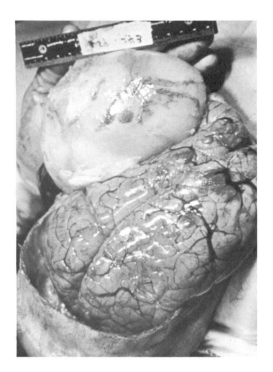

Fig. 12-6. Hydatid cyst (unilocular type) in the brain of a 7-year-old girl. (Courtesy Dr. Harold Fink, Department of Pathology, Coney Island Hospital, Brooklyn, N.Y.)

trol measures were being implemented in central Utah. In the Middle East, hydatid disease is common in sheep and cattle; among camels the infection rate approaches 100%. In Iceland, on the other hand, the disease, once prevalent, is becoming rare.

Symptomatology and pathology. Most of the hydatid cysts of the unilocular type develop in the liver, though bone, the brain, and other areas may also be invaded occasionally (Fig. 12-6). An inflammatory reaction by the host results eventually in the enveloping of the cyst by a fibrous connective tissue wall. A few dead cysts walled off in the liver are well tolerated by the host. As the cyst grows, pressure and necrosis may result in the destruction of the normal liver tissue and impaired liver function. The great danger lies in the accidental rupturing of cysts with the leakage of hydatid sand into nonwalled-off areas. New cysts may develop

nearby, or dissemination of the fluid may result in unilocular cysts being established anywhere in the body. The antigenic stimulus from this leakage may result in anaphylactic shock or at least in marked allergic reactions with a high eosinophilia. Unilocular cysts are usually quite old before being discovered in humans. They are commonly detected when x-ray examination shows a calcified cyst wall in the liver or other organ of an asymptomatic patient. Most infections in humans begin in childhood and are discovered in adult life.

Diagnosis. A history of association with dogs in an endemic area of hydatid disease, along with the detection of a slowly growing tumor mass most commonly in the liver, should lead to a presumptive clinical diagnosis. A characteristic calcified cyst wall is occasionally seen on x-ray film. The indirect hemagglutination (IHA) test and the bentonite-flocculation test (BFT) used simultaneously are the serologic tests of choice for diagnosis. A titer of 1:128 with IHA is considered significant by the Center for Disease Control diagnostic laboratory. However, it must be kept in mind that almost total cross-reactivity occurs between cysticercosis and echinococcosis. Hydatid cysts of the lung are rarely detected serologically. Recent studies suggest that a scolex antigen for use in IHA seems the most promising among antigens. The diagnosis is confirmed by the finding, at surgery, of brood capsules and scolices (hydatid sand) in the fluid of the tumor mass.

Treatment. Surgical removal is the only therapy available. Extreme caution must be exercised in enucleating the cysts to prevent rupture and leakage of hydatid sand. The injection of formalin preoperatively is recommended to kill germinative tissue, brood capsules, and scolices. Fluid can then be aspirated after a safe time, but never before the killing of the parasite. When enucleation is impossible, marsupialization may be the operation of choice. Recent studies indicate that sealing the area for surgery by freezing and then injecting a 0.5% solution of silver nitrate is very effective in killing the scolices. Reports also suggest aqueous iodine as superior to alcohol or formalin in killing scolices prior to surgery. Recent experimental studies indicate that mebendazole has a lethal effect on the germinal membrane of the hydatid cyst in white mice and retards growth of intraperitoneal cysts, as well as rendering them sterile. Intrahepatic cysts in humans (monitored by ultrasound) have shown regression in 4 to 13 months, clinical improvement, and lowering of specific IgE concentrations when treated with mebendazole in increasing doses up to a maximum of 400 to 600 mg three times a day, during courses lasting 21 to 30 days. However, in spite of the value of serial ultrasound and scanning in noting changes in size of cysts, there is no indication that size change is indicative of death of the scolices.

Echinococcus multilocularis

The adult worm *Echinococcus multilocularis* is smaller than *E. granulosus* and differs in the position of the genital pore with respect to the reproductive organs as well as the number of testes. Grossly, both species look very much alike. Eggs are identical in appearance. Foxes and various wildcats such as pumas and jaguarundi are the definitive hosts. Rodents are the natural intermediate hosts. In parts of central Europe, Siberia, the Balkans, the U.S.S.R., and on Rebun

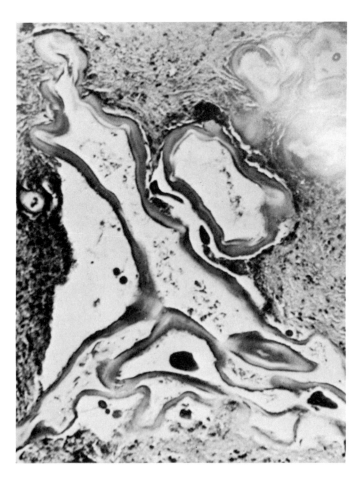

Fig. 12-7. Multilocular (alveolar) hydatid cyst. Note that each lobule shows an external laminated membrane and no scolices in this sterile cyst. (AFIP N-81099.)

Island, Japan, multilocular or alveolar cysts have been reported in humans. A few cases have also been reported in areas of South America, Australia, and New Zealand. Man is essentially a poor intermediate host. The sylvatic form is common in North Dakota. Instead of the large unilocular cyst previously described, there is a spongy mass of small vesicles filled with a jellylike matrix and enmeshed in connective tissue. Brood capsules are scattered in the mass. Growth continues from the periphery while degeneration takes place centrally. There is no walling-off by the host; thus there are resultant metastases through the lymphatics and circulation. Most alveolar cysts occur in the liver (Fig. 12-7).

In humans, multilocular or alveolar cysts are invariably fatal. Intrahepatic portal hypertension results in ascites and splenomegaly. The failure of the host to wall off the metastasizing mass renders surgery difficult and dubious since tiny bits of germinative tissue left behind may give rise to more cysts. There is no chemotherapy.

Familiarity with dogs, particularly by children, should be avoided. Only good sanitation and a sacrifice of infected animals can rid humans of this dread parasite.

Echinococcus oligarthrus

Echinococcus oligarthrus is a tapeworm of wild felines in Central and South America. The jaguarundi, puma, and jaguar have been found infected in nature. Wild rodents are the intermediate hosts. The adult tapeworm is slightly larger than *E. multilocularis* and has more hooklets, as well as more testes, in the mature proglottid. Alveolar cysts are rare in humans and are described as being less alveolar in makeup than those of *E. multilocularis*. The first reported case was in Panama.

Echinococcus vogeli

Another species, *Echinococcus vogeli*, has been reported in one patient in Colombia, South America. The patient was described as having polycystic hydatid disease. Verification was based on the recovery of the adult tapeworm from a dog that was fed cysts from the patient.

SPARGANOSIS

The plerocercoid larvae, or spargana, of species of pseudophyllidean tapeworms may infect humans and cause sparganosis. Most of the spargana reported in humans in the United States are believed to be *Spirometra mansonoides* (Fig. 12-8). Cats, dogs, and related wild animals serve as the definitive hosts, with copepods *(Cyclops)* being the first intermediate hosts. Water snakes and field mice are the chief second intermediate hosts, but a wide range of amphibians, reptiles, birds, and mammals, including humans, may be involved as a result of the accidental ingestion of copepods containing the procercoid larvae.

In humans the liberated procercoid larvae migrate through the gut wall and through the circulation reach the subcutaneous tissues and muscles where they become established and grow into spargana. Little or no host reaction occurs in the early stages. The larva is a whitish, wrinkled worm sometimes up to 14 inches in length, with an invaginated scolex at one end. Later in the infection, the area about the worm becomes edematous and painful to the touch. Death of the worm results in a marked inflammatory reaction with local eosinophilia and Charcot-Leyden crystals. Infections about the eye produce severe pain, lacrimation, and edema. Such infections are common in Southeast Asia, where frog-muscle poultices for boils and sores result in the transfer of the spargana to the wound. The ingestion of raw meat from infected frogs, snakes, fowl, or various mammals containing plerocercoid larvae can result in establishment of the larvae in humans through migration from the gut to the body tissues. Infections about the eye can be treated with injections of 2 to 4 ml of 40%

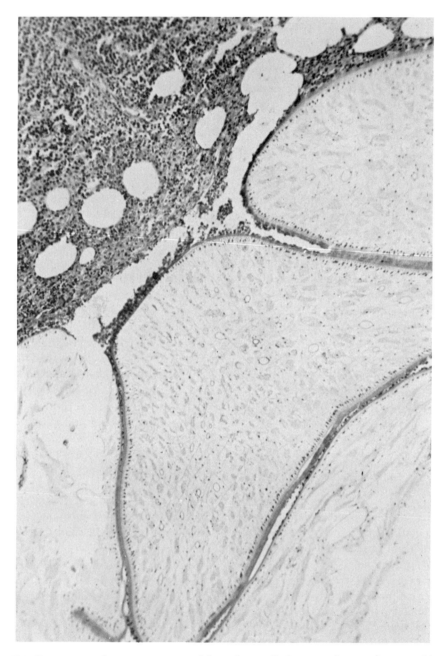

Fig. 12-8. Cross-section of sparganum, removed from chest wall of patient, showing the internal loose fibrillar network, osmoregulatory canals, and internal muscle fibers. Plasma cells, lymphocytes, histiocytes, and necrosis surround the worm. (Photograph by James J. Daly.)

ethyl alcohol with procaine (epinephrine-free). Those in the subcutaneous tissues can be removed surgically.

Proliferating spargana have been recorded. They are elongated, branching forms believed to be aberrant or degenerate worms that may separate and continue to grow, honeycombing the tissues.

REVIEW QUESTIONS

1. What is meant by the phrase somatic tapeworm?
2. What is cysticercosis? Discuss.
3. Describe a unilocular cyst. Describe a multilocular, or alveolar, cyst.
4. What two dangers exist during surgical intervention for a hydatid cyst? How can each be prevented?
5. What is sparganosis? Discuss.
6. How is hydatid disease diagnosed?
7. What is the significance of wild rodents in the transmission of hydatid disease in humans?
8. Discuss the use of mebendazole in the treatment of hydatid disease in humans.

REFERENCES

Anderson, F. L., J. R. Everett, A. G. Barbour, and F. J. Schoenfeld. 1974. Current studies on hydatid disease in Utah. Proc. 78th Annual Meeting. U.S. Animal Health Association, pp. 370-384.

Anderson, F. L., and M. V. Wallentine. 1976. Hydatid disease. National Wool Grower Magazine.

Ardehali, S., and others. 1977. Evaluation of counter immuno-electrophoresis crossed electro-immunodiffusion and agar gel diffusion for immunodiagnosis of human hydatid disease. Trans. R. Soc. Trop. Med. Hyg. 71:481-485.

Coltori, E. A., and V. M. Varela-Diaz. 1978. Detection of antibodies against Echinococcus granulosus arc 5 antigens by double diffusion test. Trans. R. Soc. Trop. Med. Hyg. 72:226-229.

Corkum, K. C. 1966. Sparganosis in some vertebrates of Louisiana and observations on a human infection. J. Parasitol. 52:444-448.

Daly, J. J., G. F. Baker, and B. R. Johnson. 1975. Human sparganosis in Arkansas. J. Arkansas Med. Soc. (May).

DeBuen, S. 1970. Cisticercosis ocular. Gac. Med. Méx. 100:137-144.

Dewhirst, L. W., J. D. Cramer, and W. J. Pistor. 1963. Bovine cysticercosis. I. Longevity of cysticerci of Taenia saginata. J. Parasitol. 49:297-300.

Hermos, J. A., and others. 1970. Fatal human cerebral coenurosis. J.A.M.A. 213:1461-1464.

Hoghooghi, N., and others. 1976. Evaluation of the slide-latex agglutination and intradermal (Casoni) tests

for echinococcosis. Am. J. Trop. Med. Hyg. 25:660-661.

Jalayer, T., and I. Askari. 1966. A study of the effect of aqueous iodine on hydatid cysts in vitro and in vivo. Ann. Trop. Med. Parasitol. 60:169-171.

Jampol, L. M., J. B. H. Caldwell, and D. M. Albert. 1973. Cysticercus cellulosae in the eyelid. Arch. Ophthalmol. 89:319-320.

Johnstone, H. E., and O. W. Jones. 1950. Cerebral coenurosis in an infant. Am. J. Trop. Med. 30:431-441.

Kagan, I. G. 1968. A review of serologic tests for the diagnosis of hydatid disease. Bull. WHO 39:25-27.

Kagan, I. G., and M. Agosin. 1968. Echinococcus antigens. Bull. WHO 39:13-24.

Kammerer, W. S., and M. V. Pérez-Esandi. 1973. The current status of the chemotherapy of hydatid disease. Bull. Pan Am. Health Organ. 7:47-52.

Kelkar, S. S., and S. E. Kotwal. 1975. Counter immunoelectrophoresis in diagnosis of hydatid disease. Lancet 1:755-756.

Kritsky, D. C., and P. D. Leiby. 1978. Studies on sylvatic echinococcosis. V. Factors influencing prevalence of Echinococcus multilocularis Leuckart 1863, in red foxes from North Dakota, 1965-1972. J. Parasitol. 64:625-634.

Leiby, P. D., W. P. Carney, and C. E. Woods. 1970. Studies on sylvatic echinococcosis. III. Host occurrence and geographic distribution of Echinococcus multilocularis in the north central United States. J. Parasitol. 56:1141-1150.

Leiby, P. C., and D. C. Kritsky. 1972. Echinococcus multilocularis: a possible domestic life cycle in central North America and its public health importance. J. Parasitol. 58:1213-1215.

Liu, I. K. M., C. W. Schwabe, P. M. Schantz, and M. N. Allison. 1970. The occurrence of Echinococcus granulosus in coyotes (Canis latrans) in the Central Valley of California. J. Parasitol. 56:1135-1137.

Loveless, R. M., F. L. Anderson, M. J. Ramsay, and B. K. Hedelius. 1977. Echinococcus granulosus in dogs and sheep in central Utah, 1971-1976. Am. J. Vet. Res. 39:499-502.

Lukashenko, N. P. 1971. Problems of epidemiology and prophylaxis of alveococcosis (multilocular echinococcosis): a general review, with particular reference to the U.S.S.R. Int. J. Parasitol. 1:125-134.

Mueller, J. F., E. P. Hart, and W. P. Walsh. 1963. Human sparganosis in the United States. J. Parasitol. 49:294-296.

Mueller, J. F., and A. J. Strano. 1974. Sparganum proliferum, a sparganum infected with a virus? J. Parasitol. 60:15-19.

Nagaty, H. F., and M. A. Ezzat. 1946. On the identity of Multiceps multiceps (Leske, 1780). M. gaigeri (Hall, 1916), and M. seriatis (Gervais, 1845), with a review of these and similar forms in man and animals. Proc. Helminthol. Soc. 13:33-44.

Orihel, T. C., F. Gonzalez, and P. C. Beaver. 1970. Coenurus from neck of Texas woman. Am. J. Trop. Med. Hyg. 19:255-257.

Polley, L. 1978. Visceral larva migrans and alveolar hydatid disease, dangers real or imagined. Vet. Clin. North Am. 8:353-378.

Rausch, R. L. 1967. A consideration of the intraspecific categories in the genus *Echinococcus* Rudolphi 1801 (Cestoda: Taeniidae). J. Parasitol. 53:484-491.

Rausch, R. L. 1967. On the occurrence and distribution of *Echinococcus* spp. (Cestoda: Taeniidae) and characteristics of their development in the immediate host. Ann. Parasitol. 42:19-63.

Rausch, R. L., and J. J. Bernstein. 1972. *Echinococcus vogeli* sp. n. (Cestoda: Taeniidae) from the bush dog, *Speothos venaticus* (Lund). Z. Tropenmed. Parasitol. 23:25-34.

Richard-Lenoble, D., M. D. Smith, and M. Liosy. 1978. Human hydatidosis: evaluation of three sero-diagnostic methods, the principal subclass of specific immunoglobulin and the detection of circulating immune complexes. Ann. Trop. Med. Parasitol. 72:553-560.

Saidi, F., and I. Nazarian. 1971. Surgical treatment of hydatid cysts by freezing of cyst wall and installation of 0.5 percent silver nitrate solution. N. Engl. J. Med. 284:1346-1350.

Schwabe, C. W., and others. 1972. Hydatid disease is endemic in California. Cal. Med. 117:13-17.

Slais, J. 1970. The morphology and pathogenicity of the bladder worms *Cysticercus cellulosae* and *Cysticercus bovis*. Dr. W. Junk, BV., Publishers, The Hague.

Stiles, C. W. 1908. The occurrence of a proliferating cestode larva *(Sparganum proliferum)* in man in Florida. Hyg. Lab. Bull. 40:7-18.

Swartzwelder, J. C., P. C. Beaver, and M. W. Wood. 1964. Sparganosis in southern United States. Am. J. Trop. Med. Hyg. 13:43-47.

Varela-Díaz, V. M., and others. 1975. Evaluation of whole and purified hydatid fluid antigens in the diagnosis of human hydatidosis by the immunoelectrophoresis test. Am. J. Trop. Med. Hyg. 24:298-303.

Varela-Díaz, V. M., and others. 1975. Evaluations of four variants of the indirect hemagglutination test for human hydatidosis. Am. J. Trop. Med. Hyg. 24:304-311.

Yarzabel, L. A., J. Leiton, and M. H. López-Lemes. 1974. The diagnosis of human pulmonary hydatidosis by the immunoelectrophoresis test. Am. J. Trop. Med. Hyg. 23:662-666.

Yarzábel, L. A., P. M. Schantz, and M. H. Lopez-Lemes. 1975. Comparative sensitivity and specificity of the Casoni intradermal and the immunoelectrophoresis tests for the diagnosis of hydatid disease. Am. J. Trop. Med. Hyg. 24:843-848.

Walls, K. W. 1979. Immunoserology of parasitic diseases. In Friedman, H., T. J. Linna, and J. E. Prier, Editors. Immunoserology in the diagnosis of infectious diseases. University Park Press, Baltimore, Md.

Wilson, J. F., M. Davidson, and R. L. Rausch. 1978. A clinical trial of mebendazole in the treatment of alveolar hydatid disease. Am. Rev. Respir. Dis. 118:747-757.

Wilson, J. F., A. C. Diddams, and R. L. Rausch. 1967. Cystic hydatid disease in Alaska. A review of 101 cases of *Echinococcus granulosus* infection. Am. Rev. Respir. Dis. 98:1-15.

World Health Organization. 1968. Echinococcosis. WHO 39(1):1-136.

CHAPTER 13

The intestinal, liver, and lung flukes

INTESTINAL FLUKES

Humans are considered to be only an accidental host of the flukes of the intestinal tract. Intestinal flukes are primarily parasites of other animals, even though, in some areas, they are quite common in humans. It is because of omnivorous food habits that humans become so frequently parasitized with these flukes. There is no other animal except the pig that offers such close competition for this rather dubious honor. The following intestinal flukes are of major medical importance:

Fasciolopsis buski
Metagonimus yokogawai
Heterophyes heterophyes
Gastrodiscoides hominis

There are other intestinal flukes parasitic in humans, but they are of minor importance. References will be made to some of them in the text.

Fasciolopsis buski

Fasciolopsis buski is the largest trematode parasitizing humans and averages up to 7 or 8 cm in length (Fig. 13-1). The eggs average 140 μm $\times$ 80 to 85 μm. This fluke has an extensive distribution in pigs in Southeast Asia. Humans vie with the pig for first place in the incidence of infection and in some villages in China, without question, hold top honors by having a 100% infection rate. In many villages in China the homes are built so that sewage drains into an adjacent pond. Night soil is used to fertilize the plants growing there. Embryonation takes place in fresh water after passage from the host. The hatched miracidia infect appropriate snail

hosts. Cercariae from the snails are deposited on vegetation in the pond, and the water plants known as red caltrop, or red ling, are commonly contaminated (Fig. 13-2). Metacercariae are often found encysted on the nuts of this plant; the Chinese eat these nuts after peeling the outer shell with their teeth. Examination of the husks of these nuts has revealed more than 200 metacercariae present on one shell. Other edible plants involved in transmission are the water chestnut, water bamboo, and water hyacinth. During the developmental period of the flukes no noticeable symptoms are present. Adults are attached to the mucosa of the small intestine and mature in 3 months, when diarrhea and abdominal pain may appear. Heavy infections are followed by severe mucous diarrhea, marked anemia, ascites, and edema of the legs and face, which may lead to prostration and death, particularly in children.

In endemic areas the clinical manifestations lead to a presumptive diagnosis that can be confirmed by finding typical operculated eggs in the stool (Fig. 13-3). Adult flukes, when recovered, are easily identified also. Hexyresorcinol given orally or by duodenal tube is the drug of choice. When given orally, hard gelatin capsules, each containing 0.1 or 0.2 gm to a total of 1 gm, are administered (Table 13-1). Pretreatment and posttreatment purgations are employed. Greater effectiveness is obtained by giving 1 gm in 20 ml of water through a duodenal tube. Tetrachloroethylene, on an empty stomach, at a dosage level of 0.10 to 0.12 ml/

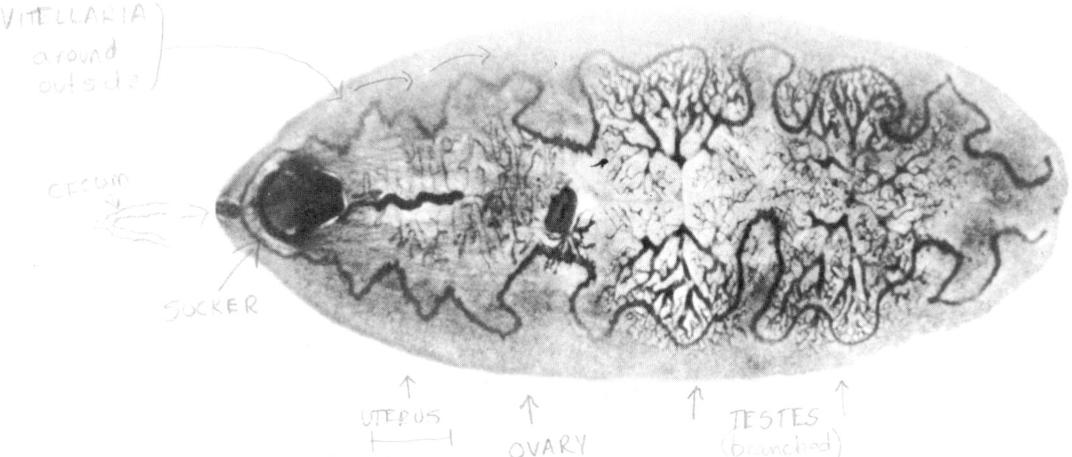

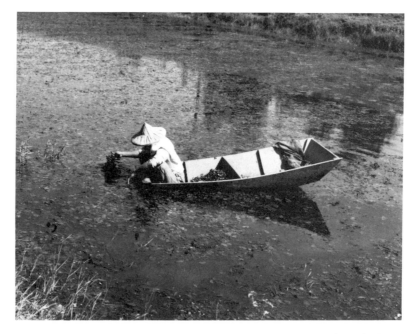

VITELLARIA
around
outside

CECUM

SUCKER

UTERUS   OVARY   TESTES
(branched)

Fig. 13-1. *Fasciolopsis buski.* Note the absence of an anterior cone. (From a nonprofit cooperative endeavor by numerous colleagues under the editorship of Dr. Herman Zaiman, Valley City, N.D.)

Fig. 13-2. A woman harvesting water caltrop, a source of metacercariae of *Fasciolopsis buski* in humans. (Photograph by Robert E. Kuntz. From Schmidt, G. D. and Roberts, L. S.: Foundations of parasitology, St. Louis, 1977, The C. V. Mosby Co.)

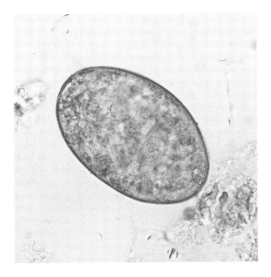

Fig. 13-3. *Fasciolopsis buski* egg. Note the morphologic resemblance to *Fasciola hepatica* egg. (Courtesy Dr. W. Henry Leigh, Department of Biology, University of Miami.)

Table 13-1. Treatment for intestinal, liver, and lung flukes

Infection	Drug	Adult dose*	Pediatric dose*
Flukes, hermaphroditic			
Opisthorchis (Clonorchis) sinensis (liver fluke)			
Drug of choice	Chloroquine phosphate[1]	250 mg (150 mg base) tid × 6 wk	Not recommended
Alternatives	None		
Fasciola hepatica (sheep or liver fluke)			
Drug of choice	Bithionol[2]	30-50 mg/kg on alternative days × 10-15 doses	30-50 mg/kg on alternate days × 10-15 doses
Alternatives	None		
Paragonimus westermani (lung fluke)			
Drug of choice	Bithionol[2]	30-50 mg/kg on alternate days × 10-15 doses	30-50 mg/kg on alternate days × 10-15 doses
Alternatives	None		
Fasciolopsis buski			
Drug of choice	Hexylresorcinol	A single dose of 1 gm in two hard gelatin capsules	*1-7 yr:* 400 mg; *8 yr:* 500 mg; *9 yr:* 600 mg; *10 yr:* 700 mg; *11 yr:* 800 mg; *12 yr:* 900 mg; *13 yr:* 1 gm
Alternatives	None		

Adverse effects of antiparasitic drugs

Chloroquine HCl and chloroquine phosphate USP (Aralen; and others)

  Occasional: pruritus; vomiting; headache; confusion; depigmentation of hair; skin eruptions; hemolysis especially with G6PD deficiency; corneal opacity; irreversible retinal injury (especially when total dosage exceeds 100 gm); weight loss; partial alopecia; extraocular muscle palsies; exacerbation of psoriasis, eczema and other exfoliative dermatitis

  Rare: discoloration of nails and mucous membranes of mouth; nerve-type deafness; blood dyscrasias; photophobia

Bithionol

  Frequent: photosensitivity skin reactions; vomiting; diarrhea; abdominal pain; urticaria

Hexylresorcinol

  Frequent: high concentrations on skin are irritant and corrosive

From The Medical Letter, Inc., 56 Harrison Street, New Rochelle, N.Y.

*The letter d indicates day.

1. Chloroquine usually does not cure, but produces temporary suppression of ova, and should be reserved for symptomatic patients.

2. In the U.S.A. this drug is available from the Parasitic Diseases Division, Center for Disease Control, Atlanta, Georgia 30333; telephone 404-329-3311.

kg, is also effective. No purgation is desired. Fats in the diet should be avoided.

Heterophyidae

Metagonimus yokogawai and *Heterophyes heterophyes* are members of a family of flukes known as the Heterophyidae, or the heterophyids. All of the members of this family are small and, in turn, produce operculated eggs that are small. The flukes vary up to 2 or 3 mm in size, and the eggs average about 20 to 35 μm in length by 10 to 20 μm in diameter. Various species of freshwater snails serve as the first intermediate host. The metacercariae are encysted under the scales in the flesh of freshwater fish. Humans are infected by eating raw fish. The heterophyids are versatile about the hosts they will infect but show unusual behavior by burrowing into the mucosa when not well adapted to their host.

M. yokogawai is primarily an intestinal fluke of dogs and cats throughout Asia and parts of Europe. It occurs sporadically in a wide variety of carnivores, including even the pelican. Human infections occur mostly in Asia and Sibera. *H. heterophyes* is also primarily a fluke of dogs and cats in the Near East, Far East, and parts of Africa where human infections also occur. Both of these flukes live in the crypts of the duodenum and jejunum and are tolerated rather well by the host, although abdominal discomfort and diarrhea may accompany heavy infection. Occasionally, eggs of both heterophyids reach the intestinal hymphatics and pass to the central nervous system or heart where granulomatous reaction may ensue. Hexyresorcinol is the drug of choice for all of the

Fig. 13-4. A typical heterophyid egg.

heterophyids. Treatment follows the same pattern outlined for *F. buski* (Fig. 13-4).

In the Philippines and Japan, other species of heterophyids not well adjusted to humans have been noted to burrow deep into the mucosa and deposit eggs into the lymphatics and blood vessels. Damage to the heart results from numerous eggs being deposited there, with acute dilatation producing symptoms like cardiac beriberi. Eggs have also been recovered from the brain and spinal cord, with central nervous system disorders present.

Amphistomes

The suborder of flukes called Amphistomata is characterized by having the ventral sucker near the posterior end. Only one member, *Gastrodiscoides hominis*, is found frequently in humans. In India the incidence is quite high in some areas where it is a common infection of pigs. The adult fluke, averaging up to 7 mm in length, lives in the cecum and colon, where it causes diarrhea, some catarrhal inflammation, and abdominal discomfort. Eggs pass out in the feces and develop miracidia. The snail is the first intermediate host, and vegetation is suspected as the chief second intermediate host. Soapsuds enemas are often more successful than chemotherapy in removing the worms. Tetrachloroethylene is the drug of choice and is administered as in the treatment for hookworms. A single adult dose of up to 5 ml is administered on an empty stomach, with the avoidance of fats in the diet made certain.

Echinostomatidae

The family of flukes, the echinostomes, like the heterophyids, has a diversified list of hosts that harbor the adult stage. The flukes are small to medium in size and occasionally are found in the human jejunum. They are characterized by a collar of spines near the anterior end. Their primary hosts are aquatic birds. Infections in humans are acquired by eating the appropriate second intermediate host, usually a mollusk. *Echinostoma ilocanum* is common in the Ilocanos of the Philippines. It averages 2.5 to 10 mm in length and 0.5 to 1.5 mm wide and has 51 collar spines. Raw snails are the source of infection for the natives. *E. malayanum*, with 43 collar spines, is common among some tribes living on the Sino-Tibetan frontier and also has been reported in Malaya and Sumatra. Other species of echinostomes occasionally appear in humans. The flukes are tolerated quite well; infections are accidental and are confined to the Orient. Nearly any vermifuge is successful in purging the host of these unwanted guests.

LIVER FLUKES

The flukes inhabiting the biliary passages of the liver are commonly referred to as liver flukes. Those of significant medical importance are as follows:

Fasciola hepatica
Opisthorchis sinensis
Opisthorchis felineus
Opisthorchis viverrini

Others of lesser importance are mentioned in the text.

Fasciolidae

The members of the family Fasciolidae are large in size and utilize vegetation as the second intermediate host. One member, *F. buski*, has already been discussed under the intestinal flukes. The liver fluke of major importance in this family is *Fasciola hepatica*.

Fasciola hepatica

Geographic distribution. *F. hepatica*, commonly known as the sheep liver fluke, is cosmopolitan throughout many sheep- and cattle-raising countries of the world. Numerous infections in humans have been reported in Cuba, southern France, and Algeria. Many other Latin American and Mediterranean countries are foci of human infections also. The fluke is common in cattle in some areas of the southern United States, and human infection has resulted.

Morphology. Adult flukes average 25 to 30 mm in length by about 13 mm in width. They are flat and leaflike, with a distinct anterior cone, which along with the branching of the intestinal ceca, serves to differentiate it from *F. buski* (Fig. 13-5).

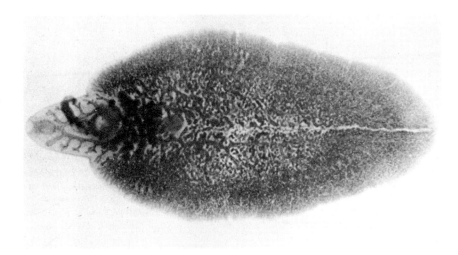

Fig. 13-5. *Fasciola hepatica.* Note the presence of the anterior cone. (From a nonprofit cooperative endeavor by numerous colleagues under the editorship of Dr. Herman Zaiman, Valley City, N.D.)

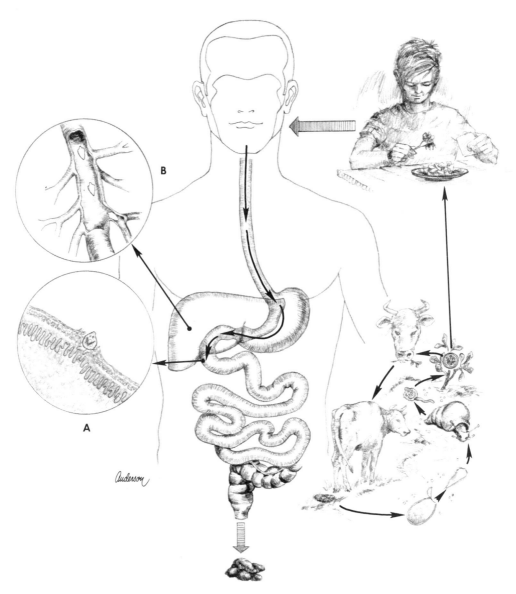

Fig. 13-6. Life cycle of *Fasciola hepatica*. Infected cattle and sheep, grazing in meadows, seed the fresh-water ponds with the eggs of *F. hepatica* from their feces. Development and hatching of the miracidia occurs with penetration of the appropriate species of snails. Asexual multiplication within the snail host results in the formation of cercariae, which, upon leaving the snail, encyst on various grasses. Water-cress and other grasses containing encysted metacercariae are eaten raw by humans in salads. Excysta-tion and penetration of the duodenal wall, **A**, by the metacercariae results in their being free in the body cavity to penetrate the liver capsule, reach the biliary ducts, and develop into adult flukes. **B**. Eggs produced pass down the common bile duct into the lumen of the intestine.

Life cycle and epidemiology. Grazing sheep and cattle seed the soil or water source with viable eggs in the feces. If the water, usually a stream, contains snails, they are infected with the miracidia, which hatch in about 2 weeks. Cercariae produced in the snail are shed and encyst as metacercariae on vegetation, commonly watercress or grass. Sheep, cattle, and other herbivores, including humans, who enjoy fresh watercress in a salad, become infected by eating the contaminated vegetation. In the intestinal tract the metacercariae penetrate the gut wall and reach the peritoneal cavity. From here many migrate to the liver, penetrate the capsule, and burrow through the liver parenchyma, until they become established in branches of the biliary ducts. As growth occurs, they move to the larger ducts and reach maturity in about 12 weeks. Eggs produced pass through the common bile duct to the intestinal canal and thence in the fecal stream to the external environment to begin another life cycle if circumstances permit. (Fig. 13-6).

Symptomatology and pathology. Digestive disturbances, fever, and pain are early symptoms. Allergic manifestations and eosinophilia follow. Peritonitis, hepatitis, and hepatomegaly occur in heavy infections. Larvae, wandering loose in the peritoneal cavity, produce necrotic foci, with eventual fibrosis. Within the bile ducts, desquamation occurs, with hyperplasia and cystic dilatation of the passages. Eggs deposited and trapped in smaller ducts become centers of inflammation and fibrosis. Extensive liver damage eventually results in cirrhosis, with a shrunken liver and portal hypertension. The prognosis is grave in heavy infections.

Diagnosis and treatment. Eggs recovered in the feces must be differentiated from those of *F. buski*, which are morphologically similar. A history of travel and eating habits will often prove helpful in this regard. Duodenal intubation may be more successful for recovering eggs in light infections. Precipitin and complement-fixation tests are helpful (Fig.

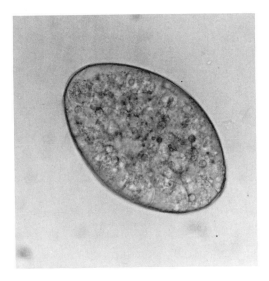

Fig. 13-7. *Fasciola hepatica* egg. Note the morphologic resemblance to *Fasciolopsis buski* egg. (Courtesy Dr. W. Henry Leigh, Department of Biology, University of Miami.)

13-7). The indirect hemagglutination test is adequate. The drug of choice is bithionol at the dosage of 30 to 50 mg/kg on alternate days for 10 to 15 doses (Table 13-1). Bithionol is frequently associated with photosensitivity skin reactions, vomiting, diarrhea, abdominal pain, and urticaria.

In Hawaii and parts of Asia, a larger, closely related fluke, *Fasciola gigantica*, is responsible for human infections.

Opisthorchidae

The members of the family Opisthorchidae are flat, elongated flukes parasitic in fish-eating animals, particularly in Europe and Asia but also in Canada and the United States. The most important member of the family parasitic in humans is *Opisthorchis sinensis*, the Chinese liver fluke. It is widely distributed in humans in the Far East, as well as in cats and dogs. Infection is not uncommon in older New York Jews who escaped Hitler's Germany by way of China.

The adult fluke averages from 10 to 25 mm in length (Fig. 13-8). It lives in the small bili-

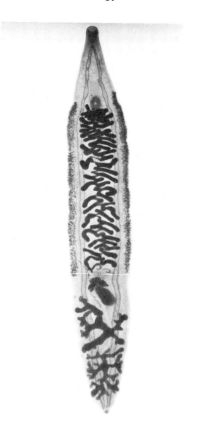

Fig. 13-8. The Chinese liver fluke *Opisthorchis sinensis*. (Photograph by Robert E. Kuntz. From Schmidt, G. D. and Roberts, L. S.: Foundations of parasitology, St. Louis, 1977, The C. V. Mosby Co.)

ary passages of the liver and, in heavy infections, also in the bile ducts, the gallbladder, and sometimes the pancreatic duct. Its life span is about 20 years. When infected raw fish is eaten, the metacercaria excysts in the intestine and migrates up the lumen until it finds the ampulla of Vater. It then moves up the bile duct to the liver. Within a month the worm becomes a mature adult.

Typical, small operculated eggs pass down the bild duct to the intestine and out of the host in the feces (Fig. 13-9). Damage to the bile ducts occurs, with thickening pericholangitic fibrosis and parenchymal granuloma with fibrosis. Heavy infections cause eventual cirrhosis of the liver. Death seldom oc-

curs directly from infection; secondary infection, malnutrition, or carcinoma may cause death when the liver flukes are numerous.

Diagnosis is made by recovery and identification of the eggs in the feces. The indirect hemagglutination test is helpful. Treatment is unsatisfactory in heavy infections. Gentian violet and related dyes were the early drugs used and have been found to be efficacious in light infections. Chloroquine phosphate, although chiefly suppressive in function, is about the best available drug today. It is given at the dosage of 250 mg three times daily for 6 weeks. As an alternative, dehydroemetine or emetine, at the dosage of 2.5 mg/kg every other day for 12 to 15 doses may be used, but the efficacy is questioned by some.

Two members of this family are also parasitic in humans, though less commonly than *O. sinensis*. They are *Opisthorchis felineus* and *O. viverrini*. *O. felineus* is common in cats chiefly, but also in dogs and other animals across Europe and Asia that, like humans, become infected by eating raw fish. *O. viverrini* occurs in Southeast Asia, mainly in Thailand and Laos. In Thailand, particularly, infections are common and often quite heavy. Both cause disease similar to but milder than that caused by *O. sinensis*.

Metorchis conjunctus is a common opisthorchid fluke of dogs, foxes, cats, minks, and raccoons over a wide area of Canada. Occasional infections have been reported in humans. The common sucker is the second intermediate host and the chief source of infections in humans. The fish are usually heavily infected.

Dicrocoelidae

Members of the family Dicrocoelidae are small, flat flukes with small eggs and are chiefly parasitic in the bile ducts and pancreatic ducts of birds and mammals. *Dicrocoelium dendriticum*, a common liver fluke of sheep and other ruminants around the

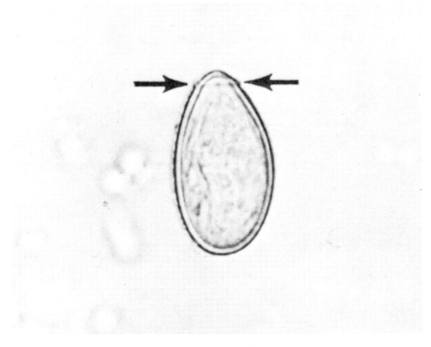

Fig. 13-9. *Opisthorchis sinensis* egg showing elevated shoulders *(arrow)* at rim of the operculum. (AFIP 72-17746.)

world, has been reported in humans. It is a very flat, lanceolate fluke measuring 5 to 15 mm by 1.5 to 2.5 mm. The eggs are brown, thick shelled, measure around 40 to 50 μm by 22 to 30 μm, and usually contain a miracidium when laid. Snails are the first intermediate host. Cercariae invade the respiratory chamber of the snail where several hundred may be encased in a "slime cyst." Several slime cysts, rolled together into a "slime ball," are dropped onto moist vegetation where they are eaten by the lowly ants. Development into metacercariae occurs, and there they await the definitive host. Humans accidentally ingest ants with vegetation and thus become infected. The metacercariae reach the liver by way of the portal circulation after invasion of the intestinal mucosa. They then find their way into the biliary passage. Damage to the liver similar to that caused by *F. hepatica* occurs, but of lesser intensity. A paucity of genuine infec-

tions has been reported from Europe, Asia, and Africa. No satisfactory treatment is known for humans.

LUNG FLUKES

Flukes parasitizing the lungs of various mammals, such as rats, pigs, opossums, and humans, belong to the genus *Paragonimus*. The speciation in some animals is fairly well established, but those parasitizing humans, tigers, and American fur-bearing animals are still debated. The consensus is that they are all the same species. *Paragonimus westermani* was first described from the lungs of a Bengal tiger. Later, when similar flukes were observed in human lungs, the name *P. ringeri* was given. The name *P. westermani* was subsequently adopted for both organisms. In North America, similar flukes common in mink and other fur-bearing animals, particularly in Michigan, are referred to as *P. kellicotti*. One human autochthonous case

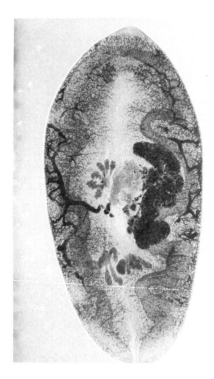

Fig. 13-10. *Paragonimus westermani* adult. (Photograph by Robert E. Kuntz and Jerry A. Moore. From Schmidt, G. D. and Roberts, L. S.: Foundations of parasitology, St. Louis, 1977, The C. V. Mosby Co.)

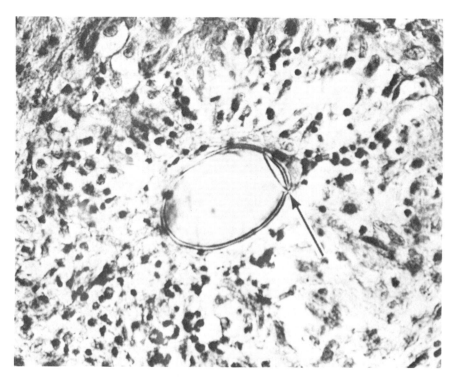

Fig. 13-11. *Paragonimus westermani* egg within a granuloma in the brain. Note the operculum *(arrow).* (AFIP 53-6071.)

of *P. kellicotti* has been reported in North America. Human infections are common in the Far East, mainly in China, Korea, Japan, the Philippines, and Taiwan, hence the name Oriental lung fluke. Endemic foci are recorded in Nigeria because of the species *P. uterobilateralis*, while in Cameron the parasite is *P. africanus*. *P. skrjabini* is reported in humans in northeast China, and *P. heterotrema* in Thailand and Laos. Unidentified species are reported in Mexico and Central America, and in South America, infections have been reported in Peru and Ecuador.

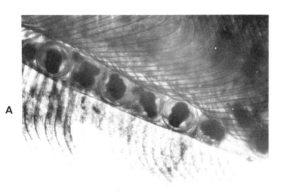

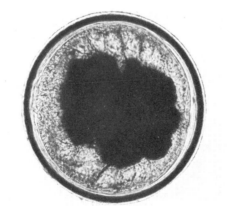

Fig. 13-12. **A,** Several metacercariae of *Paragonimus westermani* in a gill filament of a crab. **B,** A single metacercaria. The opaque mass is characteristic for this genus. (Photograph by Robert E. Kuntz. From Schmidt, G. D. and Roberts, L. S.: Foundations of parasitology, St. Louis, 1977, The C. V. Mosby Co.)

Morphology and life cycle. *P. westermani*, the cause of paragonimiasis, or endemic hemoptysis, is a reddish brown fluke, quite small in size, averaging 5 mm × 10 mm (Fig. 13-10). The typical, operculated ova measure 85 µm × 55 µm (Fig. 13-11). The adult flukes live in cystic cavities that rupture into the bronchioles. Eggs coughed up in the sputum are expectorated or swallowed. In fresh water they develop and hatch. The miracidia penetrate appropriate snails and undergo asexual multiplication. Emerging cercariae next enter suitable crabs and crayfish to form metacercariae (Fig. 13-12). When raw crab or crayfish is eaten, the metacercariae penetrate the intestinal wall and enter the body cavity. The adolescent worms remain in the body cavity, often wandering about, in and out of the liver and other organs. In about 3 weeks they penetrate the diaphragm and enter the lungs to develop into adults in 5 to 6 weeks. The tendency to wander aimlessly in the peritoneal cavity and to enter organs other than the lungs, particularly common in heavy infections, suggests that they are in an abnormal host. Fibrous inflammatory cysts are formed around entrapped worms.

Epidemiology. Paragonimiasis is essentially a zoonosis. The natural definitive hosts comprise a wide variety of fur-bearing animals around the world and thus become the reservoir hosts for humans. Crab collectors in some countries distribute their catch miles away from home base (Fig. 13-13). In the Orient, crabmeat marinated in brine, vinegar, or wine is a delicacy, and although the meat portion is coagulated, giving it a cooked appearance, the metacercariae are unharmed. Fingers and cooking utensils, frequently contaminated in food preparation, often end up in the mouth. The medicinal use of juice from crushed crabs in some cultures may also be an important factor in human infection.

Symptoms do not occurs until the stage of inflammatory reaction around the worms and

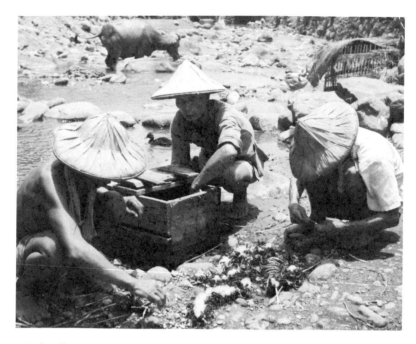

Fig. 13-13. Crab collectors in Taiwan stringing crabs for a trip to market. In this manner *Paragonimus westermani* is distributed far from its source. (Photograph by Robert E. Kuntz. From Schmidt, G. D. and Roberts, L. S.: Foundations of parasitology, St. Louis, 1977, The C. V. Mosby Co.)

eggs (Fig. 13-14). Although symptoms are most severe during the first 5 to 6 years, the worms may survive as long as 20 years, resulting in a progressive increase in symptomatic signs and pathologic findings. The onset of symptoms is usually insidious, with little fever. There is a spasmodic cough, eventually productive of thick, blood-flecked sputum. Gross hemoptysis and severe pleuritic chest pain may occur. Gradually there is progressive bronchitis, bronchiectasis, and fibrosis; there may be pleural effusion. Shortness of breath and wasting ensue. The disease may be spontaneously arrested at any stage, and the final severity is related to the worm burden. Often, paragonimiasis is mistaken for tuberculosis.

Worms in the abdominal cavity can cause symptoms related to their location, for example, hepatitis, enteritis, lymphadenitis, or draining fistulas to the outside. Involvement of the central nervous system may result in encephalomeningitis, myelitis, or focal seizures.

Symptomatology and pathology. Eosinophilic and neutrophilic infiltration is followed by formation of a fibrous connective tissue capsule around the worm. Rupture of the capsule, with the release of eggs into surrounding tissue, leads to granulomatous formation somewhat similar to that around schistosome eggs. Intracranial calcification is common in cerebral infections.

Diagnosis. Residence in an endemic area, ingestion of uncooked crabs or crayfish, and pulmonary symptoms should suggest the diagnosis. Peripheral eosinophilia may be present. Examination of the bloody or rusty part of sputum will usually reveal eggs and Charcot-Leyden crystals. Eggs may also be recovered from feces or draining cutaneous fistulas. The complement-fixation test is helpful.

Treatment. Bithionol is now the drug of

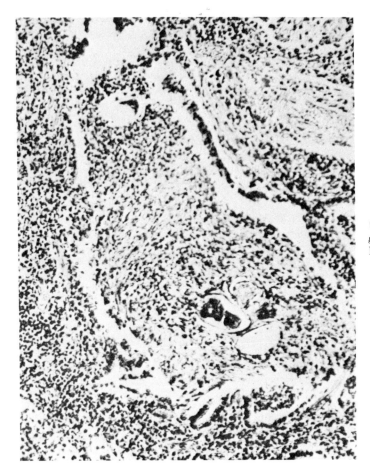

Fig. 13-14. Lung showing eggs of *Paragonimus westermani* within a granuloma in a bronchiole. (AFIP 496822.)

choice at a dosage of 30 to 50 mg/kg given every other day for 10 to 15 doses. Children should receive the same dosage (Table 13-1). Chloroquine phosphate has also been used successfully in some cases at the dosage of 250 mg three times daily for 6 weeks. The side effects of these drugs have been discussed under fascioliasis.

REVIEW QUESTIONS

1. Describe the life history pattern common to all hermaphroditic flukes.
2. Discuss the pathogenicity of the intestinal flukes, liver flukes, and lung flukes.
3. What is the treatment for the intestinal flukes? Liver flukes? Lung flukes?
4. What is the significance of heterophyid flukes not well adjusted to humans?
5. What is the geographical distribution of the echinostomes? Discuss their pathogenicity.
6. Discuss the role of the ant in fluke transmission.

REFERENCES

Ashton, W. I. G., and others. 1970. Human fascioliasis in Shropshire. Br. Med. J. 3:500-502.

Barlow, C. H. 1925. The life cycle of the human intestinal fluke *Fasciolopsis buski* (Lankester). Am. J. Hyg. Monograph Series no. 4.

Cross, J. H. 1969. Fasciolopsiasis in south-east Asia and the far east: a review. Pages 177-199. In C. Harinasuta, Editor. Proceedings of the Fourth Southeast Asian Seminar on Parasitology and Tropical Medicine, Schistosomiasis and other Snail-transmitted Helminthiasis, Manila, 1969. Bangkok.

Dutt, E. C., and H. D. Srivastava. 1966. The intermediate host of the cercaria of *Gastrodiscoides hominis* (Preliminary Report). J. Helminthol. 40:45-53.

Hadden, J. W., and E. F. Pascarelli. 1967. Diagnosis and treatment of human fascioliasis. J.A.M.A. **202:** 149-151.

Hardman, E. W., R. L. H. Jones, and A. H. Davies. 1970. Fascioliasis: a large outbreak. Br. Med. J. **3:** 502-505.

Healy, G. R. 1970. Trematodes transmitted to man by fish, frogs, and crustacea. J. Wildl. Dis. **6:**255-261.

Hou, P. C. 1955. The pathology of *Clonorchis sinensis* infestation of the liver. J. Pathol. Bac. **70:**53-54.

Hou, P. C. 1965. The relationship between primary carcinoma of the liver and infestation with *Clonorchis sinensis*. J. Pathol. Bact. **72:**239-246.

Kean, B. H., and R. C. Breslau. 1964. Parasites of the human heart. Grune & Stratton, Inc., New York, pp. 95-103.

Kean, B. H., and D. W. Hoskins. 1966. Drugs for intestinal parasitism. Pages 353-364. In W. Modell, Editor. Drugs of choice: 1966-1967. The C. V. Mosby Co., St. Louis.

Komiya, Y. 1966. *Clonorchis* and clonorchiasis. Pages 53-106. In Dawes, B., Editor. Advances in parasitology. Academic Press, Inc., New York.

Krull, W. H. 1958. The migratory route of the metacercaria of *Dicrocoelium dendriticum* (Rudolphi, 1819) Looss, 1899 in the definitive host: Dicrocoeliidae. Cornell Vet. **48:**17-24.

Krull, W. H., and C. R. Mapes. 1952. Studies on the biology of *Dicrocoelium dendriticum* (Rudolphi, 1819) Looss, 1899 (Trematoda: Dicrocoeliidae), including its relationship to the intermediate host *Cionella lubrica* (Muller). VII. The second intermediate host of *Dicrocoelium dendriticum*. Cornell Vet. **42:**603-604.

Little, M. D. 1968. *Paragonimus caliensis* sp. n. and paragonimiasis in Colombia. J. Parasitol. **54:**738-746.

Markell, E. K. 1966. Laboratory findings in chronic clonorchiasis. Am. J. Trop. Med. Hyg. **15:**510-515.

Miyazaki, I. 1974. Occurrence of the lung fluke, *Paragonimus pervianus* in Costa Rica. Jp. J. Parasitol. **23:** 280-284.

Miyazaki, I. 1974. V. Lung flukes in the world: morphology and life history. A symposium on epidemiology of parasite diseases. Pages 101-135. International Medical Foundation of Japan, Tokyo.

Miyazaki, I., and K. Nishimura. 1975. Cerebral paragonimiasis. Pages 109-132. In Hornabrook, R. W., Editor. Topics in tropical neurology. Contemporary Neurology. Series. No. 12. F. A. Davis, Co., Philadelphia.

Norton, R. A., and L. Monroe. 1961. Infection by *Fasciola hepatica* acquired in California. Gastroenterology **41:**46-48.

Nwokolo, C. 1974. Endemic paragonimiasis in Africa. Bull. WHO **50:**569-571.

Sadun, E. H. 1955. Studies on *Opisthorchis viverrini* in Thailand. Am. J. Hyg. **62:**81-115.

Sogandares-Bernal, F., and J. R. Seed. 1973. American paragonimiasis. Pages 1-56. In Cheng, T., Editor. Current topics in comparative pathobiology. Vol. 2. Academic Press, Inc., New York.

Voelker, J., and C. Nwokolo. 1973. Human paragonimiasis in eastern Nigeria caused by *Paragonimus uterobilateralis*. Z. Tropenmed. Parasitol. **24:**323-328.

Walls, K. W. 1979. Immunoserology of parasitic diseases. In Friedman, H., T. J. Linna, and J. E. Prier, Editors. Immunoserology in the diagnosis of infectious diseases. University Park Press, Baltimore, Md.

Wykoff, D. E., K. Chittayasothorn, and M. M. Winn. 1966. Clinical manifestations of *Opisthorchis viverrini* infections in Thailand. Am. J. Trop. Med. Hyg. **15:** 914-918.

Yokogawa, M. and others. 1976. Immunoglobulin E: raised levels in sera and pleural exudates of patients with paragonimiasis. Am. J. Trop. Med. Hyg. **25:** 581-586.

Yokogawa, M. and others. 1974. *Paragonimus miyazakii* infections in man first found in Kanto District, Japan, especially on the methods of immunoserodiagnosis for paragonimiasis. Jpn. J. Parasitol. **23:**167-179. (In Japanese, English summary.)

Yokogawa, M., S. Kojima, K. Araki, and H. Tomioka. 1975. Serum IgE levels in paragonimiasis. Jpn. J. Parasitol. **24**(suppl.):40. (In Japanese.)

Yokogawa, S., W. W. Cort, and M. Yokogawa. 1960. *Paragonimus* and paragonimiasis. Exp. Parasitol. **10:** 81-137.

CHAPTER 14

The blood flukes, or schistosomes

BLOOD FLUKES

The trematodes parasitizing the human bloodstream belong to the genus *Schistosoma*. Three species, collectively referred to as the schistosomes of man, are of major medical importance. These species, listed below, live in the portal system and mesenteric and vesicle venules of humans:

Schistosoma mansoni
Schistosoma japonicum
Schistosoma haematobium

The schistosomes, the cause of schistosomiasis, or bilharzia as it is commonly known in many endemic areas, are unique among the flukes parasitizing humans in that the sexes are separate, the ova produced by the females are not operculated, and there is no second intermediate host. Infection takes place by pentration of the wet skin by the cercariae (Fig. 14-1), which had emerged from the snail host. The schistosomula, which are the bodies of the cercariae, except for the forked tail, which is shed at the point of skin penetration, travel around the body through the circulation. On the portal side of the liver they grow and develop and, when adults or near adulthood, migrate against the portal flow to the mesenteric venules of the small or large intestine and the venules of the vesicle plexus. Although the location of the adult worm is species related, it is not absolute and adults of one species may be found at sites typical for another. The large male, about 1 cm in length, and the more slender female, sometimes half again as long as the male and clasped in the male's gyne-

cophoral canal, lie with their anterior ends facing the capillary bed (Fig. 14-2). In this environment they live for 30 years or more, with the female ovipositing eggs from the anteriorly located vulva. Many of the eggs, lodged in the tiny vessels like beads on a rosary, lie in front of the worms as they retreat during their egg laying. Through pressure and perhaps with the aid of histolytic enzymes elaborated by the miracidium within the eggshell, the eggs break through the vessel wall and come to lie in the surrounding tissues. Many are walled off, but some, very close to the lumen of the intestine or bladder, again by pressure or necrosis, become squeezed into the intestine or bladder and pass from the host in the feces or urine. Those that reach fresh water develop, hatch, and can perpetuate the species when appropriate snails are available. One miracidium inside the snail host, through asexual reproduction, will give rise to thousands of cercariae. From the snails come the cercariae, which, in turn, penetrate the skin of the human host.

The World Health Organization has stated that schistosomiasis is second only to malaria as the primary cause of morbidity and mortality in the tropics. Of all the tropical diseases acquired by American troops in World War II, schistosomiasis was the most important as a cause of chronic disability. Most disease was caused by *Schistosoma japonicum*, acquired during the occupation of the island of Leyte.

Schistosomiasis is spread widely over three

239

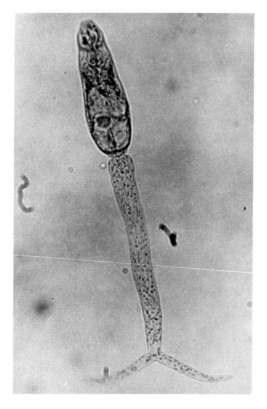

Fig. 14-1. Cercaria of *Schistosoma mansoni*. (Photograph by Warren Buss. From Schmidt, G. D. and Roberts, L. S.: Foundations of parasitology, St. Louis, 1977, The C. V. Mosby Co.)

continents, afflicting more than 200 million persons and causing considerable morbidity. It is estimated that about 400,000 infected persons, many of them Puerto Ricans, live in the United States. No risk in transmission, however, is involved, since appropriate snails are lacking and sanitation is generally good. The maintenance and spread of this disease are closely interwoven with the customs and habits of the natives in the endemic area. The age-old custom of washing clothes along the riverbank still persists, and accompanying the women are the children playing and splashing in the water. An examination of many of these washing areas will reveal suitable snail hosts that, upon microscopic study, are seen shedding cercariae. In some endemic areas the incidence is on the in-

crease because of the extension of irrigation ditches and the construction of dams, an aid to modern agriculture but a boon to the spread of infected snails along the grassy banks of the shallow canals where people still defecate, wash clothes, and walk barefooted and barelegged. An extensive control program is currently under way in Brazil, where a considerable portion of the population is afflicted. The basic approach to the problem is to simultaneously reduce the miracidia and planorbid snail populations in predefined areas through appropriately synchronized chemotherapy and planorbiciding methods. Support will be added by health education, improvement of basic sanitation, and provision of potable water.

Schistosoma mansoni

Geographic distribution and snail hosts. *Schistosoma mansoni* is coextensive with *S. haematobium* in Africa but less widely spread. It is common throughout most of tropical Africa and is hyperendemic in the Nile Delta. Several foci occur on the Arabian peninsula. A village in the Nile Delta, surveyed in 1935 and again in 1979 under similar conditions, showed an increase in prevalence of *S. mansoni* from 3.2% to 73%. *S. haematobium*, on the other hand, dropped from 74% to 2.2%. Comparable data from urine and stool examinations in the local hospital since 1972 supported this change. Changes in proportion of snail vectors appear to be related to the construction of the Aswan High Dam and the changes in the waterflow patterns of the Nile. Public health implications become apparent because hepatosplenic disease caused by *S. mansoni* is more difficult to treat and causes more morbidity and mortality than the urinary diseases caused by *S. haematobium*. In the western hemisphere, *S. mansoni* is found in Brazil, Venezuela, the Guianas, and the West Indies, extending northward to the island of Puerto Rico.

The confused state of snail taxonomy has

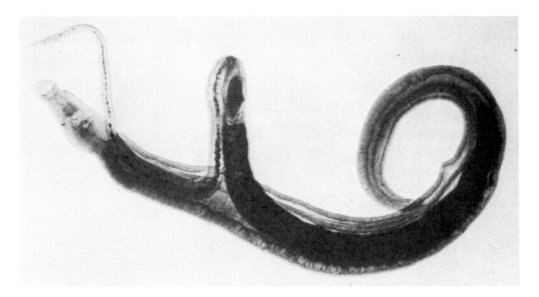

Fig. 14-2. Adult schistosomes. *Schistosoma japonicum* female clasped in the gynecophoral canal of the male. (From a nonprofit cooperative endeavor by numerous colleagues under the editorship of Dr. Herman Zaiman, Valley City, N.D.)

led to numerous generic names appearing in the literature. The genus *Biomphalaria* is commonly accepted as the snail host for *S. mansoni*. *B. glabrata* (synonym: *Australorbis glabratus*) accounts for most infections in the Caribbean islands. *S. mansoni* var. *rodintorum* is considered by many to be *S. mansoni* in rodents in Africa; *S. rodhaini*, in rodents and dogs in Africa, with its subterminal spine and transmission by planorbid snails, is considered a distinct species.

Morphology and habitat. The male worm averages 10 mm in length by about 1.1 mm in width and has a grossly tuberculated integument. The female is longer and more slender, averaging 14 mm × 0.16 mm. The eggs, when oviposited, are immature but within 10 days or so contain a miracidium (Fig. 14-3). They are ovoid and yellowish brown and have a lateral spine, a distinguishing feature of this species. In size they average 115 to 175 μm × 45 to 70 μm.

The adult worms migrate from the liver primarily to the branches of the inferior mesenteric veins in the wall of the large

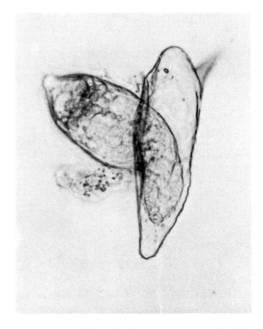

Fig. 14-3. Miracidium of *Schistosoma mansoni* breaking out of the egg shell. (Photograph by Robert E. Kuntz. From Schmidt, G. D. and Roberts, L. S.: Foundations of parasitology, St. Louis, 1977, The C. V. Mosby Co.)

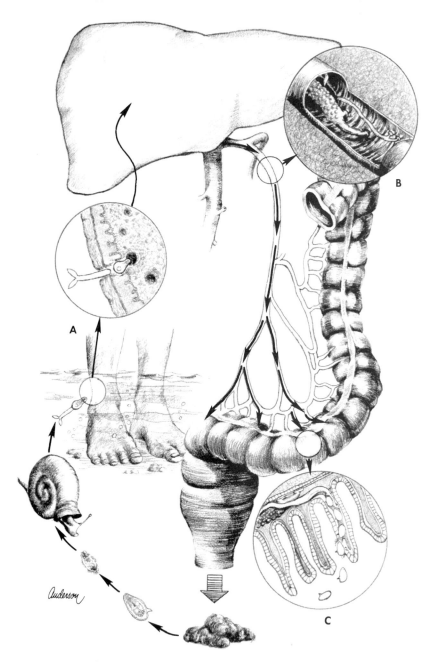

Fig. 14-4. Life cycle of *Schistosoma mansoni.* Eggs, passed in the feces, hatch in freshwater streams and yield miracidia, which penetrate appropriate species of snails. Cercariae, produced by asexual multiplication, leave the snail host and penetrate the skin of humans, **A,** exposed in freshwater streams. Schistosomula, by way of the bloodstream, eventually reach the liver where development into adulthood continues. Maturing male and female adults, in copulation, migrate against the portal flow, chiefly by way of the inferior mesenteric vein, **B,** to the small venules in the rectosigmoid area of the large intestine. Many eggs, deposited like beads in a chain, in the small venule, **C,** break out into the lumen of the intestine and pass out in the feces.

intestine. While the female is held in copulation, eggs are oviposited in small venules, commonly in the submucosal layers of the bowel wall. Some eggs, being trapped in the tissues, never reach the lumen of the intestines, whereas others penetrate the mucosa and are passed in the feces. Other eggs are carried in the portal flow to the liver, whereas still others, in the hemorrhoidal plexus, are carried by anastomoses to the inferior vena cava and thence to the heart and lungs where many are trapped in the capillary bed. Thus the possibility exists for the passage of eggs throughout the body (Fig. 14-4).

Symptoms and pathology. Symptoms can be related to the stage of infection and later to the primary area of body involvement. The first stage—the stage of invasion—is frequently asymptomatic. Some patients can recall an initial tingling sensation as the cer-

cariae penetrate the skin. This stage may be followed by a transient dermatitis and, rarely, a lymphangitis. The incubation period is otherwise usually asymptomatic until oviposition; the schistosomula are apparently poor allergens. Rarely, in heavy infections, death occurs during pulmonary migration before eggs are found in the stools. The lungs show hemorrhages, giant cell reaction, and eosinophils (Fig. 14-5).

The second stage is related to egg deposition. Schistosomes mate in the liver, migrate to the inferior mesenteric venules, and produce eggs within 6 weeks of skin penetration. An explosive onset of severe constitutional symptoms with fever, chills, and gastrointestinal complaints, frequently mimicking typhoid fever, is commonly seen within a month of infection. Much of this toxic stage has been attributed to an allergic reaction to the eggs or, possibly, to the adult parasites.

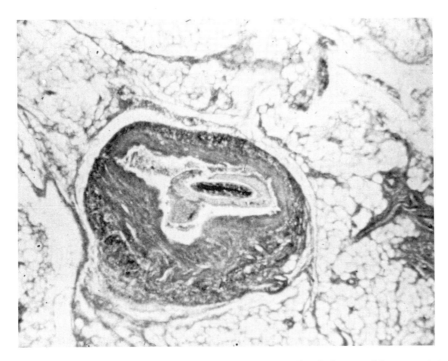

Fig. 14-5. *Schistosoma mansoni* adults in a mesenteric vein. Note the thickening of the tunica intima. (From a nonprofit cooperative endeavor by numerous colleagues under the editorship of Dr. Herman Zaiman, Valley City, N.D.)

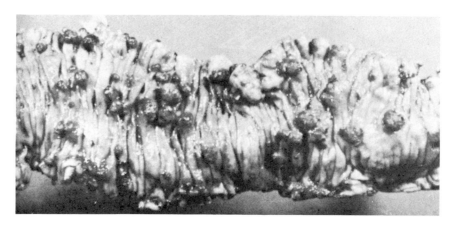

Fig. 14-6. Surgically resected colon with severe schistosomal colonic polyposis. (AFIP 76-2328.)

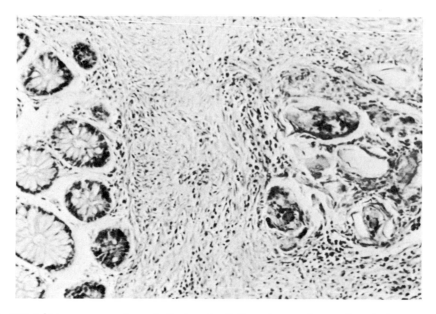

Fig. 14-7. *Schistosoma mansoni* eggs in the bowel wall. Note the granuloma with multiple eggs, one of which displays the lateral spine. (From a nonprofit cooperative endeavor by numerous colleagues under the editorship of Dr. Herman Zaiman, Valley City, N.D.)

Urticaria, angioneurotic edema, and eosinophilia are frequent. Gastrointestinal, hepatic, or pulmonary dysfunction may be prominent. In *S. mansoni* infections, dysentery, and abdominal cramps simulating amebiasis with frequent exacerbations may recur for months; ulcers and polyps (Fig. 14-6) appear in the colon. This schistosomal dysentery, often called the acute stage, may appear without preceding toxic manifestations and may be first seen within 2 months to several years after the initial infection. Egg deposition (Fig. 14-7) continues for the life of the adult worm, which averages 4 to 5 years but may be as long as 20 years.

The third stage is tissue reaction. The characteristic lesion is a pseudotubercle. Granulomas may be misdiagnosed as tuber-

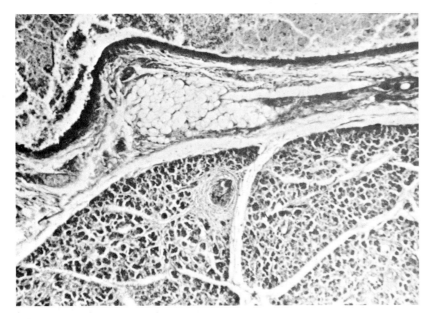

Fig. 14-8. *Schistosoma mansoni* egg in centrally located granuloma of pancreas. (From a nonprofit cooperative endeavor by numerous colleagues under the editorship of Dr. Herman Zaiman, Valley City, N.D.)

culosis. The pathologic condition is related to the eggs only; adult worms cause no disease per se. In S. *mansoni* infection, eggs may be swept along the portal circulation into the liver where granulomas result. Late in the disease periportal pipestem fibrosis may result in a clinical picture of cirrhosis, including portal hypertension and splenomegaly. Unlike other types of cirrhosis, there is little hepatocellular regeneration and no apparent increased incidence of liver carcinoma, and catheterization studies show a normal hepatic blood flow and hepatic vein pressure. However, more recent studies show that a presinusoidal block to liver blood flow occurs in association with the normal total liver blood flow. The antigenic and enzymatic secretions of the eggs induce a granulomatous cell-mediated response of lymphocytes, macrophages, and eosinophils, about 100 times the volume of the egg. During the chronic stages of infection, the granulomatous response to newly deposited eggs is much less than that to eggs in the acute

phase. Antibody blockage and suppressor T-lymphocyte and antigen-antibody complexes have been suggested as explanations for this phenomenon, raising hope for an immunologic approach to control of these diseases. Eosinophilia is known to coincide with the beginning of egg production, but in the chronic stages may be diminished. Since roughly half the cells in the egg granuloma are eosinophils, they possibly may add greatly to the tissue injury and any obstruction which follow. On the other hand, immunity to reinfection has been shown to depend on antibodies, mediated by eosinophils, and directed against the invading schistosomula. Eosinophils have been shown to act as killer cells for schistosomula in the presence of IgG antibody. Studies further indicate that neutrophils, and mononuclear leukocytes as well, damage schistosomula coated with antibody or complement. Since malnutrition and idiopathic cirrhosis are common in areas with schistosomiasis, some authors have questioned the importance of schistosomal infection in the production of cirrhosis and Egyptian splenomegaly (Fig. 14-8).

Eggs may be swept to other organs and result in primarily pulmonary or nervous system complications. Pulmonary hypertension and cor pulmonale may result from egg deposition in the lungs. With S. *mansoni* infection, the rare nervous system disease is most likely to involve the spinal cord, with a resulting clinical picture of transverse myelitis.

Schistosoma japonicum

Geographic distribution and snail hosts. *Schistosoma japonicum* is confined to the Far East, where it is highly endemic in the Yangtze River region of central China. Infections occur also in Japan, Celebes, Laos, Thailand, Cambodia, and the Philippines. This species shows very little host specificity, since it is found not only in humans in endemic areas but also in cattle, pigs, dogs, cats, goats, and various rodents. The propensity for infection of a wide variety of mammals makes control difficult; matters are made worse by the amphibious habits of some snail vectors not exposed to the molluscicides applied to

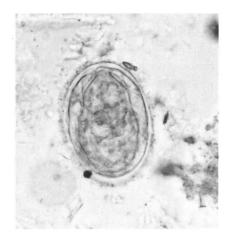

Fig. 14-9. *Schistosoma japonicum* egg. Note the sticky outer coat covered with debris. Rudimentary lateral spine not discernible. (Courtesy Dr. W. Henry Leigh, Department of Biology, University of Miami.)

the water. Amnicolid snails of the genus *Oncomelania* are the intermediate hosts of this parasite. A variety of S. *japonicum* on Formosa is not infective for humans. A schistosome recovered from the Mekong River basin, apparently different from other strains of S. *japonicum*, has been identified as S. *mekongi*.

Morphology and habitat. The adults primarily invade the human superior mesenteric veins. Consequently, the eggs, for the most part, enter the lumen of the small intestine and become well mixed with the fecal mass before their exit from the body. The male averages 12 to 20 mm × 0.5 mm. Unlike S. *mansoni*, the integument is not tuberculated. The delicate female averages 15 to 30 mm × 0.1 to 0.3 mm. The ova are the smallest of the schistosomes, from 70 to 100 μm × 50 to 65 μm. They are more rounded than the others and have a rudimentary lateral spine that is usually very difficult to see (Fig. 14-9). They are the most difficult of the *Schistosoma* ova to identify, because the outer coat is sticky and usually covered with debris. In this species, more so than in the others, many eggs laid in clusters are frequently swept past the worms in the portal flow to the liver. Other organs may be involved. The adult female produces approximately 3,000 eggs daily.

Symptomatology and pathology. Since this worm is the most prolific egg producer of the three species, extensive liver and other organ damage is more common. The phases of infection are similar to those described for S. *mansoni*, except that severe pulmonary manifestations during the invasive stage and chronic pulmonary disease resulting in cor pulmonale in the late stage are more common. Although most of the adults live in the superior mesenteric venules, they are also found elsewhere, and during the second stage at least half the patients have diarrhea, or dysentery, a tender palpable colon, and eggs in the stools. The large number of eggs in the liver is believed to explain the more frequent severe and fatal cirrhosis. *S. japoni-cum* more commonly invades the central nervous system than do the other schisto-somes; in endemic areas this infection may be the most common cause of a space-oc-cupying lesion in the brain, with fits, hemi-paresis, or other neurologic sequelae. In the Far East *S. japonicum* is considered among the more important causes of focal epilepsy.

Schistosoma haematobium

Geographic distribution and snail hosts. *S. haematobium* is found throughout large areas of Africa; it is especially abundant in the Nile Valley. It also occurs in the Near East. *S. haematobium* is primarily a human parasite,

showing little affinity for other hosts. Planor-bid snails, conical in shape, belonging to the subfamily Bulininae, are the intermedi-ate hosts. A single genus *Bulinus* and two subgenera, *Bulinus* and *Physopsis*, are the vectors involved. Related to *S. haemato-bium*, but considered by some as distinct species, are *S. bovis* in cattle, sheep, and goats, *S. matheei* in sheep, and *S. intercala-tum* in humans; the third has been reported from Zaire. *Bulinus* snails are involved in transmission. Foci of *S. intercalatum* are also reported in Gabon, Congo-Brazzaville, the Central African Republic, and Cameroon.

Morphology and habitat. The adults occur primarily in the vesicle plexus, the eggs

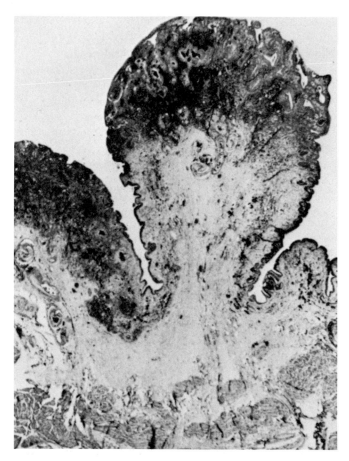

Fig. 14-10. Inflammatory polyps in the urinary bladder. Note the schistosomes in the veins. Hemorrhage, congestion, and necrosis occur at the tips of the polyps. (AFIP N-80024.)

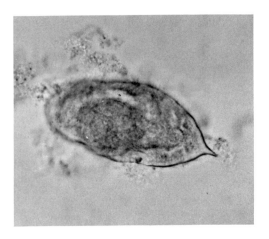

Fig. 14-11. *Schistosoma haematobium* egg. Note the terminal spine. (Courtesy Dr. W. Henry Leigh, Department of Biology, University of Miami.)

being trapped in the urinary bladder wall (Fig. 14-10). Some penetrate into the lumen of the bladder and are passed during the time of urination to perpetuate the life cycle. The adult male averages 10 to 15 mm in length by 1 mm in width while the female is about 20 mm × 0.25 mm. The eggs, measuring 115 to 170 μm × 45 to 65 μm, are the same size as those of *S. mansoni* but differ in that the characteristic spine, protruding from the shell wall, is terminal (Fig. 14-11).

The three phases described for the intestinal schistosomes also occur with *S. haematobium* but are usually less severe. Because most of the adults live in the vesicle plexus, the majority of eggs are passed to the outside

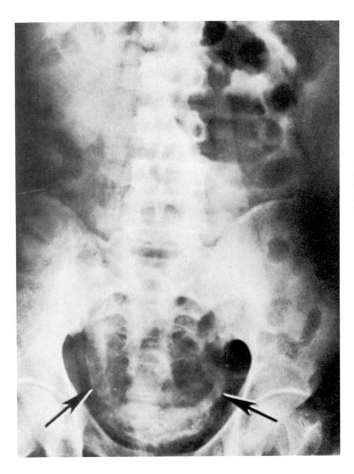

Fig. 14-12. X-ray film of pelvis with obstructive uropathy resulting from schistosomes. Note linear calcification in the base of the bladder *(arrow)* and along the dilated lower ureters. (AFIP 76-2403.)

through the urinary bladder. Eggs are also found in the stools, however.

Symptomatology and pathology. The usual initial symptoms of patients with S. *haematobium* infection are related to those of the second stage when painless terminal hematuria, gross or microscopic, with or without symptoms of cystitis, is seen. In some parts of Africa, infection is so common that hematuria is accepted as a sign of manhood in young boys (Fig. 14-12). Hematuria throughout all of micturition is rare and should suggest another etiologic factor. The third stage—reaction around eggs that have failed to transverse the bladder wall—results in pseudotubercle formation, which can often be identified at cystoscopy by physicians familiar with this disease (Fig. 14-13). Later, fibrosis of the bladder wall and calcification, visible on x-ray film of 10% to 15% of the patients, ensue. Secondary changes in the upper urinary tract may result in hydronephrosis and hydroureter, with death from

renal failure, but a surprising amount of disease, as demonstrated on intravenous pyelogram, is reversible. The existence of glomerular lesions suggests that abnormalities such as the nephrotic syndrome or proteinuria should not routinely be attributed to chronic pyelonephritis. Further studies, including renal biopsy, if not contraindicated for other reasons, are advised. Initial reports from Egypt of an increased association with bladder carcinoma have not been confirmed in other areas and suggest that the cancer may result from another factor and may be only coincidentally related to schistosomiasis.

Diagnosis of schistosomiases. During the stage of invasion, the diagnosis of schistosomiasis is largely based on a history of freshwater exposure in an endemic area. In the acute or second stage, the diagnosis can usually be made by examination of the stools in intestinal schistosomiasis, or of the urine in S. *haematobium* infection. For stool examination, specks of blood or mucus on the fecal

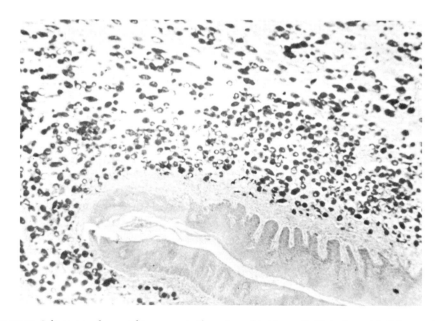

Fig. 14-13. *Schistosoma haematobium* eggs in the urinary bladder wall. Note the epithelial metaplasia. (From a nonprofit cooperative endeavor by numerous colleagues under the editorship of Dr. Herman Zaiman, Valley City, N.D.)

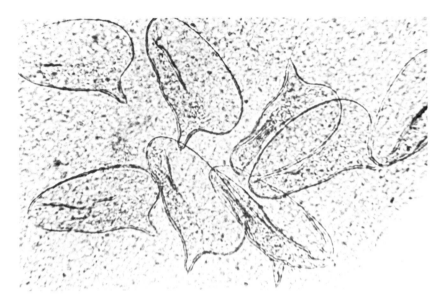

Fig. 14-14. *Schistosoma mansoni* eggs in a press preparation of bowel biopsy specimen. Note the lateral spine present. (From a nonprofit cooperative endeavor by numerous colleagues under the editorship of Dr. Herman Zaiman, Valley City, N.D.)

bolus are most likely to contain the eggs of *S. mansoni; S. japonicum* is found within the bolus. Flotation concentration procedures should not be employed since they destroy eggs. Centrifugation techniques or examination of an emulsion with unchlorinated fresh water for hatching miracidia (found swimming on top of a narrow flasked vessel) are useful when egg counts are low, particularly during late disease. In *S. haematobium* infection, microscopic examination of urine, especially that obtained after exercise, has the best yield. When eggs are difficult to find, a 24-hour sample should be examined after sedimentation; it should be made certain that the last drops from micturition are included. At least five urine or stool examinations must be made to diagnose a reasonable percentage of patients.

When stool examinations are negative, rectal biopsy or snips is the next procedure of choice. An unstained crush preparation is more satisfactory than fixed sections (Fig. 14-14). This method will be positive in nearly 100% of patients with clinically significant

S. mansoni infection, 80% of those with *S. haematobium* infection, and 65% of those with *S. japonicum* infection. Various serologic tests, such as complement fixation, hemagglutination inhibition, circumoval precipitation (precipitates around eggs in immune serum), and precipitates around cercariae are also employed. The indirect immunofluorescence (IIF) test, using parts of whole worms as antigen, is reported to be highly sensitive. However, in endemic areas where prolonged and extensive exposure to infection occurs, serologic titers bear no relationship to clinical problems and simply reflect exposure to infection. This becomes relevant in the United States where the majority of cases reported occur in the Puerto Rican population. A micro-enzyme-linked immunosorbent assay (ELISA) test for the recognition and quantification of antibodies against a specific circulating schistosomal antigen has been reported with an exceptionally high degree of sensitivity and a very high degree of specificity.

In spite of the many serologic tests available, adequate diagnosis is still a problem.

Table 14-1. Treatment for the schistosomes

Infection	Drug	Adult dose*	Pediatric dose*
Schistosoma haematobium[1]			
Drug of choice	Metrifonate[2]	10 mg/kg every other week × 3	10 mg/kg every other week × 3
Alternatives	Niridazole[2,3]	25 mg/kg/d PO (max. 1.5 gm) × 5-7d	25 mg/kg/d PO (max. 1.5 gm) × 5-7d
	Antimony sodium dimercaptosuccinate[2,4]	8 mg/kg IM given once or twice/wk for a total of 5 doses	8 mg/kg IM given once or twice/wk for a total of 5 doses
Schistomsoma japonicum[1]			
Drug of choice	Niridazole[2,3]	25 mg/kg/d PO (max. 1.5 gm) × 10d	25 mg/kg/d PO (max. 1.5 gm) × 10d
Alternative	Antimony sodium dimercaptosuccinate[2,4]	8 mg/kg IM given once or twice/wk for a total of 5 doses	8 mg/kg IM given once or twice/wk for a total of 5 doses
Schistosoma mansoni[1]			
Drug of choice	Niridazole[2,3] or Oxamniquine[5]	25 mg/kg/d PO (max. 1.5 gm) × 5-7d / 15 mg/kg once[6]	25 mg/kg/d PO (max. 1.5 gm) × 5-7d / 15 mg/kg once[6]
Alternative	Antimony sodium dimercaptosuccinate[2,3]	8 mg/kg IM given once or twice/wk for a total of 5 doses	8 mg/kg IM given once or twice/wk for a total of 5 doses

Adverse effects of antiparasitic drugs

Metrifonate
  Occasional: nausea; vomiting; bronchospasm; weakness; diarrhea; abdominal pain
Antimony sodium dimercaptosuccinate (Stibocaptate, Astiban)
  Adverse effects similar to effects of antimony potassium tartrate, but, except for rash and pruritus, less frequent and usually less severe
Antimony potassium tartrate USP
  Frequent: painful local inflammation following leakage during intravenous injection; coughing and vomiting when intravenous administration is rapid; muscle pain and joint stiffness; bradycardia
  Occasional: colic; diarrhea; rash; pruritus; myocardial damage
  Rare: liver damage; hemolytic anemia; renal damage; shock; sudden death
Niridazole (Ambilhar)
  Frequent: immunosuppression; vomiting; cramps; dizziness; headache
  Occasional: diarrhea; slight ECG changes; rash; insomnia; paresthesia
  Rare: psychosis; hemolytic anemia in G6PD deficiency; convulsions
Oxamniquine (Mansil)
  Occasional: headache; dizziness; somnolence; nausea; diarrhea; rash; insomnia; hepatic enzyme changes; ECG changes
  Rare: convulsions

From The Medical Letter, Inc., 56 Harrison Street, New Rochelle, N.Y.
*The letter d indicates day.

1. Not all patients with schistosomiasis need be treated. The decision to treat should be based upon such factors as the clinical status of the patient, viability of eggs, and concentration of eggs in urine and feces. An experienced clinician should be consulted before treatment is initiated. Hycanthone is widely used in some countries for treatment of S. *mansoni* and S. *haematobium* infections, but the drug can cause fatal hepatic necrosis and is suspected of being teratogenic and carcinogenic.
2. In the U.S.A., this drug is available from the Parasitic Diseases Division, Center for Disease Control, Atlanta, Georgia 30333; telephone 404-329-3311.
3. Niridazole is absolutely contraindicated in the presence of hepatocellular disease, portal hypertension, or a history of mental disorders or seizures.
4. Antimony sodium dimercaptosuccinate is contraindicated in renal and cardiac disease, and in hepatic disease not caused by schistosomiasis (but note that *Schistosoma* infections can cause hepatic disease). The drug should be stopped in the event of recurrent vomiting, progressive albuminuria, persistent joint pain, rash, intercurrent infection, purpura, or falling hematocrit.
5. Not available in the U.S.A.
6. For patients who contract a disease in Africa the dose should be increased to 30 mg/kg/d × 2d.

The complement-fixation (CF) test is still the most commonly used. At present, the simultaneous use of the CF test with a titer of 1:8 and the indirect hemagglutination (IHA) test with a titer of 1:16 is considered significant by the diagnostic laboratory of the Center for Disease Control.

Treatment of schistosomiases. Treatment is not necessary in all cases. The clinical evaluation of the patient, viability of eggs, and the concentration of eggs in the feces and urine are all criteria that should be used in judging the need for chemotherapy. The three major species vary in their response to the various drugs used (Table 14-1).

Niridazole (Ambilhar) causes frequent vomiting, diarrhea, cramps, dizziness, and headaches. Occasionally, slight electrocardiographic changes, rash, insomnia, and paresthesia are observed. Convulsions, psychosis, and hemolytic anemia in G6PD-deficient patients are rare. This drug is definitely contraindicated when hepatocellular disease, portal hypertension, or a history of mental disorders or seizures is present.

Antimony sodium dimercaptosuccinate (Stibocaptate, Astiban) may produce symptoms similar to those caused by antimony potassium tartrate, except for rash and pruritus, but usually less severe and less frequent. This drug is contraindicated in renal and cardiac disease and in hepatic disease not caused by schistosomiasis. Recurring vomiting, progressive albuminuria, persistent joint pain, rash, intercurrent infection, and falling hematocrit are indications to stop drug administration.

Antimony potassium tartrate causes frequent coughing and vomiting (when the intravenous drip is too rapid), muscle and joint stiffness, and bradycardia. Occasionally, colic, diarrhea, rash, pruritus, herpes zoster, renal damage, and shock occur. Liver cell damage and hemolytic anemia are rare.

Stibophen (Fuadin) may produce reactions similar to those caused by antimony potassium tartrate but usually less frequent and less severe. Occasionally, with prolonged use, heart damage may occur. Sulfhemoglubinuria and encephalopathy are rare. Stibophen, like antimony sodium dimercaptosuccinate, is contraindicated in cardiac and renal disease and in liver disease exclusive of schistosomiasis. Administration should be stopped in cases of recurring vomiting, progressive albuminuria, persistent joint pain, rash, falling hematocrit, and intercurrent infection.

Niridazole and antimony sodium dimercaptosuccinate are available from the Parasitic Disease Drug Service of the Center for Disease Control, Atlanta, Georgia.

The success of therapy is evaluated by further study of appropriate exudates for ova. Eggs found within 3 to 4 weeks of therapy may have been released prior to treatment, but positive stool or urine examinations 4 to 10 weeks after treatment indicate therapeutic failure. Even in such cases, reduction in egg

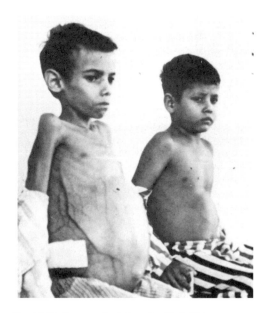

Fig. 14-15. Two youths infected with *Schistosoma mansoni*. Note the engorgement of collateral circulation of abdomen in the more advanced case. (From a nonprofit cooperative endeavor by numerous colleagues under the editorship of Dr. Herman Zaiman, Valley City, N.D.)

production may have resulted and the potential for serious sequelae is reduced.

All these drugs are contraindicated and ineffective once liver involvement is extensive (Fig. 14-15). Some patients, particularly those with *S. mansoni* infection, have benefited from a surgical procedure involving a sieve of the portal venous system into which the adult worms are flushed by a single dose of tartar emetic. Surgical extirpations of central nervous system lesions of *S. japonicum* have also met with limited success. Late-stage disease generally can be managed only supportively, and the prognosis is poor.

Disease prevention and control. The prevention of schistosomiasis becomes intricately involved in the sociocultural environment of people and for this reason presents almost insurmountable problems. If humans did not come in contact with polluted water,

infection would not occur. The primitive custom of defecating in or near canals, irrigation ditches, and streams where children frequently play and swim and women wash clothes has resulted in the increase of this disease (Fig. 14-16). In many endemic areas facilities for the disposal of human feces in a sanitary way are absent or inadequate at best (Fig. 14-17). Where *S. japonicum* is prevalent, animal reservoir hosts help to maintain the infection although human host infection may not be common.

Mass therapy has its limitations because of the difficulties in ensuring that therapy is completed, the number of relapses occurring, and the numbers who receive no treatment at all.

Snail control has received greatest attention through the use of molluscicides, engineering methods, and more recently, the

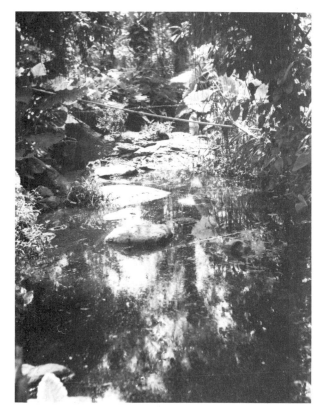

Fig. 14-16. Typical environment of a slow-running stream with protective vegetation providing an ideal habitat for *Biomphalaria*, the snail host for *Schistosoma mansoni* in Puerto Rico. (Photograph by Robert E. Kuntz. From Schmidt, G. D. and Roberts, L. S.: Foundations of parasitology, St. Louis, 1977, The C. V. Mosby Co.)

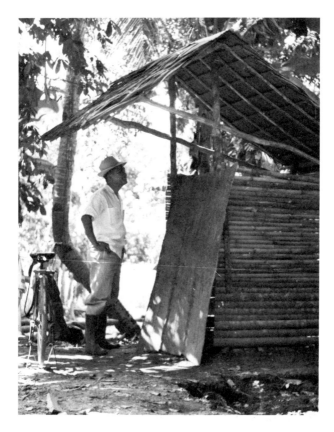

Fig. 14-17. Pit latrines, encouraged by the government in the Philippines, help prevent schistosomiasis. (Photograph by Robert E. Kuntz. From Schmidt, G. D. and Roberts, L. S.: Foundations in parasitology, St. Louis, 1977, The C. V. Mosby Co.)

use of disease agents to infect snails, certain insects, or their larvae for feeding on the young, and stocking freshwater fish that feed on molluscs. In Puerto Rico, the ampullarid snail *Marisa cornuareitis*, aside from being a competing voracious feeder, also devours the eggs and young of *Biomphalaria glabrata*.

Many factors are contributing to the growing public health problem of schistosomiasis (Fig. 14-18). Continuous irrigation of rice fields in Leyte in the Philippines favors the multiplication of the vector snail *Oncomelania quadrasi* for *S. japonicum* in these areas; the increase in manmade lakes in tropical areas is another example where cultural changes are contributing to the problem. At present, snail control through the use of molluscicides is the single most effective approach. The World Health Organization Ex-

pert Committee on Insecticides at present considers that 2',5-dichloro-4'-nirtosalicylanilide (Niclosamide) and N-tritylmorpholine (Frescon) are the safest and most effective molluscicides. Neither presents a serious toxicity hazard to humans, and concentrations in water after a single application range from 0.005 to 4 mg/liter; second treatments of water should not be done within 4 weeks of the initial application. Several authorities have stressed the need to grow strains of rice that require less water, and in the Philippines the number of snails dropped from 200 to less than one per square meter with the adaptation of intermittent applications of water.

Personal prophylaxis consists in boiling or filtering nonchlorinated water from streams, the use of ointments containing 20% benzyl benzoate or insect repellents such as dibutyl

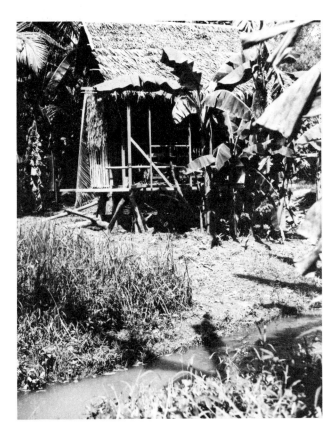

Fig. 14-18. Typical native abode in a schistosomiasis area in the Philippines. *Oncomelania* snails, host for *Schistosoma japonicum*, are found in the stream near the dwelling, which is probably contaminated with human feces as well. (Photograph by Robert E. Kuntz. From Schmidt, G. D. and Roberts, L. S.: Foundations of parasitology, St. Louis, 1977, The C. V. Mosby Co.)

phthalate to prevent skin penetration by cercariae, impregnation of clothing with repellents, and the wearing of rubber footwear when wading in streams. Research on immunization is in progress.

Schistosome (cercarial) dermatitis

Many members of the schistosome family are parasitic in birds and mammals other than humans. Their life cycles are similar to the species parasitic in humans, the definitive hosts becoming infected by exposure to the cercariae in water. These cercariae may penetrate the skin of humans bathing or swimming in these waters. About 25 species of cercariae from freshwater snails and at least 4 from marine forms are thus far implicated. In humans, an abnormal host, the cercariae are walled off in the epithelial layers and evoke an acute inflammatory response with leukocytic infiltration and edema. Severe itching follows. Papules, pustules, or hemorrhagic rash may last for a week or longer. Secondary infections are common. The dermatitis may be mild or quite severe. The phenomenon is believed to be a hypersensitivity reaction related to prior exposure to similar antigens. In many areas, particularly the northern lakes of the United States and Canada, "swimmer's itch" is the plague of bathers during the summer season (Fig. 14-19). In Michigan, the problem of "swimmer's itch" is reported to be increasing in magnitude in spite of the control measures (chiefly copper sulfate in the lakes) being used. Resort operators and park managers report adverse effects on business because patrons are worried about exposure to "swimmer's itch." Areas along the saltwater beaches of the northeastern coast, Florida,

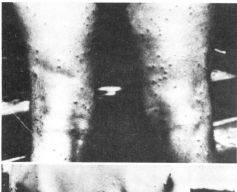

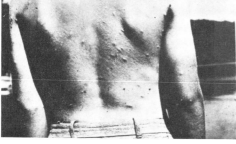

Fig. 14-19. Cercarial dermatitis, "swimmer's itch," caused by the cercariae of avian blood flukes. Note the acute inflammatory response of the host. (AFIP N-77203. From Schmidt, G. D. and Roberts, L. S.: Foundations of parasitology, St. Louis, 1977, The C. V. Mosby Co.)

southern California, and Hawaii are also plagued with the problem. Cercarial dermatitis also occurs in areas of India, Malaya, Africa, and Sumatra, as well as in the Middle East. Topical ointments to relieve the itching are the only palliatives necessary. Cercarial dermatitis, although rare, has been reported in American servicemen returning from Vietnam.

REVIEW QUESTIONS

1. How do the life history patterns of the schistosomes differ from those of the hermaphroditic flukes?
2. Discuss the major pathologic conditions in schistosomiasis.
3. What is the treatment for schistosomiasis?
4. Discuss cercarial dermatitis.
5. What are the methods presently employed in the control of schistosomiasis? Which is the most feasible?
6. Discuss the geographic distribution of the schistosomiases? How is it affected by snail population?
7. What is the role of the eosinophil in schistosomiasis?

8. Discuss the immunologic approach to the control of schistosomiasis.

REFERENCES

Anwar, A. R. E., S. R. Smithers, and A. B. Kay. 1979. Killing of schistosomula of *Schistosoma mansoni* coated with antibody and/or complement by human leukocytes in vitro: requirement for complement in preferential killing by eosinophils. J. Immunol. **122:**628-637.

Beaufils, H., P. Lebon, M. Auriol, and M. Danis. 1977. Glandular lesions in patients with *Schistosoma haematobium* infection. Trop. Geogr. Med. 30:183-191.

Bittencourt, A. L., O. Pinho, H. L. Lenzi, and I. H. C. Costa. 1979. Extragenital cutaneous lesions of schistosomiasis mansoni: report of two cases. Am. J. Trop. Med. Hyg. **28:**84-86.

Boros, D. L. 1976. Schistosomiasis mansoni: a granulomatous disease of cell-mediated immune etiology. Ann. N.Y. Acad. Sci. **278:**36-46.

Butterworth, A. E., and others. 1979. Damage to schistosomula of *Schistosoma mansoni* induced directly by eosinophil major basic protein. J. Immunol. **122:**221-229.

Byram, J. E., and A. W. Senft. 1979. Structure of the schistosome eggshell: amino acid analysis and incorporation of labelled amino acids. Am. J. Trop. Med. Hyg. **28:**534-547.

Camus, D., and others. 1977. Immunologic studies in human schistosomiasis. IV. Immunoglobulin levels, antibodies, and delayed hypersensitivity. Am. J. Trop. Med. Hyg. **26:**482-490.

Capron, A., and others. 1977. IgE and cells in schistosomiasis. Am. J. Trop. Med. Hyg. **26:**39-47.

Capron, M., and others. 1977. Immunological studies in human schistosomiasis. II. Antibodies cytotoxic for *Schistosoma mansoni* schistosomules. Am. J. Trop. Med. Hyg. **26:**248-253.

Carlier, Y., and others. 1975. Immunlogical studies in human schistosomiasis. I. Parasitic antigen in urine. Am. J. Trop. Med. Hyg. **24:**949-954.

Carlier, Y., D. Bout, and A. Capron. 1978. Further studies on the circulating M antigen in human and experimental *Schistosoma mansoni* infections. Ann. Immunol. (Inst. Pasteur) **129:**811-818.

Cha, Y. N. 1978. Inducibility of the hepatic drug-metabolizing capacity of mice infected wiht *Schistosoma mansoni*. Am. J. Trop. Med. Hyg. **27:**1181-1187.

Cha, Y. N., and E. Bueding. 1978. Recovery of the hepatic drug-metabolizing capacity in mice infected with *Schistosoma mansoni* following curative chemotherapy with the schistosomicide 4-isothiocyano-4'-nitro-dephenylamine (CGP4540). Am. J. Trop. Med. Hyg. **27:**1188-1191.

Chu, G. W. T. C. 1958. Pacific area distribution of fresh-water and marine cercarial dermatitis. Pacific Science **12:**229-312.

Colley, D. G., and others. 1977. Immune responses during human schistomiasis mansoni. I. In vitro lymphocyte blastogenic responses to heterogenous antigenic preparations from schistosome eggs, worms and cercariae. Int. Arch. Allergy Appl. Immunol. 53:420-433.

Colley, D. G., S. E. Hieny, R. K. Bartholomew, and J. A. Cook. 1977. Immune responses during human schistosomiasis mansoni. III. Regulatory effect of patient sera on human lymphocyte blastogenic responses to schistosome antigen preparations. Am. J. Trop. Med. Hyg. 26:917-925.

Cort, W. W. 1950. Studies on schistosome dermatitis Am. J. Hyg. 52:251-307.

Deedler, A. M., and P. C. Eveleigh. 1978. An indirect hemagglutination reaction for the demonstration of *Schistosoma mansoni* circulating anodic antigen. Trans. R. Soc. Trop. Med. Hyg. 72:178-180.

DeSole, G., and A. Lemma. 1978. *Schistosoma haematobium* in the Wabi Shebelle Valley of Ethiopia. Am. J. Trop. Med. Hyg. 27:928-930.

Fuller, G. K., A. Lemma, and T. Haile. 1979. Schistosomiasis in Omo National Park of southwest Ethiopia. Am. J. Trop. Med. Hyg. 28:526-530.

Gelfand, M. 1967. A clinical study of intestinal bilharziasis *(Schistosoma mansoni)* in Africa. Edward Arnold, London.

Goodgame, R. W., and others. 1978. Humoral immune responses in human hepatosplenic schistosomiasis mansoni. Am. J. Trop. Med. Hyg. 27:1174-1180.

Gremillion, D. H., R. W. Geckler, R. E. Kuntz, and R. V. Marraro. 1978. Schistosomiasis in Saudi Arabian recruits: a morbidity study based on quantitative egg secretion. Am. J. Trop. Med. Hyg. 27:924-927.

Hartman, P. E., and P. B. Hulbert. 1975. Genetic activity spectra of some antischistosomal compounds, with particular emphasis on thioxanthenones and benzothiopyranoindazoles. J. Toxicol. Environ. Health 1:243-270.

Hayunga, E. G., K. D. Murrell, D. W. Taylor, and W. E. Vannier. 1979. Isolation and characterization of surface antigens from *Schistosoma mansoni*. II. Antigenicity of radiolabeled proteins from adult worms. J. Parasitol. 65:497-506.

Hillyer, G. V., and others. 1979. Immunodiagnosis of infection with *Schistosoma mansoni*: comparison of ELISA, radioimmunoassay, and precipitation tests performed with antigens from eggs. Am. J. Trop. Med. Hyg. 28:661-669.

Hoshino-Shimizu, S., and others. 1976. Human schistosomiasis: *Schistosoma mansoni* antigen detection in renal glomeruli. Trans. R. Soc. Trop. Med. Hyg. 70:492-496.

Jobin, W. R., and A. Laracuente. 1979. Biological control of schistosome transmission in flowing habitats. Am. J. Trop. Med. Hyg. 28:916-917.

Jordon, P., and G. Webbe. 1969. Human schistosomiasis. Heineman, London.

Kagan, I. G. 1968. Serological diagnosis of schistosomiasis. Bull. N.Y. Acad. Med. 44:262-277.

Kamel, I. A., and others. 1978. *Schistosoma mansoni* and S. *haematobium* infections in Egypt. IV. Hepatic lesions. Am. J. Trop. Med. Hyg. 27:931-938.

Kelsoe, G. H., and T. H. Weller. 1978. Immunodiagnosis of infection with *Schistosoma mansoni*: enzyme-linked immunosorbent assay for detection of antibody to circulating antigen (polylysine-polysaccharide binding/worm burden and antibody relationship). Proc. Natl. Acad. Sci. 75:5715-5717.

Kitani, K., R. Miura, and M. Iuchi. 1979. Crossreactivity of schistosome antigens between *Schistosoma mansoni* and *japonicum*. Tohoku J. Exp. Med. 127:151-156.

Kuntz, R. E., T. C. Huang, and J. A. Moore. 1979. African baboon *(Papio cynocephalus)* infected with three strains of *Schistosoma mansoni*. J. Parasitol. 65:463-464.

Kuntz, R. E., T. C. Huang, and J. A. Moore. 1979. American opossums *(Didelphis marsupialis)* exposed to different strains of *Schistosoma mansoni*. Proc. Helminthol. Soc. Wash. 46:275-277.

Kuntz, R. E., J. A. Moore, and T. C. Huang. 1979. Distribution of egg deposits and gross lesions in nonhuman primates infected with *Schistosoma haematobium* (Iran). J. Med. Primatol. 8:167-178.

Laracuente, A., R. H. Brown, and W. Jobin. 1979. Comparison of four species of snails as potential decoys to intercept schistosome miracidia. Am. J. Trop. Med. Hyg. 28:99-105.

Laughlin, L. W., and others. 1978. Bacteriuria in urinary schistosomiasis in Egypt: a prevalence survey. Am. J. Trop. Med. Hyg. 27:916-918.

Lehman, J. S., Jr., and others. 1975. The association of Schistosomiasis mansoni and proteinuria in an endemic area: a preliminary report. Am. J. Trop. Med. Hyg. 24:616-618.

Lewert, R. M., M. G. Yogore, Jr., and B. L. Blas. 1979. Lymphocyte responsiveness to phytohemagglutinin and to worm and egg antigens in human schistosomiasis japonica. Am. J. Trop. Med. Hyg. 28:92-98.

Lewert, R. M., M. G. Yogore, Jr., and B. L. Blas. 1979. Schistosomiasis japonica in Barrio San Antonio, Basey, Samar, the Philippines. I. Epidemiology and morbidity. Am. J. Trop. Med. Hyg. 28:1010-1025.

Lunde, M. N., E. A. Ottesen, and A. W. Cheever. 1979. Serological differences between acute and chronic schistosomiasis mansoni detected by enzyme-linked immunosorbent assay (ELISA). Am. J. Trop. Med. Hyg. 28:87-91.

Machado, J. A., and others. 1978. Peripheral lymphocytes in patients with intestinal schistosomiasis mansoni. Trans. R. Soc. Trop. Med. Hyg. **72**:441.

Maddison, S. E., and others. 1978. *Schistosoma mansoni* infection in intact and B cell deficient mice: the effect of pretreatment with BCG in these experimental models. Am. J. Trop. Med. Hyg. **27**:966-975.

Maddison, S. E., and I. G. Kagan. 1979. Adoptive transfer of protective immunity in experimental schistosomiasis in the mouse. J. Parasitol. **65**:515-519.

Madwar, M. A., J. M. O'Shea, J. A. Skelton, and J. F. Soothill. 1978. Complement components and immunoglobulins in patients with schistosomiasis. Clin. Exp. Immunol. **34**:354-358.

Mahmoud, A. A. 1977. Current concepts: schistosomiasis. N. Engl. J. Med. **297**:1329-1331.

Maldonado, J. F. 1967. Schistosomiasis in America. Editorial Científico Médica, Barcelona. Spain.

McLaren, M., and others. 1978. Studies on the enzyme-linked immunosorbent assay (ELISA) test for *Schistosoma mansoni* infections. Ann. Trop. Med. Parasitol. **72**:243-253.

McMahon, J. E. 1978. Treatment of schistosomiasis: factors affecting chemotherapy and reflections on ideal drug treatment. Trop. Geogr. Med. **30**:161-174.

Most, H., and others. 1950. Schistosomiasis japonica in American military personnel: clinical studies of 600 cases during the first year after infection. Am. J. Trop. Med. **20**:239-299.

Mostofi, F. K., Editor. 1967. Bilharziasis. International Academy of Pathology Special Monograph. Springer-Verlag New York, Inc., New York.

Nash, T. E. 1978. Antibody response to a polysaccharide antigen present in the schistosome gut. I. Sensitivity and specificity. Am. J. Trop. Med. Hyg. **27**:939-943.

Nash, T. E., E. A. Ottesen, and E. W. Cheever. 1978. Antibody response to a polysaccharide antigen present in the schistosome gut. II. Modulation of antibody response. Am. J. Trop. Med. Hyg. **27**:944-950.

Negrón-Aponte, H., and W. R. Jobin. 1979. Schistosomiasis control in Puerto Rico: twenty-five years of operational experience. Am. J. Trop. Med. Hyg. **28**:515-525.

Otteson, E. A., and others. 1977. Immunoglobulin and complement receptors on human eosinophils and their role in cellular adherence to schistotomules. Am. J. Trop. Med. Hyg. **26**:134-141.

Ottesen, E. A., and others. 1978. The acquisition and loss of antigen-specific cellular immune responsiveness in acute and chronic schistosomiasis in man. Clin. Exp. Immunol. **33**:38-47.

Pelley, R. P., and G. V. Hillyer. 1978. Demonstration of a common antigen between *Schistosoma mansoni* and *Fasciola hepatica*. Am. J. Trop. Med. Hyg. **27**:1192-1194.

Pelley, R. P., K. S. Warren, and P. Jordan. 1977. Purified antigen radioimmunoassay in serological diagnosis of schistosomiasis mansoni. Lancet **2**(8042):781-785.

Pelley, R. P., and K. S. Warren. 1978. Immunoregulation in chronic infectious disease: schistosomiasis as a model. J. Invest. Dermatol. **71**:49-55.

Phillips, S. M., and D. G. Colley. 1978. Immunology of *Schistosoma mansoni* infection: workshop report III. Am. J. Trop. Med. Hyg. **27**:1058-1060.

Phillips, S. M., and D. G. Colley. 1979. The immunlogy of schistosomiasis: workshop report III. Am. J. Trop. Med. Hyg. **28**:914-915.

Phillips, T. M., and C. C. Draper, 1975. Circulating immune complexes in schistosomiasis due to *Schistosoma mansoni*. Br. Med. J. **2**:476-477.

Pinon, J. M., A. Sulahian, and G. Dropsy. 1978. The use of ELIEDA (Enzyme-linked-Immuno-Electro-Diffusion-Assay) in the study of humoral antibodies in human schistosomiasis. Trans. R. Soc. Trop. Med. Hyg. **72**:492-495.

Ruiz-Tiben, E., J. R. Palmer, and F. F. Ferguson. 1969. Biological control of *Biomphalaria glabrata* by *Marisa cornuarietis* in irrigation ponds in Puerto Rico. Bull. WHO **41**:329-333.

Salih, S. Y., A. Voller, and A. W. Woodruff. 1978. Serum immunoglobulin concentrations in human *S. mansoni* and *S. haematobium* infections in the Sudan, with special reference to the effect of chemotherapy. Tropenmed. Parasit. **29**:269-274.

Santoro, F., and others. 1977. Mother-child relationship in human schistosomiasis mansoni. I. Parasitic antigens and antibodies in milk. Am. J. Trop. Med. Hyg. **26**:1164-1168.

Santoro, F., B. Vandemeulebrooke, and A. Capron. 1978. The use of the radioimmunoprecipitation-peg. assay (RIPEGA) to quantify circulating antigens in human and experimental schistosomiasis. J. Immunol. Methods **24**:329-337.

Seed, J. L., M. C. Pratt, and J. L. Bennett. 1979. The effects of chronic disulfiram treatment on mice infected with *Schistosoma mansoni*. Am. J. Trop. Med. Hyg. **28**:508-514.

Senft, A. W., and others. 1979. Species specificity of the immediate hypersensitivity to schistosomal proteolytic enzyme. Parasite Immunol. **1**:79-89.

Senft, A. W., and S. E. Maddison. 1975. Hypersensitivity to parasite proteolytic enzyme in schistosomiasis. Am. J. Trop. Med. Hyg. **24**:83-89.

Sher, A., and others. 1977. Immune responses during human schistosomiasis mansoni. II. Occurrence of eosinophil-dependent cytotoxic antibodies in relation to intensity and duration of infection. Am. J. Trop. Med. Hyg. **26**:909-916.

Shookoff, H. C. 1961. Clinical aspects of Manson's schistosomiasis. N.Y. J. Med. **61**:3864-3873.

Smith, M. D., and others. 1975. Circulating immune complexes in schistosomiasis. Br. Med. J. **2**:274.

Sodeman, W. A., Jr. 1979. A longitudinal study of schistosome vector snail populations in Liberia. Am. J. Trop. Med. Hyg. 28:531-538.

Sornmani, S., and others. 1973. Mekong schistosomiasis. I. Life cycle of *Schistosoma japonicum*, Mekong strain in the laboratory. Southeast Asian J. Trop. Med. Public. Health 4:218-225.

Stunkard, H. W., and M. C. Hinchcliffe. 1952. The morphology and life history of *Microbilharzia variglandis* (Miller and Northrup, 1926) Stunkard and Hinchcliffe, 1951, avian blood-flukes whose larvae cause "Swimmer's Itch" of ocean beaches. J. Parasitol. 38:248-265.

Tachon, P., and R. Borojevic. 1978. Mother-child relation in human schistosomiasis mansoni: skin test and cord blood reactivity to schistosomal antigens. Trans. R. Soc. Trop. Med. Hyg. 72:605-609.

Tiboldi, T. 1979. Reversibility of histopathological changes in the ovaries in acute murine schistosomiasis mansoni after niridazole treatment. Am. J. Trop. Med. Hyg. 28:1026-1030.

Van DerSchalie, H., and H. Blankespoor. 1977. Potential use of solar energy for snail-host control. The Biologist 59:16-24.

Waksman, B. H., and J. A. Cook. 1975. A report of a conference on newer immunologic approaches to schistosomiasis. Am. J. Trop. Med. Hyg. 24:1037-1039.

Walls, K. W. 1979. Immunoserology of parasitic diseases. In Friedman, H., T. J. Linna, and J. E. Prier, Editors. Immunoserology in the diagnosis of infectious diseases. University Park Press, Baltimore, Md.

Walls, R. C. 1976. An analysis of the current status of the schistosome dermatitis problem in Michigan. Sterkiana 63-64:1-64.

Warren, K. S. 1978. The pathology, pathobiology, and pathogenesis of schistosomiasis. Nature 273:609-612.

Warren, K. S., and others. 1979. Schistosomiasis hematobia in Coast Province Kenya: relationship between egg output and morbidity. Am. J. Trop. Med. Hyg. 28:864-870.

Warren, K. S., and V. A. Newill. 1968. Schistosomiasis. The Press of Case Western Reserve University, Cleveland, Ohio.

Webster, J. T., and others. 1975. Suppression of delayed hypersensitivity in schistosome-infected patients by niridazole. N. Engl. J. Med. 292:1144-1147.

Weiss, W., D. Stürchler, and F. M. Dietrich. 1978. Radioallergosorbent and indirect fluorescent antibody tests in immunodiagnosis of schistosomiasis. Lancet 2(8012):1231-1233.

Wilson, M., J. Fired, R. M. McQuay, and A. J. Sulzer. 1977. Evaluation of the indirect immunofluorescence and complement fixation tests for the serodiagnosis of schistosomiasis. Am. J. Trop. Med. Hyg. 26:1159-1163.

World Health Organization. 1967. Schistosomiasis. Measure of the public health importance of bilharziasis. WHO Technical Report Series no. 349. Geneva, Switzerland, pp. 1-81.

Wright, C. A., V. R. Southgate, and R. J. Knowles. 1972. What is *Schistosoma intercalatum?* Fisher, 1934? Trans. R. Soc. Trop. Med. Hyg. 66:28-56.

CHAPTER 15

Laboratory diagnosis of the protozoa and helminths

The diagnosis of protozoan infections of humans is dependent primarily on direct microscopic identification in the laboratory. When the parasites cannot be demonstrated, techniques such as immunoserology (Tables 15-1 and 15-2), biochemical tests, culture, and animal inoculation may be helpful.

The immunoserology of the parasitic diseases is a rapidly developing field. More effective methods for serodiagnosis are becoming available. The Center for Disease Control laboratory has available useful tests for 18 diseases (Table 15-1). New procedures have been developed involving the indirect hemagglutination (IHA), the enzyme-linked immunosorbent assay (ELISA), the indirect immunofluorescence (IIF), and the fluorescent immunoassay "X" (FIAX) tests. Serologic tests performed at the Center for Disease Control for the diagnosis of parasitic diseases are listed in Table 15-2, with their respective diagnostic titers.

INTESTINAL PROTOZOA

The intestinal canal is the chief route by which many protozoa parasitizing humans make their exit from the body. Obviously, the simplest means of establishing the presence of such parasites is to examine the feces.

Careful attention should be given to the collection and subsequent examination of the stool. Specific instructions should be given to the patient, nurse, or other attendant, to write the *time of passage* on the stool con-

tainer along with the name, date, and any other information needed. The specimen should be collected by *direct passage* into a clean container, avoiding contamination with urine, and brought directly to the laboratory. Urine, like water, will destory trophozoites present. Half-pint-sized, waxed cardboard cartons with overlapping lids are preferable because they eliminate the contamination which may easily occur when reusable containers with water containing free-living protozoa are used (Fig. 15-1). Pint- or quart-sized cartons may be necessary if larger samples are to be examined. The specimen should be covered *immediately* after passage to prevent deposition of fly eggs, larvae, or other possible contaminants.

If examination within 1 or 2 hours is not feasible, preservation is necessary to maintain the diagnostic stages of the protozoa present. Immediate refrigeration will sustain trophozoites from bacterial action for short periods of time, but motility characteristics may also be lost in the process. Cysts, on the other hand, will keep well for several days or weeks if drying of the specimen is prevented. It is advisable, however, insofar as trophozoites are concerned, to preserve part of the specimen in polyvinyl alcohol (PVA) fixative (see Appendix A), and the remainder in 5% formalin, or only part in formalin and part kept in the refrigerator as indicated previously. In place of PVA, merthiolate-iodine-formaldehyde (MIF) fixative-stain may be

Table 15-1. Immunodiagnostic tests for parasitic diseases

Parasitic diseases	Complement fixation	Agglutination tests				Indirect immuno-fluorescence	Immuno-diffusion	Immuno-electro-phoresis	Countercurrent electro-phoresis	Intradermal
		Bentonite flocculation	Indirect hemag-glutination	Latex	Direct agglu-tination					
Amebiasis	1	2	1	2	3	1	1	1	2	2
Chagas' disease	1		1	2	2	1	3	2	3	3
African trypano-somiasis	2		3			2	2			
Leishmaniasis	1		1	3	3	2	3	3	3	1
Malaria	2		1	2		1	1	3		
Pneumocystis	1			3		2				
Toxoplasmosis	1		1	3		1	3			1
Ancylostomiasis	3		1	2		3		3		2
Ascariasis	3	1	1			2	2	3		2
Clonorchiasis	1		1					3		1
Cysticercosis	2		2	2		2	2	3	3	3
Echinococcosis	1	1	1	2		1	2	1	3	1
Fascioliasis	1	3	1	2		2	3	3	3	2
Filariasis	2	1	1	3		1		3		2
Paragonimiasis	1	3	3				3	3		1
Schistosomiasis	1	2	1	3		1	2	3		1
Toxocariasis	3	1	1			2	3	3		2
Trichinellosis	1	1	1	1		1	2	2		1

Modified from Walls, K. W.: Immunoserology of parasitic diseases. In Friedman, H., Linna, T. J., and Prier, J. E., Editors. Immunoserology in the diagnosis of infectious diseases. University Park Press, 1979, Baltimore, Md.

*1, evaluated 2 test; 2, experimental test; 3, reported in the literature.

Table 15-2. Serologic tests performed in the Parasitology Division, Center for Disease Control, for the diagnosis of parasitic diseases

Disease	Tests*	Respective diagnostic titers
Amebiasis	IHA	$\geq 1:128$
Chagas' disease	CF, IHA	$\geq 1:8,\ \geq 1:128$
Leishmaniasis	DAT	$\geq 1:64$
Malaria	IIF	$\geq 1:64$
Pneumocystosis	IIF	$\geq 1:16$
Toxoplasmosis	IIF, IgM-IIF, IHA	$\geq 1:256,\ \geq 1:16,\ \geq 1:256$
Ascariasis	IHA,† BFT,† ELISA	$\geq 1:128,\ \geq 1:5,\ \geq 1:32$
Filariasis	IHA,† BFT†	$\geq 1:128,\ \geq 1:5$
Toxocariasis	IHA,† BFT,† ELISA	$\geq 1:128,\ \geq 1:5,\ \geq 1:32$
Strongyloidiasis	IHA	$\geq 1:64$
Trichinellosis	BFT	$\geq 1:5$
Paragonimiasis	CF	$\geq 1:8$
Schistosomiasis	IIF	Positive or negative
Cysticercosis	IHA	$\geq 1:128$
Echinococcosis	IHA	$\geq 1:128$
Babesia	IIF	$\geq 1:256$

From Department of Health, Education, and Welfare, Public Health Service, Center for Disease Control. Revised April 1979.

*IHA, Indirect microhemagglutination; CF, complement fixation; DAT, direct agglutination; IIF, indirect immunofluorescence; BFT, bentonite flocculation; ELISA, enzyme-linked immuno-specific assay.

†Both tests must be diagnostically positive for clinical purposes.

used (see Appendix A). The purpose of the PVA is to fix and preserve trophozoites of the amebas, but poorer results are obtained with cysts; however, MIF fixes and preserves trophozoites and cysts equally well.

Immediate examination of the specimen after passage is desired to capture the motility characteristics of trophozoites. The diagnosis of frank amebic dysentery, for example, will be relatively easy when this is done. The custom of some technicians to "warm" the dysenteric stool to preserve the motility characteristics of *E. histolytica* is not necessary and may prove detrimental by enhancing bacterial destruction of the organisms. The use of slides, coverslips, and reagents at room temperature (about 22° C) is sufficient for sustaining motility characteristics. When shipping by mail is necessary, stools may be preserved in MIF or part in PVA and part in 5% formalin.

The stool analysis consists of two parts, a macroscopic and microscopic examination.

Macroscopic examination

The consistency of the stool may furnish valuable information (Fig. 15-2). A watery, loose, soft stool is most likely to contain motile trophozoites and should be examined as soon as possible—at least within half an hour after passage—to utilize most effectively motility characteristics of the organisms. Diarrheal stools caused by amebiasis are usually offensive in odor, abundant in fecal material, and acidic in reaction, but occasionally, in dysentery, they may appear to be pure blood. Examine all stools with the aid of an applicator stick. Small flecks of blood and mucus, which may contain trophozoites of *E. histolytica*, should be selected for prompt microscopic examination. The applicator stick may also reveal hidden worms that might otherwise be completely overlooked within the fecal mass. Part of the fecal mass may be washed thoroughly, and strained through wire sieves of graded sizes in a search for worms.

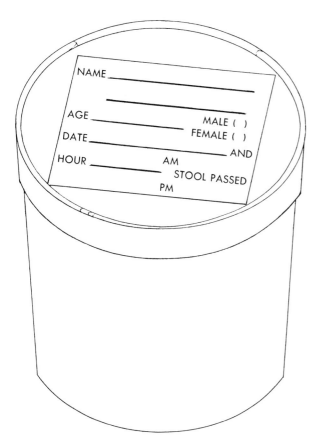

NAME_____

_____

AGE_____   MALE ( )

DATE_____   FEMALE ( )

_____ AND

HOUR _____ AM

STOOL PASSED

PM

Fig. 15-1. Cardboard carton container with overlapping lid for collection of fecal specimen. (From Melvin, D. M., and Brooke, M. M.: Laboratory procedures of intestinal parasites. 1934. CDC 75-8282, Atlanta, Georgia.)

Microscopic examination

The microscopic examination may be divided into three phases—direct saline smear, direct iodine-stained smear, and concentration.

Direct saline smear

Emulsify a small portion of feces from an applicator stick in a few drops of saline (0.85%) solution on a glass slide, cover with a coverslip, and examine microscopically (specimens containing oil droplets, barium, bismuth, and iron are unsatisfactory and should be discarded since they produce confusing artifacts or obscure the organisms). The ratio of feces to saline depends on the stool consistency and should result in a mount thin enough so that print can be easily read through it. It is best for beginners to make extra thin smears. After experience is acquired in distinguishing various artifacts from protozoa, the density of the smear may be increased as desired. Wet mounts may be ringed with melted paraffin-Vaseline (1:1) mixture, or nail polish, resin, or a similar substance to prevent drying for a prolonged period of study (Fig. 15-3).

Beginning at any one corner of the coverslip, cover the entire area using the *low-power* (16 mm) objective. Proper adjustment of the transmitted light is important.

All protozoa, as well as helminth ova and larvae, can be detected. Protozoan trophozoites and cysts will appear as glassy, clear, hyaline bodies, particularly noticeable as one begins to raise the objective out of focus (Fig. 15-4). Motility can be seen in the trophozoites. As organisms are found, examination by use of the high, dry (4 mm) objective will reveal greater detail. If no organ-

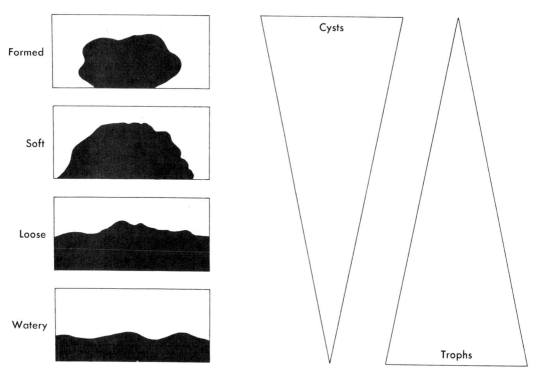

Fig. 15-2. Consistency of feces and distribution of cysts and trophozoites. (From Melvin, D. M., and Brooke, M. M.: Laboratory procedures for the diagnosis of intestinal parasites. 1934. CDC 75-8282, Atlanta, Georgia.)

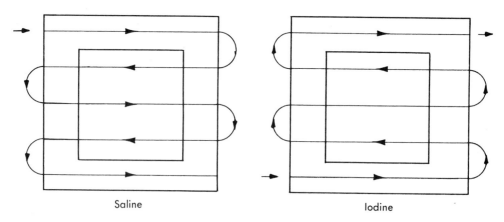

Fig. 15-3. Saline and iodine wet mounts sealed with paraffin-Vaseline (1:1) mixture. (Modified from Melvin, D. M., and Brooke, M. M.: Laboratory procedures for the diagnosis of intestinal parasites. 1934. CDC 75-8282, Atlanta, Georgia.)

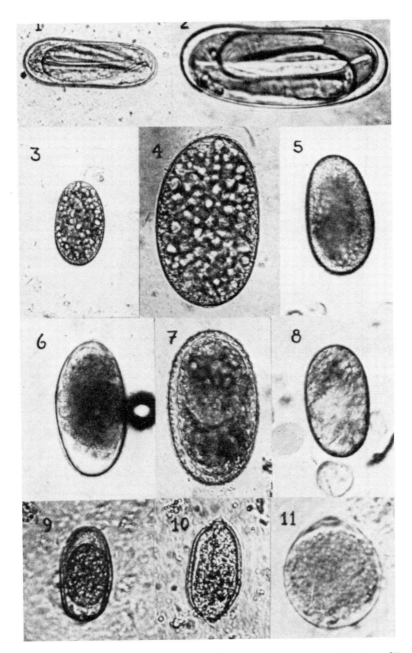

Fig. 15-4. Microscopic pseudoparasites encountered in human stool examinations. 1-2, Eggs of *Heterodera marioni* (nematodes in vegetables); 3-8, eggs of *Tyroglyphus* (mites) in various stages of development; 9-10, vegetable cells confused with helminth ova; 11, pine pollen grain. (From Kouri, P., and Basnuevo, J. G.: Lecciones de parasitología medicina tropical. Tomo II. Helmintología Humana. Ed. 3. 1949. La Habana, Cuba.)

isms are found in the direct saline smear, the direct iodine-stained smear may be omitted and the concentration procedure employed next.

Direct iodine-stained smear

Since it is usually impossible to identify protozoan cysts with certainty in a direct saline smear, some staining procedure must be employed. Emulsify a small portion of feces, as previously, in a few drops of iodine solution on a glass slide, place coverslip, and examine as described earlier.

Several iodine solutions have been recommended (see Appendix A). The cytoplasm of the protozoan cysts will stain a light brown to yellow; glycogen present will take on a more intense brownish coloration. The nuclei, with the chromatin granules and karyosomes, become dark brown and appear as refractile masses. Chromatoidal bodies, unfortunately, are less discernible than in saline preparations. Trophozoites are usually distorted beyond recognition.

In place of iodine, MIF (see Appendix A) may be substituted. This method has the added advantage of preserving and staining trophozoites as well as cysts. The staining reaction occurs in the following two parts:

1. An initial iodine stain in which cysts and trophozoites stain from a yellowish green to a yellowish brown.
2. A subsequent eosin stain that gradually replaces the iodine and persists. Nuclear and cytoplasmic elements vary in staining intensity with species, age, and stage of the protozoan parasites. Helminth eggs and larvae also stain and remain morphologically characteristic. At time of completion of staining, the cytoplasm of all trophozoites and cysts takes the eosin stain. Nuclear membranes appear to stain dark red to jet black, whereas nuclear chromatin remains essentially unstained as in the simple iodine stain.

Concentration

Protozoan cysts, when present in small numbers, may be missed completely in the direct smear examination. When one or more parasites are readily apparent, other species that are detected only by concentration tech-

nique may be present. Thus a concentration procedure should be used on all stools whether or not the direct smear is positive.

All concentration techniques employ the principle of either flotation or sedimentation. Trophozoites are destroyed in both procedures except when the MIF concentration method is used.

Flotation procedures. Though various salt and sugar solutions may be used in most instances, zinc sulfate (sp gr, 1.18) is the solution of choice for protozoan cysts and many helminth ova. All depend on the principle of having a specific gravity greater than that of the organism to be recovered. The *zinc sulfate flotation technique* (modified) is described here:

1. Make an emulsion of feces in tap water and filter the suspension through two layers of wet gauze.
2. Centrifuge 1 to 2 minutes at about 1,500 rpm. Decant supernatant.
3. Add a few milliliters of tap water, reemulsify sediment, and fill tube with tap water. Centrifuge as before. Decant supernatant.
4. Repeat washings until supernatant is fairly clear. Decant.
5. Add a few milliliters of $ZnSO_4$ (sp gr, 1.18); reemulsify and fill tube with $ZnSO_4$. Centrifuge as before.
6. Carefully remove test tube to rack and remove organisms from top film by wire loop, pipette, or coverslip.
7. Prepare unstained and iodine-stained smears and examine microscopically.

NOTE: It is very important that the $ZnSO_4$ solution have a specific gravity of exactly 1.18. Check solution with hydrometer after first dissolving 400 gm of salt in 100 ml of water. Add water or salt as needed to adjust specific gravity to exactly 1.18.

Sedimentation procedures. Sedimentation techniques, usually involving centrifugation to hasten the sedimentation of organisms, are based on the principle that much fecal debris, along with soluble material, can be removed by extraction from the sediment. Such procedures are preferred to flotation techniques in that the recovery of more species of parasites is possible, since all will sediment but not all will float. Also, in some sedimentation procedures the organisms are in a better state of preservation and are more abundant than with flotation methods.

The *Formalin-ether sedimentation technique* (modified) is the most popular of many such techniques available (see Appendix A) and is described here:

1. Comminute a portion of feces in tap water and strain the emulsion through two layers of wet gauze.
2. Centrifuge at 1,500 rpm for 1 to 2 minutes. Decant supernatant.
3. Add a few milliliters of tap water, reemulsify sediment, and fill tube with tap water. Centrifuge as before. Decant supernatant.
4. Repeat washings until supernatant is fairly clear. Decant.
5. Add a few milliliters of 5% formalin, reemulsify and fill tube three-fourths full with 5% formalin. Allow suspension to stand 5 minutes. Killing and fixation of organisms take place. The preserved material may be kept indefinitely or the procedure continued.
6. Resuspend the sediment and overlay with about 3 ml of ether. Stopper and shake vigorously.
7. Centrifuge as before for 1 to 2 minutes. Four layers will result, as follows: a topmost layer of ether, a ring of debris, a solution of formalin, and sediment in the bottom containing the organisms.
8. Ring the plug of fecal debris with an applicator stick and decant the three top layers.
9. Remove sediment to a slide and prepare unstained and iodine-stained smears. Examine microscopically.

MIF preserved specimens may also be concentrated in the same manner as the formalin-ether technique described previously, by substituting the MIF specimen for the formalin and beginning the procedure at step 5.

Special stains such as Quensel's and buffered methylene blue (see Appendix A) are useful in revealing the nuclear characteristics of the trophozoites of the amebas. The presence of *Dientamoeba fragilis* may be demonstrated by making an aqueous mount (tap or distilled water) of the fecal specimen. This method is used to destroy *Blastocystis hominis*, a common yeast in feces, and to identify *D. fragilis*. While other trophozoites disintegrate completely, *D. fragilis* swells, ruptures, and then regains a spherical shape enclosing small particles in brownian movement. This phenomenon can be microscopically observed immediately after making the aqueous mount.

If facilities permit and time is available, cultivation (see Appendix A) may be used to good advantage when dealing with fresh specimens. The modified Boeck and Drobohlav's medium consists of a solid egg base with an overlay of Locke's solution. It supports and maintains the growth of most of the intestinal protozoa. The materials for preparing it are usually readily available in most laboratories. An added advantage is that fresh serum is not required. Balamuth's egg infusion medium, satisfactory for most intestinal protozoa, is an all liquid medium to which liver has been added. Storage for several months without much deterioration is one of its advantages. Cleveland and Collier's medium for cultivating the intestinal protozoa consists of a solid liver infusion agar slant with an overlay of physiological saline and fresh horse serum. According to some workers, it is more specific for *E. histolytica* than for the other protozoa. Permanent stained smears should be made of organisms recovered by cultural methods and should be examined under oil immersion.

Instances arise when permanent stained smears of the fecal specimen are necessary for diagnosis or medical-legal reasons. Such preparations afford a permanent record, and frequently small organisms missed by routine wet preparations are found on the stained slide when examined under oil immersion. The PVA method of fixation is recommended as the effective way to preserve fecal specimens for staining by any of the usual staining procedures since the films are permeable to most of the stains employed. It is important to remember that PVA fixed slides must be thoroughly dried and then placed in 70% alcohol containing iodine (port wine color) for about 20 minutes to remove the mercuric chloride crystals. Since PVA serves as both an adhesive and a fixative, diarrheic stools and sediment from cultures may be placed on slides with no fear of losing the material during the staining process. The classic, long iron-hematoxylin method, while giving excellent results, is also time consuming and requires critical attention in the destaining procedure. The present scarcity of hematoxylin has resulted in greater use of shorter methods such as the trichrome and chlorazol black E procedures (see Appendix A).

The trichrome staining method is rapid and simple in technique and gives satisfactory results for routine use. No mordant is necessary before staining as in the long iron-hematoxylin procedure. The stain solution is stable and can be used repeatedly; the only concern is that a rest period is necessary after repeated use. Strength returns upon standing in 3 to 8 hours after open air evaporation. Staining time is longer for PVA fixed material than for fresh materials fixed by other methods.

The chlorazol black E staining technique combines fixation and staining in the same solution. No destaining is necessary. The procedure is more satisfactory with fresh fecal smears than with PVA fixed material. The stock solution may be kept indefinitely, and dilutions for use made as needed. Repeated use of the working solution will "wear out" the stain as indicated by the slides appearing visibly red rather than greenish black. Such red slides, however, can be restained in fresh stain. Each liter of stain must have the optimal staining dilution and time determined. Protozoa in tissue sections may also be stained with chlorazol black E. Sections are treated in the same manner as other tissue slides for removal of the paraffin. Thickness of 5 to 7 μm give good staining results.

Repeatedly negative examinations of formed stools for protozoa, in suspected cases, can be followed by the examination of postcathartic specimens; this procedure will frequently flush out the organisms lying in the cecum. Saline cathartics, preferably buffered sodium biphosphate or sodium sulfate, should be used for purgation. Agents such as bismuth, mineral oil, or magnesia compounds are not satisfactory, since oil globules confuse the examiner, and crystalline debris from bismuth and magnesia compounds often obscure the organisms or distort the appearance of trophozoites. In diarrheal or cathartic stools or material collected at sigmoidoscopy, trophozoites are usually recovered when protozoa are present, and so direct saline smears should be examined as soon as possible. Since trophozoites of the amebas may be difficult to identify, permanent stained slides should also be examined under oil immersion for identifying characteristics.

When protozoan infection is strongly suspected, repeated stool examinations should be made before concluding that the tests are negative. Since the protozoa are cyclic in appearance and are more abundant at some times than others, *at least* three stool examinations should be made, spread 2 to 3 days apart. Cultivation, postcatharsis examination, and sigmoidoscopy should be employed as necessary. Repeated scrapings from the rectal mucosa may reveal trophozoites of *E. histolytica* in a few chronic cases of idiopathic colitis.

TISSUE AND BLOOD PROTOZOA

Protozoa invading the body tissues present a more difficult problem in diagnosis. Techniques peculiar to location of protozoa must be employed when recovery is desired.

The aspirate from a liver abscess should be collected in serial containers. Only the last portion drawn (which is frequently reddish in color) should be used for examination; it represents pus nearest the cyst wall that is most likely to contain trophozoites. When amebas are not readily apparent, treating the aspirate from an amebic abscess with streptodornase, a proteolytic enzyme, will free the ameba for microscopic examination or culture inoculation. Ten units of the enzyme are added to each 1 ml of aspirate and incubated for 30 minutes at 30° C with repeated shaking. Centrifugation for 5 minutes at 100 rpm may reveal the organisms in the sediment.

Leishmania parasites are most abundant in the border of the lesion and normal tissue. They can be recovered by aspiration of a mixture of tissue juice and cells from the indurated edge of the lesion. Dab smears, dried on a slide and stained with Wright's or Giemsa, will reveal the organism in large mononuclear cells or ruptured out of these cells from trauma in making the smear. Similar staining techniques are employed for the study of bone marrow, liver, and spleen aspirates. Occasionally, infected mononuclear cells of the bloodstream may be seen when an examination of the buffy coat is made.

Citrated blood is centrifuged at 750 rpm for 5 minutes. The thin creamy layer (buffy coat) between the red cells and the plasma is removed with a capillary pipette, placed on a slide, dried, and stained with Giemsa or Wright's (see Appendix B). This buffy coat may also be used for inoculation into hamsters or for culture on various blood agar based media (see Appendix B). Bone marrow, liver, and spleen aspirates may be handled in a similar manner.

Napier's aldehyde test and Chopra's antimony test (see Appendix B) are both nonspecific reactions not dependent on an antigen-antibody reaction but solely indicative of an increase in the euglobulin fractions of the blood protein, a condition that may occur in other diseases as well. However, both are considered valuable serologic tests for the diagnosis of kala-azar. In endemic areas, these tests are considered quite reliable, particularly when both are strongly positive simultaneously.

Trypanosoma cruzi, in the trypomastigote stage, can be detected in the peripheral blood only in early infections or during exacerbations of the disease. Frequently, the number of organisms may be so small that detection by examination of a wet mount or stained slide is not possible and concentration is desirable. Fractional centrifugation of a large blood sample is effective in concentrating a few parasites when present. Citrated blood is centrifuged at 900 to 1,000 rpm for 3 minutes. The supernatant is trans-

ferred to a second tube and centrifuged at 1,500 rpm for 10 minutes. The transfer is repeated with centrifugation at 1,800 to 2,000 rpm for 15 to 20 minutes. The sediment may be examined directly as a wet mount for living organisms or stained with Giemsa on a slide. The sediment, if handled aseptically, may be used for animal inoculation and culture. The culture of blood, bone marrow, lymph node, spleen, and liver aspirates on blood agar based media (see Appendix B) will reveal epimastigotes (crithidial forms). Xenodiagnosis, the feeding of clean triatomid bugs on the suspected patient with the subsequent examination of the bug's feces several weeks later for trypomastigotes (trypanosomal forms), is the method of choice in endemic areas of South America.

The African trypanosomes, when few in number, may be concentrated by the fractional centrifugation technique described for *T. cruzi*. *T. b. gambiense* and *T. b. rhodesiense* can be detected in peripheral blood smears during febrile attacks as well as in lymph node aspirates. Thick smears made from the layer between the plasma and leukocytes of centrifuged blood are stained with Wright's or Giemsa. Some workers employ bone marrow aspirates. The inoculation of guinea pigs and rats (the latter free of *T. lewisi*) with suspected material is sometimes effective. Culture on artificial media such as Weinman's medium (see Appendix B) is seldom used. During the central nervous system phase of the Gambian disease, the spinal fluid may reveal active trypomastigotes.

The diagnosis of malaria depends on the recovery and identification of the erythrocytic stages of the parasites in thin and thick blood films. (The exoerythrocytic stages occurring in the parenchymal cells of the liver have been demonstrated only under experimental conditions and, at present, do not offer a means of routine diagnosis.) The thick blood film is the technique of choice; it is said that 5 minutes spent examining a thick smear is equivalent to one-half hour on a thin film. A drop of blood placed on the slide is spread to form a dime-sized smear by using the edge of a second slide. Immediately after preparation, such smears should be turned film side down in a slide box and protected from dust while drying. Pretreatment before staining by dipping the smear into a methylene blue phosphate solution (see Appendix B) will lyse the red cells. Thick smears stained with Giemsa will reveal the malarial parasites free of the lysed red blood cells. The lysis of the red cells destroys many characteristics useful in identification of the various species of malaria recognizable in thin film. However, with practice, proficiency can be attained in identifying the various species. After the parasites are found, it is necessary to know the variations of forms possible and to decide what pattern is applicable. A minimum of 50 microscopic fields of a positive thick blood smear should be examined before making the decision on which species is involved. In heavy infections, readily apparent in thin smears, parasitized red cells may prove more useful for species identification for the inexperienced. It is important to examine repeated blood smears over a period of time before concluding that the patient does not have malaria.

In recent years, fluorescent antibody tests have achieved some popularity in the diagnosis and study of tissue protozoa, particularly malaria. Cross reactivity makes it possible to test the suspected patient's sera against similar but nonidentical parasites. For example, readily available slides of monkey malaria with large numbers of parasitized red blood cells are first layered with the patient's sera in various dilutions. Fluorescein-labelled antihuman gamma globulin is then layered onto the red cells.

Under fluorescent microscopy, the degree of fluorescence can be graded, and high titers are suggestive of recent infection. Such techniques are used primarily for studies of antibody response but may also be helpful in diagnosing patients with low-grade parasitemia and in detecting the source of transfusion malaria.

Animal inoculation is probably the best procedure for demonstrating the presence of *Toxoplasma gondii* since material from the patient seldom shows the organism on direct examination. White mice are the animals of choice. The leukocyte layer of centrifuged blood, concentrated spinal fluid, and lymph gland fluid are usually used as the inoculum. About 0.5 ml is injected intraperitoneally or intracerebrally, and the animals are observed for symptoms of ascites and general debility. Within a few days the peritoneal fluid should be examined by stained smear since the organisms fluorish readily in this environment. Dab smears of brain tissue may also be prepared and stained with Giemsa. Triturated brain tissue or peritoneal fluid may be blind passaged (aseptically) to other mice if examinations of the first animals are negative. Serology is discussed on p. 262.

Free-living soil amebas such as *Naegleria* and *Acanthamoeba* can be isolated from the spinal fluid of infected patients by using the fractional centrifugation technique described for the trypanosomes. The amebas will grow in the usual tissue culture systems. Good growth of *Naegleria* has been reported in 2% Bacto-Casitone with 10% fresh horse, calf, or rabbit serum, transferring being done every 5 days. Intracerebral inoculation of suspected spinal fluid sediment or tissue emulsion into white mice (11 to 13 gm) will bring up the infection. Histological sectioning of mouse brain tissue as well as microscopic examination of mouse spinal fluid will reveal organisms.

Although duodenal aspiration is not a routine procedure for parasite examination, at times it will reveal *Giardia lamblia* and *Strongyloides stercoralis*. In addition to drainage, duodenal material may be collected by using a nylon thread coiled in a weighted gelatin capsule, which the patient swallows. One end of the thread is taped to the cheek of the patient. As the thread unwinds, the capsule dissolves in the stomach and the weighted string is carried by peristalsis into the duodenum. After 3 to 4 hours the string is retrieved, the weight being released and passed out in the feces. Bile-stained mucus is scraped off the string and examined microscopically in a saline wet mount. An iodine preparation can be made also, if desired. Material, preserved in 5% formalin, may be examined at any future time. The routine method for the diagnosis of *Trichomonas vaginalis* infection (see p. 53) is the microscopic examination of the vaginal exudate in a saline preparation. More positive results, however, are obtained by culture methods (see Appendix B).

INTESTINAL WORMS

Diagnosis of the worm infections of humans, like most of the protozoan infections, is dependent primarily on microscopic examination. Recovery of worms, visible to the naked eye, from the feces or body tissues may occur sometimes. Techniques such as immunoserology, biochemical tests, animal inoculation, and culture may be useful adjuncts. Special techniques are described in Appendixes A and B.

Like the protozoa, many worms use the intestinal canal as the route of exit from the body and appear in the feces in the egg, larva, or adult stage. Worms living in the biliary passages of the liver, the bronchioles of the lung, and the bowel venous plexuses may also pass their ova into the fecal stream as do the intestinal lumen dwellers themselves.

The techniques applicable for the collection and examination of the feces for protozoa are likewise applicable for most of the helminths. Greater attention should be paid to the examination of the unstained smears because iodine, in some instances, renders some eggs more obscure by the staining reaction. In most instances, concentration techniques are best confined to sedimentation procedures, because some eggs such as those of infertile *Ascaris* and operculated ova do not float in zinc sulfate (sp gr, 1.18), whereas the schistosome eggs may be distorted.

Since many worms are prolific egg producers, the presence of these eggs in the feces affords an excellent means of diagnosis. Four important criteria should be kept in mind when examining eggs: size, shape, color, and stage of development.

For practical purposes, worm eggs may be grouped into 3 *sizes:* small, medium, and large. Small eggs average up to 35 μm the medium size are 50 to 70 μm whereas the large eggs are 100 μm or longer. These are rough estimates, and borderline ranges may occur. However, this method serves to separate some eggs from others that otherwise might be quite similar in appearance. Within egg-size range, specific measurements by means of an ocular micrometer may be necessary at times.

The *shape* of the egg may be unique to the species. The flattened side of the pinworm egg, for example, illustrates this point as does the lateral spine on *Schistosoma mansoni* and the terminal spine on *S. haematobium*. The whipworm egg is typically barrel shaped with polar plugs.

The *color* of the egg at times may be helpful in identification. *Ascaris, Hymenolepis diminuta,* and the whipworm ova, for example, pick up bile pigments as they pass down the intestinal tract and thus present a yellow-to-orange coloration when found in the feces. *H. nana* and hookworm ova, on the other hand, are never stained and so appear clear and colorless.

Eggs are eliminated from the body in varying *stages of development,* from single celled ova to eggs containing well-developed larvae. In some cases, hatching may take place within the intestinal tract or in the feces shortly after passage. Thus *Ascaris* and whipworm ova are in a single-cell stage when passed in freshly voided feces, whereas the cyclophyllidean tapeworm ova contain an embryo within. Pinworm ova oviposited in the perianal folds of the skin contain "tadpole" larvae. *Strongyloides* presents hatched rhabditiform larvae in fresh feces, but delay in passage may result in the presence of the advanced filariform stage. With a knowledge of the time of passage of the stool specimen, as well as the life history of the parasite, one can deduce which species the stage of development present might preclude.

A quantitative determination of eggs in the feces offers a means of evaluating the worm burden (see Appendix A). When adult worms are recovered, identification usually presents no problem, in most instances, to the well-trained technician. The search for adult worms in the feces may be aided by the sifting of the fecal mass, suspended in water, through sieves of graded sizes. In this manner, adult worms, such as pinworms, hookworms, whipworms, and segments of tapeworm, may be obtained.

TISSUE WORMS

The diagnostic stages of many worms, depending on their location in the body, may be recovered from various body tissues and fluids. The blood stream is the source of most microfilariae. Wet mounts of fresh blood will quickly reveal their presence, thrashing about among the red blood cells. Thick blood smears, as used in the diagnosis of malaria, will permit species identification when stained with Giemsa (see Appendix B). Since the microfilariae of *Onchocerca volvulus* and *Dipetalonema streptocerca* are found in the skin, thin sections of pinched skin sliced with a razor blade or scalpel without drawing blood will reveal the organisms when examined microscopically in a saline mount. In the Americas, where nodules of *O. volvulus* predominate in the head and neck

region, biopsies are most conveniently performed over the trapezius or deltoid muscles to obscure scarring. Muscle biopsy specimens for *Trichinella* larvae, when pressed between glass slides and examined microscopically will reveal the parasites, if present. However, digestion of portion of the biopsy specimen in artificial gastric juice (see Appendix A) is recommended to ensure a more certain diagnosis. Immunoserology (see text on *T. spiralis*), however, is more commonly employed.

The examination of sputum, as well as the feces, for eggs of *Paragonimus westermani* is indicated. Reports indicate the rare appearance of *Echinococcus* cyst material and schistosome eggs in the sputum. Collected sputum for helminths is mixed with 5 volumes of 5% sodium hydroxide and left standing for 2 to 3 hours with occasional mixing. After centrifugation at 2,000 rpm for 2 minutes the sediment is examined.

The presence of viable schistosome ova in the feces can be readily detected by the egg-hatching technique for miracidia (see Appendix A). Although the last 5 to 10 ml of urine from the bladder at times may reveal the heaviest concentration of *Schistosoma haematobium* ova, such is not always the case, and the entire specimen should be examined. Cysticerci, when removed from the subcutaneous tissues, should be dissected and the scolex evaginated and examined for hooks to substantiate the diagnosis. Liver biopsies may confirm the diagnosis of visceral larva migrans although this is not a recommended routine procedure. The rectal punch biopsy method for the diagnosis of *Schistosoma mansoni* infections is highly effective for revealing eggs when stool examinations are repeatedly negative. The technique is painless and, in the hands of a competent proctologist, easy to perform. A slide press examination of the tissue biopsy specimen will reveal both viable and dead ova.

Gross morphologic characteristics are usually sufficient for the identification of most adult worms. Microscopic examination of cuticular markings or uterine branching in tapeworm proglottids may be necessary at times. The latter is easily accomplished by pressing segments between glass slides and counting the lateral uterine branches or locating eggs in packets in uterine sacs.

REVIEW QUESTIONS

1. What are the essential parts of a stool examination for intestinal protozoa? For intestinal helminths?
2. How is the time of passage of a stool specimen, in relation to the time of examination, of importance in making the diagnosis?
3. Discuss the significance of the size, shape, color, and stage of development of worms eggs?
4. Describe how to make a thick blood film. Why is it preferred to a thin smear and why is it more difficult to prepare?
5. What is the significance of finding amastigotes in a dab smear from internal organs of the body?
6. What are the merits and drawbacks of the ZnSO₄ flotation and the formalin-ether sedimentation techniques?
7. Discuss the diagnosis of the schistosomes.
8. Discuss the status of the serodiagnosis of parasitic diseases.

REFERENCES

Ash, L. R., and others. 1977. Procedures suggested for use in examination of clinical specimens for parasitic infection: a statement by the subcommittee on laboratory standards, committee on education. American Society of Parasitologists. J. Parasitol. **63**:959-960.

Beal, C. B., P. Viens, R. G. L. Grant, and J. M. Hughes. 1970. A new technique for sampling duodenal contents. Am. J. Trop. Med. Hyg. **19**:349-352.

Beaver, P. C. 1950. The standardization of fecal smears for estimating egg production and worm burden. J. Parasitol. **36**:451-456.

Beemer, A. M. 1947. Supravital staining of amoebae and some observations on laboratory diagnosis. S. Afr. Med. J. **21**:550-552.

Blagg, W. E. L., and others. 1955. A new concentration technic for the demonstration of protozoa and helminth eggs in feces. Am. J. Trop. Med. Hyg. **4**:23-28.

Brooke, M. M., and M. Goldman. 1949. Polyvinyl alcohol-fixative as a preservative and adhesive for protozoa in dysenteric stool and other liquid material. J. Lab. Clin. Med. **34**:1554-1560.

Chopra, R. N., J. C. Das Gupta, and J. C. David. 1927. The antimony test in the diagnosis of kala azar. Indian Med. Gas. **62**:688-691.

Eveland, L. K., M. Kenney, and V. Yermakov. 1975. The value of routine screening for intestinal parasites. Am. J. Public Health **65**:1326-1327.

Garcia, L. S., and L. R. Ash. 1979. Diagnostic parasitology: clinical laboratory manual. Ed. 2, The C. V. Mosby Co. St. Louis.

Gleason, N. N., and G. R. Healy. 1965. Modification and evaluation of Kohn's one-step staining technique for intestinal protozoa in feces or tissue. Am. J. Clin. Pathol. **43**:494-496.

Kagan, I. G., and L. Norman. 1976. Serodiagnosis of parasitic diseases: manual of clinical immunology. American Society of Microbiology, Washington, D.C.

Kim, C. W. 1975. The diagnosis of parasitic diseases. Prog. Clin. Pathol. **6**:267-288.

Lobel, H. O., and I. G. Kagan. 1978. Seroepidemiology of parasitic diseases. Annu. Rev. Microbiol. **32**:329-347.

Mazzotti, L. 1951. Observations based on cutaneous biopsies in onchocerciasis. Am. J. Trop. Med. **31**:624-627.

Melvin, D. M., and M. M. Brooke. 1974. Laboratory procedures for the diagnosis of intestinal parasites. Department of Health, Education, and Welfare, Center for Disease Control, Atlanta, Georgia.

Morkey, R. L. 1950. A vaseline swab for the diagnosis of *Enterobius* eggs. Am. J. Clin. Pathol. **20**:493.

Napier, L. E. 1921. Kala-azar. Indian Med. Gaz. 401-404.

Novy, F. G., and W. J. MacNeal. 1904. On the cultivation of *Trypanosoma brucei*. J. Int. Dis. **1**:1-30.

Ritchie, L. S. 1948. An ether sedimentation technique for routine stool examinations. Bull. U.S. Army Med. Dept. **8**:326.

Sapero, J. J., and D. K. Lawless. 1953. The MIF stain-preservation technic for the identification of intestinal protozoa. Am. J. Trop. Med. **2**:613-619.

Sehgal, S. C., V. K. Vinayak, and U. Gupta. 1977. Evaluation of Kato thick smear technique for the detection of helminthic ova in feces. Indian J. Med. Res. **65**:509-512.

Sodeman, T. M., and N. Dock. 1976. Laboratory diagnosis of parasitic fungal diseases of the central nervous system. Ann. Clin. Lab. Sci. **6**:47-55.

Stoll, N. R. 1923. Investigations on the control of hookworm disease. XV. An effective method of counting hookworm eggs in feces. Am. J. Hyg. **3**:59-70.

Telemann, W. 1908. Eine Methode sur Erleicherung der Auffindung von Parasiteneiern in den Faeces. Deutsch. Med. Wochenschr. **34**:1510-1511.

Tobie, J. E., and others. 1951. The efficiency of the zinc sulfate technic in the detection of intestinal protozoa by successive stool examinations. Am. J. Trop. Med. **31**:552-560.

Walker, A. J. 1963. Manual for the microscopic diagnosis of malaria. Ed. 2. Pan American Health Organization Scientific Publication no. 87, U.S. Government Printing Office, Washington, D.C.

Walls, K. W. 1979. Immunoserology of parasitic diseases. In Friedman, H., T. J. Linna, and J. E. Prier, Editors. Immunoserology in the diagnosis of infectious diseases. University Park Press, Baltimore, Md.

Weller, T. H., and G. J. Damin. 1945. An improved method of examination of feces for diagnosis of in-

testinal schistosomiasis. Am. J. Clin. Pathol. **15**:496-500.

Wheatley, W. B. 1951. A rapid staining procedure for intestinal amoebae and flagellates. Am. J. Clin. Pathol. **21**:990-991.

Wilcox, A. 1960 Manual for the microscopic diagnosis of malaria in man. Public Health Series Publication no. 796, U.S. Department of Health, Education, and Welfare, Public Health Service, U.S. Government Printing Office, Washington, D.C.

Yaeger, R. G. 1960. A method of isolating trypanosomes from blood. J. Parasitol. **46**:288.

PART THREE

Medical arthropodology

CHAPTER 16

Introduction to the arthropods

The phylum Arthropoda, which includes the insects and their allies, contains over four times as many species of organisms as the remainder of the entire animal kingdom. Of all the invertebrates, the arthropods are the most highly organized. Three outstanding characteristics serve to distinguish them from their lowly brethren. At some period in their life history all show the following features:

Jointed appendages
Chitinized exoskeleton
Hemocele

The arthropods are of medical importance because of the role they play in causing diseases either through the transmission of disease-producing agents or the direct action through the innoculation of poison or invading tissue. The five classes categorized as being of medical importance on the basis of either the number or the severity of the illnesses that they cause are listed below:

Chilopoda—centipedes
Pentastomida—tongue worms
Crustacea—crabs, crayfish, and copepods
Arachnida—spiders, scorpions, mites, and ticks
Hexapoda—insects

FREQUENCY OF ARTHROPOD-RELATED DISEASES IN THE UNITED STATES

The arthropod diseases of major importance in terms of frequency and severity in the United States are shown in Table 16-1.

Scabies and pediculosis are currently epidemic in the United States and in many other parts of the world. It is estimated, based on pediculicide sales, that in 1976 approximately six million cases of pediculosis occurred in the United States. Envenomization is also a serious clinical entity, and reports are almost certainly inadequate. Severe illness and death from insect stings, particularly from the Hymenoptera, are common, and more than 400 fatal reactions were recorded by the American Academy of Allergy over a 10-year period. Honeybees accounted for 44% of the 400 deaths, wasps for 26%, yellow jackets for 18%, and 12% were unclassified. Seventy-eight percent of the 400 deaths had resulted from four or fewer stings, a finding which suggested an allergic basis for the fatal reaction and emphasized the need for appropriate desensitization of individuals susceptible to severe reactions. Members of these classes affect humans by being pests, inoculating poisons, invading tissues, or transmitting disease agents.

PESTS

Rare indeed is the individual who, at some time or another in his life, has not had some experience with an arthropod. Most of us are quite familiar wiht the red bugs, or chiggers, which are most annoying because of our sensitiveness to their secretions. The bites of the mosquito and a great variety of other insects are all too familiar to us. In the jungles and virgin forests large beasts roaming wild are less a threat to humans than are the untold numbers of tiny arthropods that make life unbearable for the person who travels there.

Table 16-1. Descriptive epidemiologic features of urban-pest-associated diseases in the
United States, 1970-1979

Disease	Prevalence	Severity	Geographic distribution	Population affected
Scabies	Poorly documented; ~3% patients visiting dermatologists have scabies	Mild; occasionally disabling	All areas	All; crowding a factor
Western equine encephalitis	~50 cases per year of proven encephalitis	Severe; ~2% fatal, 15% in outbreaks	Western and north central states	Rural and small-town young children most severely affected
Eastern equine encephalitis	<5 cases per year of proven encephalitis	Quite severe; 50% fatal	Eastern seaboard; Texas to New Hampshire	Typically rural-suburban; near marsh
St. Louis encephalitis	>200 cases per year of proven encephalitis	Severe; ~7% fatal	All areas except New England	Both urban and rural; most >40 years old
Arthropod envenomization	Undetermined, probably high	>40 reported deaths yearly	All areas	Both urban and rural
California encephalitis	~100 cases per year of proven encephalitis	Death uncommon; mild neurologic impairment frequent	Most north central states; few eastern and southeastern states	Children in wooded areas, including urban-suburban
Rocky Mountain spotted fever	~800 cases per year of reported infection	Moderate to severe; 5% fatal (1977)	Most of U.S.; highest prevalence in south Atlantic states	Especially children and young adults participating in outdoor activities
Pediculosis	Poorly documented studies of outbreaks in N.Y., Ga., and Fl. showed 8% prevalence in schoolchildren in 1973-74	Mild	All areas	Especially schoolchildren (head lice); crowding a factor

Adapted from Kappus, K. D. Bureau of Epidemiology, Center for Disease Control, Atlanta, Ga.

INOCULATION OF POISONS

Though the secretions of many arthropods are, in a scientific sense, poisonous to our system, we have limited the significantly poisonous arthropods to a smaller group.

The centipedes, varying in their toxicity according to species, for the most part are not dangerous, but very small children and the very aged may show marked sensitivity to their bites. Death is rarely attributable to them. Among the spiders, the black widow is well known as a poisonous species. Scorpions, quite common in the southern United States, can cause severe pain and systemic disorders through the inoculation of their poisons. Paralysis is caused by the injection of toxin from gravid female ticks embedded in the flesh of the host.

TISSUE INVADERS

Although some of the arthropods already mentioned are actually tissue invaders, for convenience we can limit this group to certain arthropods that are especially notorious for their ability to invade tissues.

The tongue worms are degenerate, worm-like arthropods that, in their larval stages, may be found free or encysted in the viscera of humans.

Though ticks and mites, for the most part, are actually tissue invaders, only a select few are discussed, since the others are of concern chiefly as vectors for disease-producing agents. The itch mite, *Sarcoptes scabiei*, is undoubtedly the best known.

The most important of the tissue invaders are those insects that, during the larval stage of their life cycle, invade the human tissues and produce the disease known as myiasis.

DISEASE TRANSMISSION AND DISSEMINATION

As stated previously, it is chiefly as vectors of disease-producing agents that arthropods are of medical importance. Transmission is accomplished in two ways—mechanical and biologic.

Mechanical transmission

Arthropods frequently act as passive agents in the transmission of pathogenic agents. The agents are like hitchhikers, bearing no relationship whatever with the vehicle carrying them. Houseflies are notorious as mechanical transmitters of bacteria, viruses, and protozoa. The importance of any particular arthropod as a mechanical vector depends on the degree to which the structures of its body facilitate the carrying of disease agents (internally and externally) and the extent to which its habits bring it in contact first with the agents and then with humans. Any arthropod capable of breaking the human skin is a potential mechanical transmitter of a blood- or tissue-disease agent.

Biologic transmission

Many times arthropods act as essential hosts of the agents being transmitted. With-

Table 16-2. Important vector-borne diseases and control measures

Disease	Main vectors	Present	Future prospects
		Control measures	
Chagas' disease (American trypanosomiasis)	Reduviid bugs (*Rhodnius prolixus*, *Triatoma maculata*)	Residual spray of insecticides indoors[1]	Improved housing
Sleeping sickness (African trypanosomiasis)	Tsetse flies (*Glossina* sp)	Selective clearing and habitat management; adulticides[2]	Permanent preventive measures through *Glossina* eradication using genetic methods and remote possibility of immunization
Leishmaniasis	Sandflies (*Phlebotomus* spp)	Residual spraying[3] or peri-domestic fogging[4]	Improvement in living conditions
Onchocerciasis	Blackflies (*Simulium* sp)	Larvicide application to breeding sites[5]	None in the immediate future
Schistosomiasis	Freshwater snails as intermediate hosts	Molluscicide application[6] and habitat management	Environmental control through source reduction, excreta disposal, and piped water supply
Tick-borne rickettsioses	Ticks	Repellents; area dusting[7]	Vaccine; antibiotics; body inspection and removal of ticks

Disease	Vector	Chemical control	Other control measures
Epidemic typhus	Lice	Dusting of clothes, bedding, and body with insecticides[8]	Improvement of living conditions; health education
Plague	Fleas	Insecticide dusting of rodent runways or burrows[8]	Environmental control; improved sanitation and housing conditions
Malaria	Anopheline mosquitoes	Indoor residual insecticides and to a limited extent larvicides[10], chemotherapy	Remote possibility of immunization; integrated vector control; environmental control
Wuchereria and Brugia filariasis	Mosquitoes (Culex, Anopheles, Aedes, Mansonia spp)	Urban sanitation; larvicides[11]; chemotherapy	Remote possibility of immunization; integrated vector control; environmental control
Dengue and dengue haemorrhagic fever	Mosquitoes (Aedes spp)	Larvicides applied to water containers[12], source reduction and sanitary measures; ultra low volume insecticide application[13] or fogging	Environmental control; improved water supply and elimination of water storage; source reduction; vaccine a remote possibility; genetic control of mosquitos a remote possibility
Yellow fever	Mosquitoes (Aedes sp)	Vaccination; larvicides[12], Ultra low volume insecticide application or fogging[13]	Remote possibility of genetic control of mosquitos
Encephalitis (Japanese, Venezuelan equine, western equine, eastern equine)	Mosquitoes (Culex spp, Aedes spp)	Ultra low volume applications of insecticide in risk areas[13]; vaccination available for Japanese encephalitis	Water management in irrigated rice fields; biologic control and use of fish

Source: WHO publications.

1. Dieldrin and HCH generally used at 1 g/m² and 0.5 g/m² respectively. Propoxur and fenitrothion also effective.
2. DDT, dieldrin, and endosulfan sprayed from ground or air.
3. Chlorinated hydrocarbons, DDT, HCH.
4. Malathion or fenitrothion as a 2–4% solution.
5. Temephos at about 1 ppm.
6. Niclosamide or Baylucide.
7. DDT or carbaryl (5%), chlordane, fenthion (3%), malathion or ronnel, propoxur, naled.
8. DDT 10%, malathion or lindane 1% temephos dust 2%, permethrin 1%.
9. DDT 10% HCH or dieldrin, Diazinon 2%, Malathion 5%, fenitrothion 2%.
10. DDT, malathion, fenitrothion, propoxur at 2 g/m²; temephos at 1 ppm.
11. Fenthion or chlorpyrifos.
12. Temephos at 1 ppm.
13. Malathion or fenitrothion at 300–500 ml/ha.

out these specific hosts, the agents themselves, in many instances, would die off. The arthropod may serve as a culture tube in which the organism merely increases in number. An excellent example is the plague bacillus in the gut of the flea. A variation is propagation of the organism in addition to a movement along its life cycle. This variation is illustrated by the malaria parasite, in which multiplication not only takes place, but the sporozoites leaving the host are different morphologically from the gametocytes ingested. Still another variation is illustrated by the filarial worms, in which cyclic development takes place without propagation, since only one infective larva leaves the host for each microfilaria taken in.

Transovarian transmission. Some arthropods, notably the mites and ticks, may transmit disease agents to their offspring by invasion of the ovary or the developing egg. This is commonly referred to as transovarian transmission and is well illustrated by the disease scrub typhus, whereby such transmission is essential to the perpetuation of the rickettsia that, otherwise, would die off, since the adult mites are not parasitic and the larvae are chiefly one-time-only hosts.

Dissemination

Stowaway arthropods may become established in their new environment or live long enough to pass the disease agents they may carry to local vectors or reservoir hosts. The introduction of various disease-bearing arthropods to various countries of the world through commerce has accounted for the introduction and spread of many disease agents. Rat-infested ships of early days accounted for the spread of the rat fleas, the vector of the plague bacillus. In the United States, for example, transfer to the local fleas and rodent population has taken place and we now have plague indigenous to our soil, with sporadic outbreaks occurring in humans. Around 1930, *Anopheles gambiae*, the near-perfect vector for malaria, was acci-

dentally introduced into Brazil. It soon proved its reputation by causing an epidemic of malaria in that country, and deaths occurred before the foci were eradicated.

With the advent of the jet age, the picture becomes even more complicated, for no one part of the world is out of touch with another, and the chances for the dissemination of disease-laden arthropods become more menacing.

DISEASE CONTROL

A wide variety of both specific and nonspecific methods have been used to prevent and control arthropod infections and transmission. Yellow fever and envenomization are good examples in which specific host protection is achieved. Thus, in yellow fever, through the use of a live, attenuated vaccine, we have an outstanding example of protection through immunization. Similarly, with bee and wasp stings the individual who is known to be susceptible to the stings of the Hymenoptera can be desensitized specifically against these and thus avoid possible life-threatening situations.

The use of chloroquine in malaria chemoprophylaxis and the use of therapeutic drugs in other arthropod-borne diseases are examples whereby the appropriate drug can prevent either the occurrence of an infection or, through early treatment, the secondary person-to-person spread. A sizeable and powerful number of drugs exist now, which are highly effective for both the control and treatment of diseases caused by arthropods and other parasites. These are summarized in Table 16-2.

Use of chemical sprays, also a principle strategy against the arthropod agent, is widespread to prevent infection and transmission. A variety of chemicals are used to control *Sarcoptes scabiei* and the various types of sucking lice that can cause human pediculosis. One percent gamma benzene hexachloride, a persistent organochlorine pesticide, is used all over the world. Other organochlorine insecticides and the organophosphate and carbamate insecticides are used both as adulticides and larvicides, with the purpose of preventing and controlling dissemination of the arthropod vector.

In addition to host- and agent-control strategies, environmental control measures existed long before the advent of chemicals. The knowledge and skills of agriculture and engineering have been used from the beginning of civilization to reduce the sources of insect breeding and to set up barriers between insects and man. The drainage of the marshes outside Rome and the development of quarantine laws are two outstanding examples of earlier nonspecific measures for environmental manipulations to control arthropod diseases. There are presently innumerable programs for control of arthropod diseases, and the major emphasis is on source reduction. Urban yellow fever was banished from tropical American cities by destroying or removing the artificial water containers in and around houses. Clearing of vegetation in strategic areas frequented by man has been effective in disease control. Removal of garbage and wastes from homes, restaurants, and industrial plants, adequate sewage systems, and removal of stabled animals has reduced the former scourge of flies from urban environments.

Intervention strategies have focused on the wearing of protective clothing, the use of screens, and recent improvements in the efficacy of chemical repellents.

REVIEW QUESTIONS

1. What are three chief characteristics of an arthropod?
2. What are the classes of arthropods of medical importance?
3. In what ways are arthropods of medical importance? Given an example of each.
4. Discuss the kinds of disease transmission.
5. Give examples of control strategies in relation to host, agent, and environmental strategies.

REFERENCES

Barnard, J. H. 1973. Studies of 400 Hymenoptera sting deaths in the United States, J. Allergy Clin. Immunol. **52:**259-264.

Belding, D. L. 1965. Textbook of parasitology. Ed. 3. Appleton-Century-Crofts, New York.

Faust, E. C., P. F. Russel, and R. C. Jung. 1970. Clinical parasitology. Ed. 8. Lea & Febiger, Philadelphia.

Gordon, R. M. 1962. Entomology for students of medicine. Blackwell Scientific Publications, Oxford, England.

Horsfall, W. R. 1962. Medical entomology: arthropods and human disease. The Ronald Press Co., New York.

James, M. T., and Harwood, R. F. 1969. Herms's Medical entomology. Ed. 6. MacMillan, Inc., New York.

Miles, J. A. R. 1964. Some ecological aspects of the problem of arthropod-borne animal viruses in the western Pacific and south-east Asia regions. Bull. WHO **30:**197-210.

Pan American Health Organization. 1972. Vector control and the recrudescence of vector-borne diseases. Scientific Publication no. 238. Pan American Sanitary Bureau, Washington, D.C.

Smith, K. G. V., Editor. 1973. Insects and other arthropods of medical importance. British Museum Publications, Ltd., London.

Taylor, R. H. 1967. Catalogue of arthropod-borne viruses of the world. U.S. Department of Health, Education, and Welfare, Public Health Service. Publication no. 1760.

CHAPTER 17

Centipedes, tongue worms, crustaceans, and arachnids

CENTIPEDES (CHILOPODA)

The centipedes, classified by some authors with the millipedes, are characterized by having a long, slender, segmented body with a single pair of legs per segment, except for the last two. The appendages of the first body segment are modified into poison claws. Millipedes, on the other hand, are nonpoisonous and have two pairs of legs per segment in the abdominal region.

The chief habitat of centipedes is a dark, dingy, damp environment such as under logs, debris, rubbish, and old buildings. The poison injected, for the most part, is not harmful in cases occurring in the temperate regions, but in the tropics and subtropics, the species of *Scolopendra* may inflict a painful bite (Fig. 17-1). Within a few hours the symptoms subside, however. A large species in the tropics, *S. gigantea*, in addition to producing a necrotic lesion, may cause systemic reactions such as fever, nausea, vomiting, and headache. Ammonia or baking soda applied to the area will relieve irritation. In uncomplicated cases no deaths have been attributed to *S. gigantea* bites.

TONGUE WORMS (PENTASTOMIDA)

Tongue worms are degenerate, wormlike arthropods, the adults of which live in the lungs and air passages of their definitive hosts, whereas the larvae and nymphs occur free or encysted in the viscera of the intermediate host, including humans. The adult worms are white, elongate, and either flattened or cylindrical, with the body serrated or divided into conspicuous rings resembling true segments. One species, *Linguatula serrata*, occurs in the nasal passages and frontal sinuses of dogs, cats, foxes and other carnivores where they suck blood. The eggs, which are swallowed and passed out in the feces, survive well in the outside environment and, when ingested by humans and other animals, hatch in the intestinal tract so that the embryos or larvae are liberated. The larvae burrow through the intestinal wall and invade the mesenteric lymph nodes and visceral organs where encapsulation takes place. Development to the nymphal stage occurs, after which they await transport to the definitive host to become adults. Autopsies reveal visceral infections rather common in Europe, and one authentic case of an adult invasion of human nasal passages is recorded (Fig. 17-2).

Species of the genus *Porocephalus* (*Armillifer*) occur commonly in the lungs of various snakes. Human infections with encysted larvae (Figs. 17-2 and 17-3) or nymphs are common in Africa, where snakes are handled frequently and python meat is considered a delicacy. Contaminated water and vegetables are other sources of infection. In the United States a few authentic cases of visceral infections have been reported in humans, presumably from eating rattlesnake meat.

Most tongue worm infections are reported in Europe, Africa, South America, and Central America. Light infections, usually seen in humans, are not serious, and most have been recorded at the time of autopsy as incidental findings. When severe infections have occurred, diagnosis has been made on clinical grounds. The prognosis is serious if the nymphs escape from their cysts and migrate. Three cases of cancer in patients with tongue worm infections and the high frequency of the primitive cancer of the liver

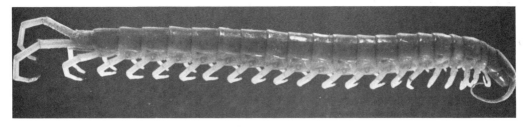

Fig. 17-1. Centipede (*Scolependra* sp). Note the presence of one pair of legs per segment. (Courtesy Dr. W. Henry Leigh, Department of Biology, University of Miami.)

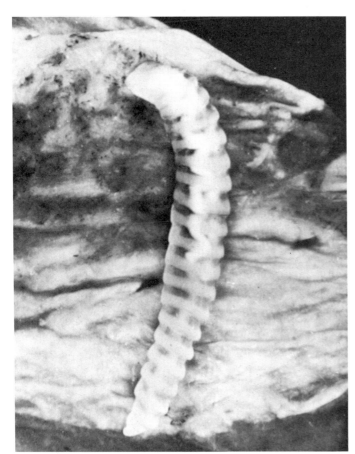

Fig. 17-2. Nonencysted larva of *Armillifer armillatus* (tongue worm) attached to the abdominal surface of the human diaphragm. (AFIP 72-4558.)

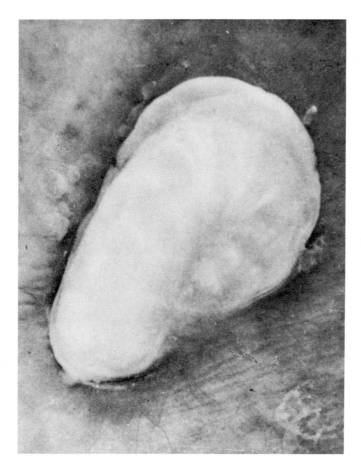

Fig. 17-3. Encysted larva of *Armillifer armillatus* (tongue worm) on surface of liver of a patient. (AFIP 72-4561.)

in Africans with a high prevalence of nymphal pentastomiasis of the liver suggest a possible relationship worthy of further investigation.

CRUSTACEANS (CRUSTACEA)

The crustaceans are primarily gill-breathing arthropods of both fresh water and salt water. Those of medical importance are found in fresh water and serve as intermediate hosts of various worms previously discussed.

The copepods, or water fleas, are represented by the genera *Cyclops* and *Diaptomus* (Fig. 17-4). Species of *Cyclops* are the intermediate hosts of *Dracunculus medinensis*, the guinea worm, *Dibothriocephalus latus*, the broad fish tapeworm, and *Gnathos-*

toma spinigerum, an occasional nematode in humans. Species of *Diaptomus* are the intermediate hosts of *D. latus*.

The larger crustaceans, called decapods, include crabs and crayfish, which serve as the second intermediate hosts of the lung fluke *Paragonimus westermani*.

Thorough cooking of fish and shellfish is the most effective means of preventing infection by *D. latus* and *P. westermani;* the boiling of water or prevention of its contamination by *Cyclops* sp is effective against *D. medinensis.*

ARACHNIDS (ARACHNIDA)

The members of this class are characterized by having four pairs of legs in the adult stage, two pairs of mouth parts, and no an-

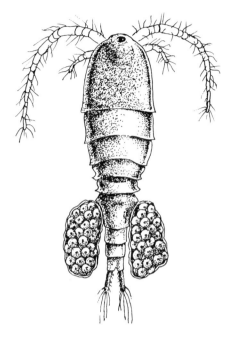

Fig. 17-4. Copepod or water flea (*Cyclops* sp).

tennae. Spiders, scorpions, mites, and ticks are the members of medical importance.

Spiders

A number of spiders throughout the world are poisonous to humans. The most important are the species belonging to the genus *Latrodectus.* They are small spiders whose venom is quite toxic. Various species are found in Europe, New Zealand, Australia, Africa, the Philippines, the West Indies, North America, and South America. Other genera also occur, predominately in South America but also in Africa and Australia. *Loxosceles laeta*, widely distributed in the southern part of South America, presents a serious clinical as well as public health problem in areas of Chile, Uruguay, and Argentina. In the United States, *Loxosceles reclusa* (Fig. 17-5) is probably the chief agent responsible for bites in the midwest. The spider is often found indoors—in basements, attics, closets, storage areas, barns, and the like. Individuals are often bitten when putting on an outer garment that was hanging in a closet or storage area. Initially there is very little discomfort, but in 2 to 8 hours the area of the bite becomes painful. Localized swelling, nausea, and other manifestations develop, and if the amount of venom inoculated is large, systematic reaction may be severe with death following. A necrotic lesion develops, with sloughing and granulomatous reaction occurring (Figs. 17-5 and 17-6). Corticosteroids alleviate the symptoms and possibly help to control necrosis (Fig. 17-6).

The black widow spider, *Latrodectus mactans,* so called because the female is black except for the orange-to-scarlet hourglass marking on her abdomen and because she frequently devours her male escort when hungry, is the most dangerous species in the United States and Canada (Fig. 17-7). These spiders live in cracks and crevices of old buildings, wood piles, junk heaps, privies, and similar habitats. The unwitting stranger who pokes his arm into such places or is caught by surprise on an outdoor privy is usually the one to be bitten. Black widow spiders haunt dark, dingy places predominantly, and people are seldom bitten in broad daylight. Of interest, however, is the case of a gas station being inspected for spiders. Black widows had literally taken over the premises, a modern all-metal station. They were found in the standards, signs, tire racks, and miscellaneous items for sale in the station house, not to mention the window of the gas pump—a far cry from the usual habitat of the black widow.

Sharp pain accompanies the bite, with systemic symptoms following. Agonizing pains, increasing in intensity, spread over the abdomen and trunk. The patient often becomes weak, dizzy, thirsty, and nauseated. Death is rare but may occur in the very young or aged and is usually caused by respiratory or circulatory failure. The toxin elaborated by the spider is probably a toxalbumin acting as a peripheral neurotoxin. Analgesics and bed rest suffice in most cases.

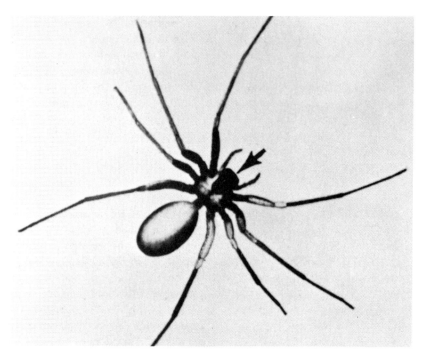

Fig. 17-5. *Loxosceles reclusa*, the brown recluse spider. Note the violin-shaped area on the anterior surface of the back *(arrow)*. (AFIP 75-5876-6.)

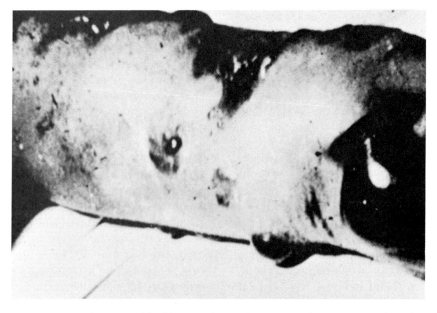

Fig. 17-6. Dermatitis, characterized by blisters, edema, ulcerations, and gangrene, resulting from the bite of the brown recluse spider, *Loxosceles reclusa*. (AFIP 75-5876-1.)

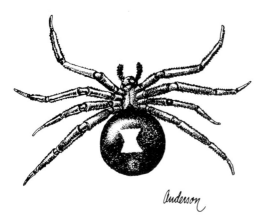

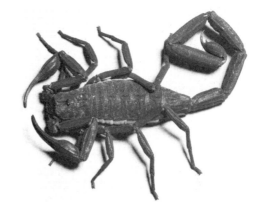

Fig. 17-7. Female black widow spider *(Latrodectus mactans).* Note the hourglass marking on the abdomen.

Fig. 17-8. Scorpion *(Centruroides* sp). Note the terminal spine. (Courtesy Charles M. Bailey, Biomedical Communications, University of Miami School of Medicine.)

A solution of 10 ml of 10% calcium gluconate given intravenously may be necessary in severe cases. Specific antivenom, if available, should be used.

Scorpions

Scorpions are characterized by the extension of the abdomen into an elongated, curved tail with a poisonous spine on the end (Fig. 17-8). They are distributed throughout the tropical and subtropical regions of the world. Most of the species in the United States produce no more ill effects than does a bee sting. The sting of the large *Centruroides* sp in Arizona may be very serious. Antivenom is available at the Poisonous Animals Research Laboratory, Arizona State College, Tempe, Arizona. In Mexico, primarily in the state of Durango, the death rate each year from scorpion stings is appreciable. Scorpions, wherever they are found, are nocturnal in their habits and during the day hide under rocks, logs, or any protective covering. Within the home they are frequent visitors of clothes closets, often taking up residence in shoes. In the tropics it is a good practice to shake shoes well before putting them on.

The venom from the scorpion is clear and colorless and is believed to be a toxalbumin that affects the nervous system and also causes pulmonary disorders. A radiating, burning sensation is experienced at the time of the sting. Numbness, muscle twitching, and itching follow quickly. Muscle spasms and convulsions may appear in severe cases. As with a snakebite, a tourniquet should be applied immediately to slow down absorption of the venom. Suction also should be applied to remove as much venom as possible from the sting. Symptomatic treatment, such as ice packs and freezing, may be employed. Procaine hydrochloride (Novocain) or epinephrine injected into the area of the wound will also give relief. Shock and pulmonary edema should be combated, if necessary. Antivenom should be administered in severe cases.

Mites and ticks

The order Acarina comprises mites and ticks. The head, thorax, and abdomen are fused together into a single structure. Sexes are separate. Four stages of development occur in their life histories: egg, larva, nymph, and adult. Mites are terrestrial and aquatic, and some species are parasites of animals and plants; ticks are only terrestrial and are parasites of animals, exclusively.

Mites

As compared with ticks, mites are small and have the hypostome hidden and unarmed (without hooks). For the most part, they are free living; the floor of the forest is covered with them, but some species, as mentioned previously, are parasites. A few are of medical importance.

Sarcoptes scabiei, commonly known as the itch mite, causes mange by burrowing into the skin (Fig. 17-9). It is a small mite, the male averaging between 200 and 250 μm in length, whereas the much larger female averages 300 to 450 μm. The impregnated female excavates tortuous tunnels in the epidermis, especially between fingers and toes, and in the groin, external genitalia, and axillary regions. As she burrows, she lays eggs and defecates. The eggs hatch in the tunnels, and the nymphs start new tunnels and undergo development. Some may come to the surface and start new tunnels from there. The life cycle takes about 1 to 2 weeks.

Initially the infection is mild, and few if any symptoms are present, but after a few weeks the skin becomes sensitized and an intense itching begins. A humoral immune response is indicated by the increased levels of IgG and IgM and a decrease in the IgA level. Circulating antigen antibody complexes have been suggested as the explanation for scabies. Scratching spreads the infection and, in breaking the skin, paves the way for secondary invaders (Figs. 17-10 and 17-11). Scabies is acquired primarily in military installations, prisons, mental institutions, and the like. The nature of the lesion and the rash are suggestive of the disease, but a certain diagnosis depends on recovering the mite from its burrow with a needle. The treatment of choice is the topical application of 10% crotamiton, usually after a hot,

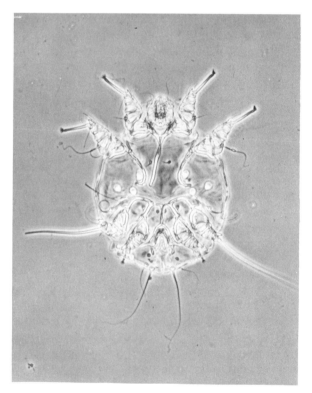

Fig. 17-9. *Sarcoptes scabiei*, the itch mite. (Photograph by Jay R. Georgi.)

soapy bath. As alternatives 1% gamma benzene hexachloride (once), 12% to 25% benzyl benzoate, or sulfur in petrolatum may be used topically.

The hair follicle mite, *Demodex folliculorum*, is a small, elongated, wormlike parasite that lives in the hair follicles and the sebaceous glands around the face. The burrows are shallow, and only a very slight reaction occurs. A dry erythema may be present. The mites present themselves in blackheads, acnes, or localized keratitis. Generally speaking, the parasite is innocuous and no treatment is required.

Red bugs, or "chiggers," as they are commonly called in the southern states, are familiar to nearly everyone. They are larval mites of the family Trombiculidae. Various species occur around the world, but the culprit causing so much discomfort in the United States is *Eutrombicula alfreddugèsi*. The adults are free living, whereas the larval stages are parasitic principally on turtles, snakes, rabbits, and ground birds. When humans enter their domain, the mites have no scruples about feeding on them, also. The mites may stay for a few days or a month. They invade persons working in the yard,

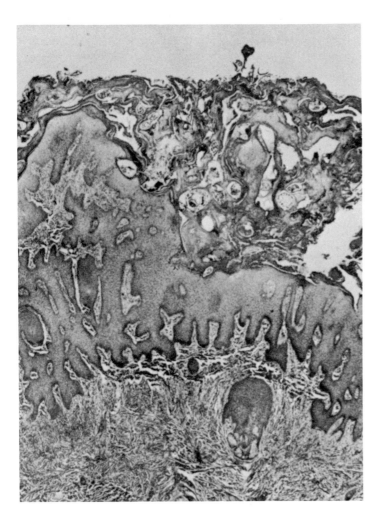

Fig. 17-10. Skin from a patient with scabies. Note the sections of many *Sarcoptes scabiei* in the hyperkeratotic horny layer. (AFIP 73-5339.)

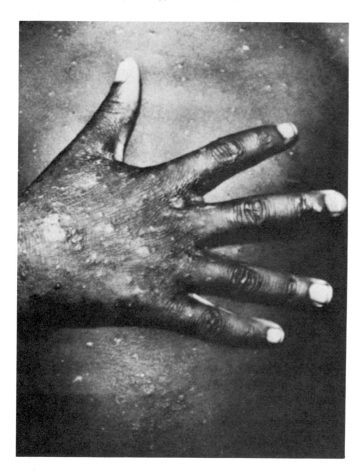

Fig. 17-11. Scabies of the hand. Lesions complicated by scratching and secondary bacterial infection. (AFIP 68-7834-20.)

weeding, and cutting grass. Oddly enough, the larval forms do not invade the skin but secrete a tube or stylostome from the mouth to the skin surface. Through this tube passes saliva that aids in dissolving dried skin and epidermis.

Sensitization results in intense itching and scratching. Alcohol or camphor helps to allay the itching. Various cream deodorants and nail polish are also effective. In Japan and the Far East, scrub typhus or tsutsugamushi fever, a rickettsia disease, is carried by the larval mite *Trombicula akamushi* and related species. The rickettsia organisms have been found in the salivary glands of the larvae. A high mortality in humans is common.

The family Dermanyssidae contains various mites that live on rats, chickens and other poultry, and various animals. Most of those invading humans are associated with an itching dermatitis caused by the bites of the adults. The chicken mite, *Dermanyssus gallinae*, which attacks humans and other animals, has been found to harbor the viruses causing St. Louis encephalitis and western equine encephalitis. The rat mite, *Liponyssus (Bdellonyssus) bacoti*, also associated with an urticaria in humans in the United States, is the vector for *Rickettsia typhi*, the cause of endemic typhus, chiefly from rat to rat but occasionally to humans. It is also the vector for rickettsial pox and Q fever.

Many mites, belonging mainly to the families Tyroglyphidae and Glycyphagidae, are pests of stores, warehouses, and grain mills. They are particularly common in hay, grains, sugar, dried fruits, cheese, and cereals. In contact with humans they cause allergic responses commonly referred to as "grocer's itch," "copra itch," or "miller's itch." Those on cheese and vegetables are ingested and, when numerous, cause gastrointestinal symptoms. Eggs and mites in all stages of development are frequently found in the feces. A famous German cheese is said to owe its delicious flavor to the myriads of mites deliberately seeded in it. After several partakings, it is said, one becomes accustomed to the mites in the intestines, and further disturbances are abated. However true this may be, one can hardly recommend the contamination of food with mites, if for no other reason than an esthetic one. Individuals so invaded, however, invariably have some gastrointestinal disturbances. Mites have been reported in other areas such as the lungs, ears, and urinary tract.

Ticks

The ticks are large and easy to recognize. Contrasted to the mites, which are usually hairy, the ticks are rather bare, except for markings. Two families are present and commonly referred to as the "soft" and "hard" ticks.

The soft ticks, the Argasidae, are distinguished by a leathery cuticle that covers the body. Numerous tubercles or granulations are scattered over this cuticle. No plates or shields are present. The hard ticks, or Ixodidae, have a dorsal shield or scutum covering almost the entire back in the males, but only a small portion anteriorly in the females. Ornamentation may be present and such hard ticks are said to be "ornate." The mouth also is anterior in position, whereas in the argasid ticks it is ventral. The ixodid ticks feed only once as adults and then drop off the host, whereas the argasids feed repeatedly. Although the ixodids feed only once as adults, they actually feed several times during development. When the eggs hatch on the ground, the young larvae, commonly

called "seed ticks," climb up on blades of grass, twigs, and similar places and wait for a host to come by. The slightest motion causes them to stretch out and cling to the first host at hand. They feed for a few days, fall off, and molt, becoming eight-legged nymphs. These nymphs, in turn, climb up on vegetation and await the passerby. After another feeding period they again fall to the ground, molt, and become adults. The adults repeat the process and feed on a host. Mating takes place and the final feeding results in tremendous engorgement.

Argasidae. In the family Argasidae are the following three genera of medical importance: *Argas*, *Ornithodoros*, and *Otobius*. Members of the *Argas* genus are primarily parasites of birds, but occasionally they parasitize mammals (Fig. 17-12). They cause painful bites on humans. The genus *Otobius* contains a species, *O. megnini*, found in the southwestern United States and Mexico, which, in the nymph stage, invades the ears of horses, domestic animals, and sometimes children. The spiny nymphs may remain attached for months. Members of the genus *Ornithodoros* attack mammals primarily. *O. moubata*, in Africa, lives primarily in human habitation and seems to prefer feeding on humans, pigs, and warthogs. *O. coriaceus*, found in California, causes painful and serious bites but also is important as a vector for relapsing fever. Various species of *Ornithodoros* harbor the agents causing Q fever, tularemia, tick-bite fever, and Russian encephalitis. *O. moubata*, mentioned previously, transmits Q fever by its bite.

Argasid ticks, being intermittent feeders, are best controlled by attacking their hiding places. Their habits are much the same as bedbugs; they hide in cracks and crevices of walls and come out at night for feeding on their hosts. Benzene hexachloride (BHC) is an effective spray.

Ixodidae. Numerous species in this family attack humans and are important as transmitters of various disease agents. Some ticks

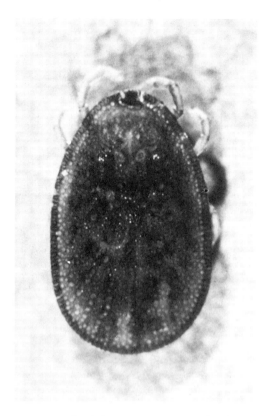

Fig. 17-12. Soft tick *(Argas persicus)*. Note the absence of a dorsal plate and the capitulum hidden beneath the anterior extremity. (From a nonprofit cooperative endeavor of numerous colleagues under the editorship of Dr. Herman Zaiman, Valley City, N.D.)

also may cause paralysis, which occurs in the United States, as well as in other countries, and is associated chiefly with *Dermacentor andersoni* and *D. variabilis* in North America. The female ticks, apparently, are the only ones involved and, when attached to the back of the neck or base of the skull, presumably elaborate, from the eggs, a toxin that causes an ascending paralysis, beginning in the legs and moving up to include the arms, chest, and neck. If the heart and respiration are not affected, recovery will follow after removal of the tick; otherwise, death may ensue. Female ticks located at the base of the skull or back of the neck and along the spinal column cause the most severe paralysis. Paralysis may occur from ticks located

elsewhere on the body but is uncommon and less severe. The prevalence of *D. variabilis*, throughout many areas of the United States, and *D. andersoni*, in the Rocky Mountain area, should warn the physician of the importance of always making a thorough examination of the body, particularly of the head, neck, and spinal column for embedded ticks (Fig. 17-13). Long hair serves as an excellent hiding place for a tick.

Hard ticks are of importance chiefly as vectors or transmitters of a variety of diseases caused by bacteria, viruses, and rickettsia. Numerous strains of *Rickettsia* spp are the causative agents of the spotted fevers, described under various names such as Rocky Mountain spotted fever, Bullis fever, Sao Paulo fever, fievre Boutonneuse, Choix fever, and Pinto fever. *D. andersoni* in the west and *D. variabilis* on the eastern seaboard and across parts of the U.S. are the chief vectors in this country. *Amblyomma americanum*, the lone-star tick, so called because of a small white spot on the scutum of the female is the chief vector in the southwest. Even if a person is bitten by an infected tick, disease may still be prevented. A tick must remain attached to the body for 4 to 6 hours before the rickettsiae are reactivated and the person becomes infected. Therefore anyone in a hazardous area should inspect the body and clothing every few hours for ticks and remove them properly (Fig. 17-14). Other species are involved in various parts of the world in transmitting to humans as well as maintaining infections among animals in nature such as rabbits and rodents. Q fever, a rickettsial disease most prevalent in the United States on the west coast, although transmitted chiefly by fomites and therefore airborne, may also be tick transmitted and is maintained in sylvatic form by hard ticks. Colorado tick fever, a viral disease, is associated chiefly with *D. andersoni* in the United States. Far-Eastern spring-summer encephalitis, a viral infection, is transmitted by a variety of hard ticks

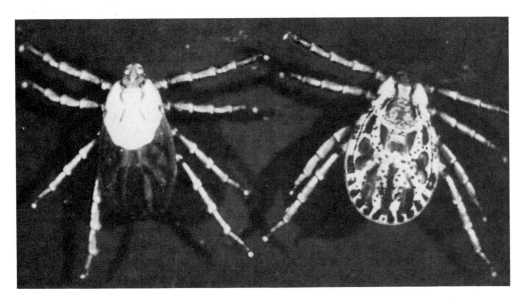

Fig. 17-13. Hard ticks *(Dermacentor andersoni).* Note scutum on the male on the right covers more surface than that on the female. (From a nonprofit cooperative endeavor of numerous colleagues under the editorship of Dr. Herman Zaiman, Valley City, N.D.)

Fig. 17-14. Technique for removing a tick embedded in the skin.

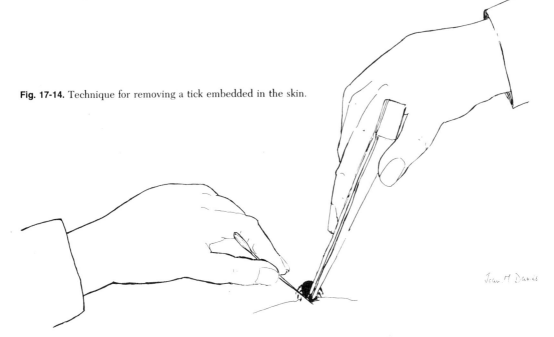

and is maintained in them through transovarial transmission. Tularemia, caused by *Francisella tularensis*, although transmitted by various arthropods as well as by contact with infected animals, is associated with a variety of hard ticks, chiefly *D. andersoni, D. variabilis,* and *A. americanum* in the United States. In the heavily wooded and sparsely settled Lyme area of Connecticut, what appeared to be juvenile articular rheumatism was diagnosed in a number of children. The disease was seasonal, appearing in spring and autumn. Adults, also, were found to be frequent victims, with neurologic, cardiologic, and renal effects, cryoprecipitates, and other changes in the blood and skin lesions. All indications point to "Lyme arthritis" as being a tick-borne disease. *Ixodes dammini*, the vector for *Babesia microti*, the cause of babesiosis in animals and man, is believed to be the tick involved. The arthritis may persist for months, and may develop some time after the clinical illness.

In addition to being excellent vectors for various disease agents and the cause of paralysis as well, ticks in themselves cause very painful bites. If the capitulum is broken off, as frequently happens when improper attempts are made to remove them, secondary infections may occur, with inflamed sores, ulcers, and even systemic poisoning (Fig. 17-14). Numerous ticks may also cause anemia in the host when present for a sustained period of time.

REVIEW QUESTIONS

1. How are centipedes, tongue worms, and crustaceans of medical importance?
2. Discuss the symptomatology and treatment for spider bites and scorpion stings.
3. How are mites of medical importance? Give examples of each.
4. What is tick paralysis? Discuss.
5. What important diseases are tick borne?
6. What is Lyme arthritis? Discuss.

REFERENCES

Arthur, D. R. 1962. Ticks and disease. Pergamon Press, Inc., New York.

Baker, E. W., and G. W. Wharton. 1952. An introduction to acarology. Macmillan, Inc., New York.

Bozeman, F. M., and others. 1967. Ecology of Rocky Mountain spotted fever. II. Natural infection of wild mammals and birds in Virginia and Maryland. J. Trop. Med. Hyg. **16**:48-59.

Bygbjerg, I. C., and M. P. Rask. 1978. Pentastomiasis and cancer of the colon. Trans. R. Soc. Trop. Med. Hyg. **72**:54-55.

Cloudsley-Thompson, J. L. 1958. Spiders, scorpions, centipedes and mites. Pergamon Press, Inc., New York.

Costa, J. 1952. Tick paralysis on the Atlantic seaboard. Am. J. Dis. Child. **83**:336-347.

D'Amour, F. E., F. E. Becker, and W. Van Riper. 1936 The black widow spider. Quart. Rev. Biol. **11**:123-160.

Fain, A. 1975. The Pentastomida parasitic in man. Ann. Soc. Belg. Med. Trop. **55**:59-64.

Harves, A. D., and L. E. Millikan. 1975. Current concepts of therapy and pathophysiology in arthropod bites and stings. Part 2. Insects: review. Int. J. Dermatol. **14**:621-634.

Johnson, C. G., and K. Mellanby. 1942. The parasitology of human scabies. J. Parasitol. **34**:285-290.

Levi, H. W., and A. Spielman. 1964. The biology and control of the South American brown spider, *Loxosceles laeta* (Nicolet), in a North American focus. Am. J. Trop. Med. Hyg. **13**:132-136.

Mapp, E. M., H. M. Pollack, and L. H. Goldman. 1976. Roentgen diagnosis of *Armillifer armillatus* infestation (porocephalosis) in man. J. Natl. Med. Assoc. **68**:198-200.

Orkin, M., H. I. Maibach, L. C. Parish, and R. M. Schwartzman. 1977. Scabies and pediculosis. J. B. Lippincott Co., Philadelphia.

Oswald, N. C. 1975. Scattered calcified larvae of *Porocephalus* or tongue worm in the lungs of a Nigerian who also had carcinoma of the bronchus. Med. Biol. Illustration **25**:20.

Prathap, K., K. S. Laws, and J. M. Bolton. 1969. Pentastomiasis: a common finding at autopsy among Malaysian aboriginies. Am. J. Trop. Med. **18**:20-27.

Schöttler, W. H. A. 1954. On the toxicity of scorpion venom. Am. J. Trop. Med. **3**:172-178.

Self, J. T., H. C. Hopps, and A. Olufemi Williams. 1975. Pentastomiasis in Africans. Trans. Geo. Med. **27**:1-13.

Steere, A. C., and others. 1977. Erythema chronicum migrans and Lyme arthritis: the enlarging clinical picture. Ann. Intern. Med. **86**:685-698.

Steere, A. C., and others. 1977. Lyme arthritis: an epidemic of oligoarticular arthritis in children and adults in three Connecticut communities. Arthritis Rheum. **20**:7-17.

Steere, A. C., T. F. Broderick, and S. E. Malawista. 1978. Erythema chronicum migrans and Lyme arthritis: epidemiologic evidence for a tick vector. Am. J. Epidemiol. **108**:312-321.

VanNeste, D., and J. Salmon. 1978. Circulating antigen antibody complexes in scabies. Dermatologica **157**:221-224.

Wallis, A. C., S. E. Brown, K. O. Klotes, and A. J. Main. 1978. Erythema chronicum migrans and Lyme arthritis: field study of ticks. Am. J. Epidemiol. **108**:322-324.

CHAPTER 18

Insects (Hexapoda)

The Hexapoda is the largest and undoubtedly the most important of all the classes of arthropods. Insects are chiefly terrestrial arthropods that breathe by means of tracheas, a system of tubes ramifying throughout the body and opening to the outside by means of spiracles, the latter being of diagnostic value in the larval forms. The bodies of insects are readily divisible into three parts, which are the head, thorax, and abdomen. Six legs are present, hence the name Hexapoda (six feet).

The significance of insects as pests and inoculators of poisons is well known. As mentioned previously, nearly everyone, at one time or another, has come in contact with arthropods as pests. Insects are chiefly the ones that cause so much nuisance. Wasps, bees, some ants, and many caterpillars are well known for their stings, or stinging hairs (in the case of the caterpillars), and the urticaria resulting therefrom.

It is as vectors of disease agents, however, that the insects are most famous. Since most damage is inflicted at feeding time, it is important to learn something about their mouthparts. For the sake of convenience, we can divide them into three general types, remembering, however, that this is an artificial classification for the purpose of simplification since many gradations exist between the following broad types:

1. Primitive chewing mouthparts
2. Mouthparts modified for lapping and sponging
3. Mouthparts modified for piercing and sucking

The type of mouthparts present in any given insect influences markedly its role as a vector of a disease agent when transmission occurs through the anterior station or mouth end. In only a few instances are disease agents transmitted by defecation. Those insects having primitive chewing mouthparts, for example, confine themselves chiefly to eating epidermis and debris on the skin surface.

As the mouthparts undergo modification, however, better adaptation to breaking of the skin occurs. Some flies, for example, are able to rasp the skin and by abrasion eventually draw blood. Mouthparts adapted for lapping and sponging are excellent mechanical transmitters of disease agents. Among the more specialized insects, we find mouthparts, again in all gradations, adapted for piercing and sucking. The mosquito, for example, with mouthparts modeled after the hypodermic needle and syringe, can inject disease-laden saliva and, in turn, draw in disease-laden blood.

Although there are over 30 orders of insects, only five are of major medical importance. Coleoptera, Hymenoptera, and Lepidoptera, of lesser medical importance, are also considered.

COLEOPTERA

A number of beetles serve as intermediate hosts for some helminths that occur occasionally in humans. *Gongylonema pulchrum* (see p. 181), *Moniliformis moniliformis* (see p. 194), and *Hymenolepis diminuta* (see p. 204), in this text. Some, known as blister beetles, may cause an irritation and blistering of the skin upon contact (Fig. 18-1).

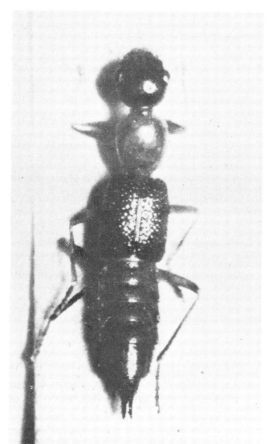

Fig. **18-1.** *Paederus laetus,* a blister beetle in Central America. (AFIP 80041-A.)

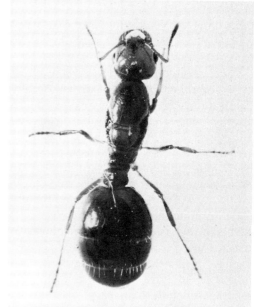

Fig. **18-2.** Fire ant (*Solenopsis* sp). Common in southern states. (Courtesy Florida Department of Agriculture and Consumer Services, Division of Plant Industry. Photo by V. Jane Windsor.)

HYMENOPTERA

The order Hymenoptera comprises the bees, wasps, hornets, and ants. Individuals vary in their reaction to the sting of these insects. The modified ovipositor of the female and worker also serves as a stinging apparatus. Anaphylactic shock from bee stings has resulted in death in some instances. Quite noticeable in the southern United States is the fire ant, *Solenopsis* sp (Fig. 18-2), which, true to its name, causes a fiery, burning sensation after its sting. Children may require parenteral use of epinephrine for severe allergic reactions, while adults require diphenhydramine HCl (Benadryl) (Fig. 18-3). Pesticides such as rotenone, chlordane, mirex,

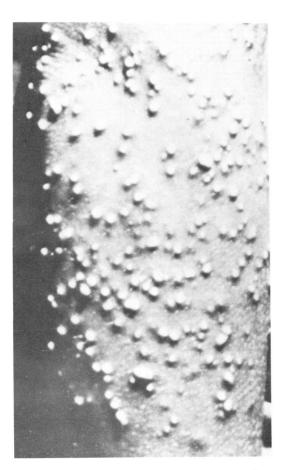

Fig. 18-3. Severe reaction to numerous stings from *Solenopsis invicta*, the fire ant. (AFIP 75-14977.)

and pyrethyrins are recommended for the control of the numerous Hymenoptera.

LEPIDOPTERA

The caterpillars of many butterflies and moths possess urticating hairs (Figs. 18-4 and 18-5). Contact with human skin causes, in some instances, a severe dermatitis. Prevalent in the southern states are the puss moth and saddle-back moth so frequently encountered by gardeners and others working around the hibiscus, palms, and other vegetation. Treatments such as warm baking soda, amonia water, and calamine lotion are palliative, at least for a time.

ORTHOPTERA

The order Orthoptera comprises the cockroaches, which, because of their habits, have been under suspicion as mechanical vectors of disease agents (Fig. 18-6). They have primitive mouthparts adapted for chewing. Their importance lies only in the possible mechanical transmission of disease agents. They have filthy habits, feeding on man's food and defecating in their wake. In their foraging for nourishment, they will eat anything, even feces. A great variety of bacteria pass through their alimentary tract. *Entamoeba histolytica* cysts have been recovered in a viable state from their excrement. In addition to being potential mechanical vectors of disease agents, they can also serve as the intermediate host for *Hymenolepis diminuta* and one of the spiny-headed worms occasionally parasitic in humans.

HEMIPTERA

The order Hemiptera comprises the true bugs. The basal portion of one pair of wings is thickened and leathery, while the terminal half is membranous. The wings of the second pair are completely membranous. In some species the wings are vestigial. Many bugs have "stink glands," which emit an unpleasant odor. Mouth parts are adapted for piercing and sucking.

Bedbugs

The bedbug has been kept under constant surveillance, being suspected of transmitting nearly every disease under the sun, but thus far never having been found guilty. Experimentally it can be infected with a wide variety of organisms. Those who have to contend with these pests know them for their painful bites and the peculiar pungent odor that they emit. It has been stated that Pliny the Elder recommended inhalation of seven bedbugs ground up in water for reviving one from fainting—a good substitute, perhaps, when spirits of ammonia is not available. Much to the disgust of good housekeepers

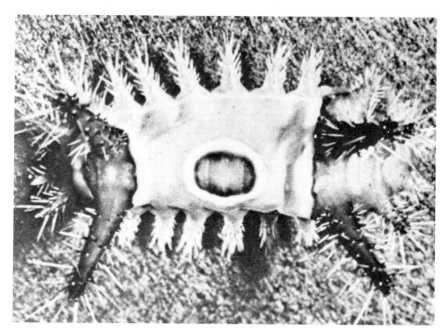

Fig. 18-4. Saddleback moth (caterpillar), *Sibine* sp, cause of dermatitis and necrosis. Note the prominent barbed, rigid netting hairs (source of irritant). (AFIP 75-5876-3.)

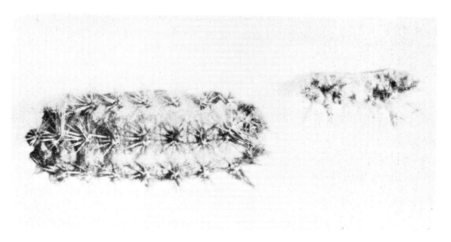

Fig. 18-5. Urticating moths (caterpillars), *Monema flavescens* (left) and *Parasa* sp (right). Stinging hairs (not visible) are located on small knobs on the body segments. (AFIP N-81367.)

all over the world, bedbugs have become domesticated and apparently are here to stay. A fresh blood meal stimulates them to defecate and the fact that they frequently adhere to clothing while biting undoubtedly diminishes their chance of defecating on the skin and near the wound or scratch present.

Infectious agents, if present, are passed only in the feces (Fig. 18-7).

Triatomid bugs

The triatomid bugs are found mainly in North and South America. The family status is somewhat in dispute; some consider the

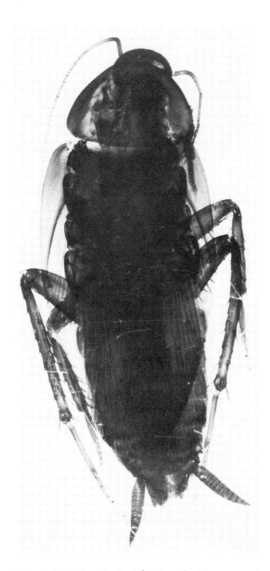

Fig. 18-6. Cockroach (*Periplaneta* sp). Common pest. (Courtesy Department of Epidemiology and Public Health, University of Miami School of Medicine.)

triatomids as a subfamily called Triatominae in the family Reduviidae, whereas others give them full family status as the Triatomidae. They are members of a large group commonly known as the "cone-nose bugs," "assassin bugs," "barbers," "reduviid bugs," and so on. The triatomids stand out as a group because of the fact that they feed on the blood of vertebrates. These bugs, quite large in size, are often brightly colored, fast

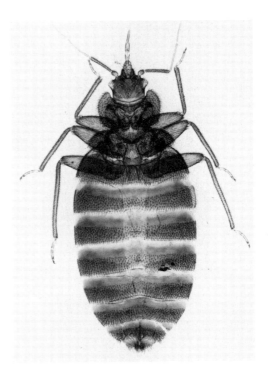

Fig. 18-7. Bedbug (*Cimex lectularius*). Common pest. (Courtesy Dr. W. Henry Leigh, Department of Biology, University of Miami.)

runners, and swift fliers. They are most prevalent in the tropics and subtropics but their range extends into temperate regions also. They are numerous throughout the southern United States down to Argentina. They are most active at night and spend the daylight hours hiding in cracks and crevices of wood piles, adobe brick huts, shanties, and such suitable places. When attacking humans, they leave their lairs in the dark and frequently alight on the eye, sucking blood through the conjunctiva. Their bite is painless and, on being engorged, they defecate. Through the feces, *Trypanosoma cruzi* is deposited on the spot and the organisms either penetrate intact tissue or enter through the puncture wound. Over 60 species of triatomids (reduviids) have been found capable of transmitting *T. cruzi* (Fig. 18-8). In the United States, where authentic human infections have been reported, several species of bugs have been found naturally

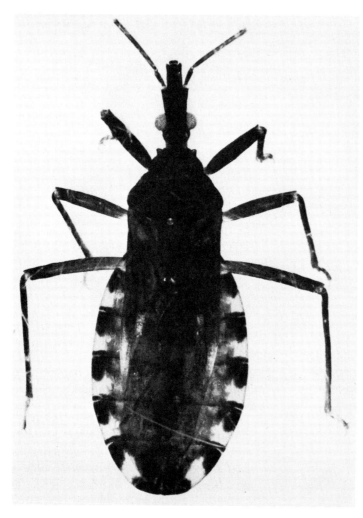

Fig. 18-8. Triatomid bug (Reduviidae). Vector of *Trypanosoma cruzi*. (Courtesy Department of Epidemiology and Public Health, University of Miami School of Medicine.)

infected. In Central and South America, another trypanosome, *T. rangeli*, has been found in humans. It is transmitted by the triatomid bug, *Rhodnius prolixus*. This bug is unique in that, though transmission may occur through the normal route, the posterior station, it may also occur through the anterior station.

SUCKING LICE (ANOPLURA)

Lice may be found in military camps, jails, mental institutions, and the like, where one is unable to choose one's companions, and facilities for cleanliness are not always to one's liking. Perhaps because they are most prevalent in places of not particularly good social standing, such as jails and mental institutions, a stigma is attached to the individual who, unfortunately, comes to harbor some of these guests. Lice, however, are not respecters of persons or social strata. After much cajoling, it has been possible to have medical students sheepishly admit to being hosts of some of these pests.

The sucking lice, or Anoplura, are exclusively mammalian parasites, and humans, being mammals, have lice. The mouthparts of the sucking lice are adapted for piercing and sucking.

Two genera infest humans, *Pediculus* and

hairy parts of the body, becoming the fore-runners of *Phthirus pubis*. The advent of clothing also afforded the opportunity for a new adaptation, and thus the body louse, *Pediculus humanus corporis*, came into his own domain, taking up residence in garments and returning to the host when mealtime dictated. Though *Pediculus humanus capitis* and *Phthirus pubis* glue their eggs, or nits, to the hair shaft of the host (Fig. 18-10), the body louse chooses the fibers of the clothing for its offspring. The forerunner of the modern day rocket may well have been the young louse, for the nymph makes its exit from the egg casing by taking in gulps of air, passing the air through the body and out the anus to build up pressure for its eventual takeoff.

Though the head louse to some extent is also involved, *P. humanus corporis* is the principle vector of epidemic typhus, trench fever, and relapsing fever. During World War I, soldiers in the trenches became very familiar with body lice, commonly referring to them as "cooties," or "graybacks." Since World War II, epidemic typhus (*Rickettsia prawazekii*) has become less of a public health problem although reservoir sources of infection remain in parts of Asia, Africa, and Latin America. Transmission occurs by deposition of louse feces on injured skin, by crushing the insect on the skin, and possibly by the insect bite itself. Trench fever is believed to be another louse-borne rickettsia disease. Relapsing fever caused by the spirochete *Borrelia recurrentis* is transmitted by crushing lice on the skin. Spirochetes permeate the body tissues of the louse and are not trasmitted by the insect bite.

Phthirus pubis, commonly known as the "crab louse" because of its appearance, acquired some endearing (though doubtlessly unprintable) nicknames by the servicemen of World War II. Notorious as pests, they have not been found to be the transmitter of any diseases to humans (Fig. 18-11).

Topical applications of various analgesics

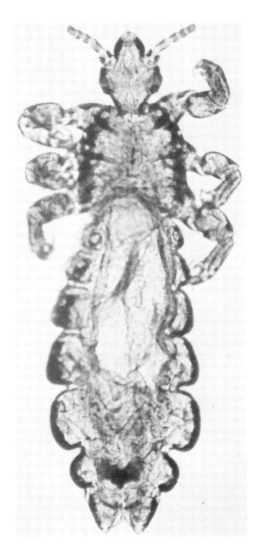

Fig. 18-9. Body or head louse *(Pediculus humanus)*. Principle vector of epidemic typhus, trench fever, and relapsing fever. (Courtesy Turtox.)

Phthirus. No doubt all of the human varieties are descendents of a common species. With man's flight from nudity and the subsequent restriction of hair to the head, axilla, and pubis, except for the hairy throwbacks to our ancestors, the lice, likewise, underwent refinements (Fig. 18-9). Some became adapted to the hairs of the head, giving rise to our present-day *Pediculus humanus capitis*, whereas others adapted to the remaining

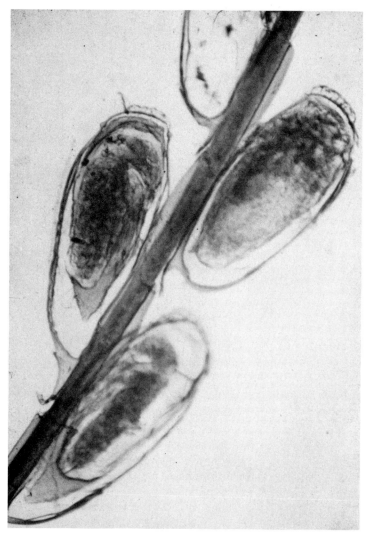

Fig. 18-10. Lice eggs (nits) on hair shaft. (Courtesy Turtox.)

alleviate the itching from the bites of lice. Sterilization of clothing is effective against *P. humanus corporis.* During World War II, DDT dusting was very effective in delousing prisoners of war, displaced persons, and others, but during the Korean conflict resistant strains made their appearance. Benzene hexachloride (BHC) has proved to be an effective agent, but resistant strains have likewise been observed. Thus, the search for more effective lousicides continues.

The drug of choice, at present, for both *Pediculus capitis* and *humanus* and *Phthiris*

pubis is 1% gamma benzene hexachloride (lindane) applied once topically. An alternative is topical applications of pyrethrins with piperonyl butoxide or 0.03% cupric oleate. For eyelashes infested with crab lice, ophthalmic ointment containing 0.25% physostigmine or ophthalmic ointment of yellow oxide of mercury is recommended.

FLEAS (SIPHONAPTERA)

The fleas also have mouthparts adapted for piercing and sucking. Over a thousand species have been described but, fortunately,

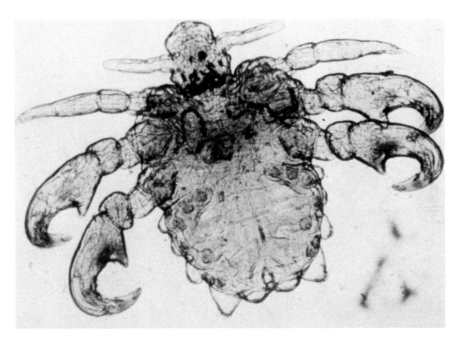

Fig. 18-11. Crab louse *(Phthirus pubis)*. Common pest. (From a nonprofit cooperative endeavor of numerous colleagues under the editorship of Dr. Herman Zaiman, Valley City, N.D.)

the ones of medical importance are limited in number. Their bodies are compressed laterally to allow for quick passage between the hairs or feathers of the host. Though deprived of wings, their powerful legs give them jumping ability unexcelled by any other animal, thus enabling them to move with great speed and agility. If a man were able to jump as well, he could leap over most buildings with the greatest of ease. Annoying though they are as pests, the bite being quite painful, their chief importance lies in the fact that they transmit two important human diseases, bubonic plague and endemic typhus. Fleas associated with human dwellings are mainly in three categories:

1. Human fleas—*Pulex irritans*
2. Cat and dog fleas—*Ctenocephalides* sp
3. Rat and mouse fleas—*Xenopsylla cheopis* and various other genera

Pulex irritans, justly deserving of its name, is primarily a flea of humans but adapts itself to other hosts as well. It probably originated in Europe but has since spread around the world. It is relatively rare in the tropics. It is not important as a disease transmitter in most instances.

The dog and cat fleas belong to the genus *Ctenocephalides. C. canis* and *C. felis* are the species, respectively. They readily pass from one host to another, and in homes where the animals have been removed, the fleas left behind readily utilize humans as a source of nourishment. They are intermediate hosts of *Dipylidium caninum* and transmit this dog tapeworm to children primarily.

The fleas of rats, mice, ground squirrels, and other rodents are accidental parasites of humans. Their importance lies in their spreading of plague and endemic typhus. *Xenopsylla cheopis* is the most important species in epidemic plague transmission (Fig. 18-12). This species attacks humans more readily then do most of the other rodent fleas. *Nosopsyllus fasciatus* is the most common flea on domestic rats in temperate

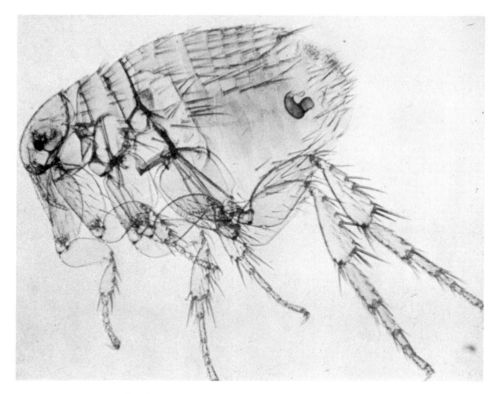

Fig. 18-12. Flea *(Xenopsylla cheopis* ♀*).* Important vector of plague. (From a nonprofit cooperative endeavor of numerous colleagues under the editorship of Dr. Herman Zaiman, Valley City, N.D.)

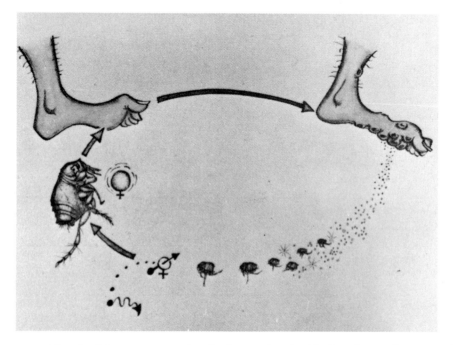

Fig. 18-13. Life cycle of *Tunga penetrans.* Eggs hatch in sandy soil. Male dies after copulation. Female hops about contacting the skin of warm-blooded animals, including man. (AFIP 70-7303.)

regions. *Leptopsylla segnis* is also common on rats and mice and is next in importance to *X. cheopis* in the southern United States.

Another flea worth mentioning, though not listed previously, is the stick-tight flea of poultry, *Echidnophage gallinacea*. Aside from being a potential plague disseminator not only chiefly among birds but also among rodents, it sometimes becomes a nuisance when attacking children. *Tunga penetrans*, the sand flea, chigoe, chigger, or jigger (not to be confused with the red bug, or chigger, see p. 289) found in tropical America and Africa, is a small flea living in sandy, shaded

soil and lying in wait for a bare foot to pass by (Fig. 18-13). They attack a wide range of the toenails. The females produce eggs that they retain and, as a result, blow up to tremendous size. The wounds become painful, inflamed, and frequently secondarily infected (Fig. 18-14). In the tropics, where tetanus is common, the wound becomes an excellent portal of entry for this and other organisms. Death from gas gangrene and tetanus is common.

DIPTERA

The order Diptera is the most important of all because it contains many members that are the normal vectors for a wide variety of disease agents. The Diptera are characterized by having two pairs of wings, one pair of which, the halteres, is vestigial and is used for balance. Without becoming involved too

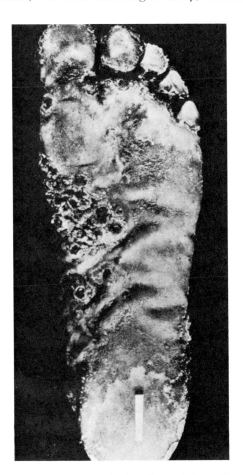

Fig. 18-14. Tungiasis. Multiple and irregularly confluent craters on nonpressure areas of the foot. Patient died of tetanus. (AFIP 70-4321.)

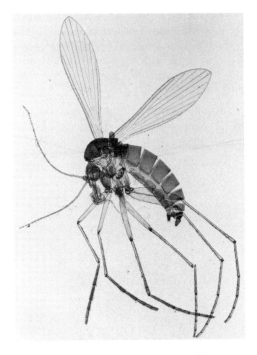

Fig. 18-15. *Phlebotomus* sp. Vector of *Leishmania* spp. (Photograph by Jay R. Georgi. From Schmidt, G. D. and Roberts, L. S.: Foundations of parasitology, St. Louis, 1977, The C. V. Mosby Co.)

deeply in the classification of these flies, we might mention some of the more important members and the diseases they transmit.

Phlebotomus flies

In addition to the transmission of the leish-maniases, discussed under the Protozoa, phlebotomus flies, commonly called sand flies, are transmitters of pappataci fever, an arboviral disease prevalent in countries around the Mediterranean and parts of Asia, and bartonellosis (Oroya fever, verruca peruana), an acute febrile disease, which at times is fatal. The etiologic agent is *Bartonella bacilliformis.*

Phlebotomus flies are very small and are able to pass through the mesh of ordinary mosquito netting. Predominately night biters, they are very annoying considering their small size. Because of their minute size and variety of hiding places, control is difficult. Their short flight range, avoidance of winds, and inability to withstand a stiff breeze offer some compensation for the difficulties involved in other means of control (Fig. 18-15).

Biting midges

Biting midges represent an assortment of tiny flies commonly known as gnats, punkies, biting midges, and so on (Fig. 18-16). The

majority attacking humans belong to the genus *Culicoides*. Some species are the vectors for *Mansonella ozzardi* and *Dipetalonema perstans*, the filarial worms of man. Only the female sucks blood. In the southern states bordering the Atlantic Ocean and the Gulf of Mexico, *Culicoides* make life miserable during the warm evenings for they are able to pass through the fine mesh of ordinary window screening. The cleaning and drainage of swamps markedly reduce their number. Fortunately, those in the United States are not infected with the filarial worms of humans.

Black flies

The black flies, or buffalo gnats, belong to the genus *Simulium*. They have rasping mouthparts and are common around the lake regions of the northern United States and Canada where they make life miserable for the hunter and fisherman. In bad outbreaks they kill large numbers of animals by sucking blood and would do the same to humans if given the chance. They are diurnal in their feeding habits, which makes matters worse. *Simulium* is peculiar in that the flies breed

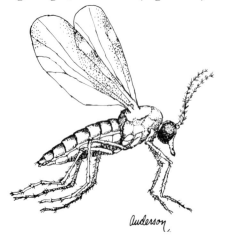

Fig. 18-16. Biting midge, or punky (*Culicoides* sp).

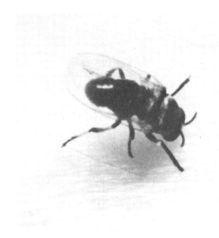

Fig. 18-17. *Simulium damnosum* (black fly or buffalo gnat). Vector of *Onchocerca volvulus* in Africa. (AFIP 68-2763-1.) (From Schmidt, G. D. and Roberts, L. S.: Foundations of parasitology, St. Louis, 1977, The C. V. Mosby Co.)

in fast-running streams, often at great depths. One species, for example, along the Danube breeds at depths to 190 feet. In Mexico, Central America, and South America, as well as in Africa, some species are the intermediate hosts for the filarial worm *Onchocerca volvulus* (Fig. 18-17).

Tabanid flies

The family Tabanidae comprises the horse flies, deer flies, mango flies, and gadflies. They are mainly animal pests, but many species attack humans and also inflict painful bites. Only the females are bloodsuckers. They are strictly diurnal and many are large and beautifully colored. Since they pass from one host to another while feeding, the soiled proboscis is a potential mechanical transmitter of various blood diseases.

Chrysops, the deer fly, is a vector for tularemia and also the intermediate host of the filarial worm *Loa loa* (Fig. 18-18).

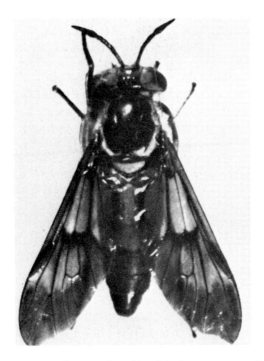

Fig. 18-18. *Chrysops silesia* (deer fly). Common vector of the eye worm, *Loa loa*. (AFIP 72-4516.)

Muscoid flies

The superfamily Muscoidea includes a miscellaneous group of various families of flies. For a simplified presentation, references are made only to the genera, and family ties are omitted. For a better understanding of this group a division into the following three subgroups will be convenient:

1. Skin-piercing flies
2. Nonpiercing or contaminating flies
3. Myiasis-producing flies

Actually, these flies are either bloodsucking or nonbloodsucking, but since members of both groups can cause myiasis, which is an important disease of humans, it is deemed advisable to consider the myiasis-producers as a distinct group. Therefore, they are omitted in the discussion of the first two groups.

Skin-piercing flies. Included in the skin-piercing group are the species of *Glossina* associated with the transmission of the African sleeping sickness (trypanosomiasis) (Fig. 18-19). The stable fly, *Stomoxys calcitrans*, also in this group, is a pest of humans all over the world. Often mistaken for the house fly, it is a true bloodsucker and produces a painful bite. In congested areas of Africa, their hopping from one host to another with a soiled proboscis results in the mechanical transmission of trypanosomiasis. Other blood infections can also be transmitted in this manner. Horn-flies, small blackish flies about half the size of houseflies, also on occasion become pests of humans by annoying them with their bites.

Nonpiercing or contaminating flies. The nonpiercing or contaminating group includes a host of genera having fleshy, lapping, nonpiercing mouthparts. The most common is the ordinary housefly, *Musca domestica*. Because of their living and feeding habits, they have excellent opportunities to mechanically transmit disease agents to humans through the disease exudates, feces, and decomposed matter they carry. Envision, for example, the common housefly with its

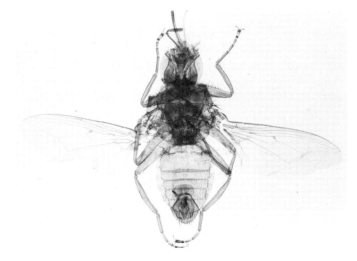

Fig. 18-19. *Glossina* sp (tsetse). Vector of African trypanosomiasis. (Photograph by Warren Buss. From Schmidt, G. D. and Roberts, L. S.: Foundations of parasitology, St. Louis, 1977, The C. V. Mosby Co.)

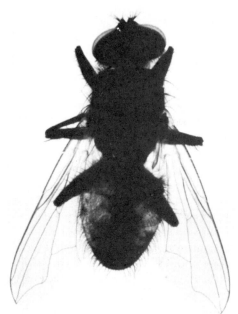

Fig. 18-20. House fly *(Musca domestica)*. Common pest and potential mechanical vector of various disease agents. (Courtesy Department of Epidemiology and Public Health, University of Miami School of Medicine.)

spongy proboscis and sticky feet, picking up disease-laden feces from the latrine down the lane and flying in the open window on a sunny day and walking over the mashed potatoes and vegetables one is enjoying for the noonday meal (Fig. 18-20). The eye gnat has been incriminated as a carrier of such diseases as yaws and pinkeye (acute contagious conjunctivitis). By means of the spines of the proboscis, abrasion of the tissue occurs even though biting does not. There is an endless number of flies in this overall group, for the most part beautifully colored and identified as flesh flies, latrine flies, blowflies, and others, all potential mechanical vectors of disease agents.

Myiasis-producing flies. Myiasis is the term applied to the disease produced by fly larvae, or maggots, that live parasitically in human tissues. As mentioned previously, the muscoid flies in this group may be the skin-piercing or nonpiercing type. Clinically, myiasis may be classified according to the part of the body involved. Thus, we speak of nasal, intestinal, urinary, and cutaneous myiasis. Most of the myiasis-producing flies are in the contaminating group. When the species involved normally feed on decaying vegetable and animal matter, such as garbage, manure, and dead animals, the condition is known as accidental myiasis. A number of families, which include the bluebottle and greenbottle flies, flesh flies, house flies, and their relatives, are in this category. Contaminated food or water is the usual source of infestation.

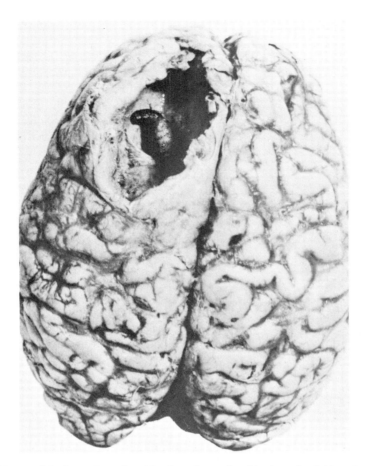

Fig. 18-21. Myiasis of the brain. Several warbles (larvae) were found in the scalp of this patient. Larva in the cavity bored through the anterior fontanelle. Child died of malaria, and larva were found at autopsy. (AFIP N-50807.)

Unprotected food is frequently the site for egglaying by many flies. When eaten, not all eggs and maggots are destroyed in the stomach, particularly when the acidity is low. When the maggots are established in the gastrointestinal tract, which is not uncommon, the person may present symptoms. This fact emphasizes the importance of keeping foodstuffs, particularly pies, custards, and the like, covered to protect the consumers against intestinal invasion. In one case, living nymphal stages of termites were recovered from a patient's feces in an all-metal, sterile bedpan, and were sent by an alert medical student for identification. After a second passage of a batch of termites, the patient was relieved of abdominal pain and eventually returned home. The patient's husband reported that swarming termites were common in the house during mating season.

On rare occasions maggots have even been reported in the female urinary tract. It is difficult to understand how they would arrive there, unless, in tropical countries where women may sit in contaminated areas, maggots gain entrance through the vulva and migrate to the urethra. The Congo floor maggot, *Auchmeromyia luteola*, is common in tropical Africa and attacks only humans. The flies lay eggs on the dirty soil of the hut floor,

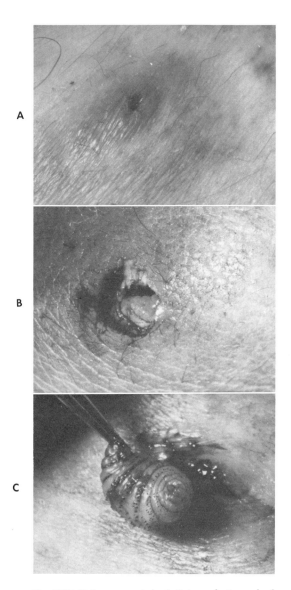

and at night the maggots crawl up through the mats to bite the hosts and suck blood. One fly, *Dermatobia hominis,* has an intriguing way of disseminating its eggs. It catches a mosquito or other fly on the wing and glues its eggs to the belly of the insect. When the mosquito bites a human, the warmth of the skin causes the eggs to hatch. The larvae crawl into the puncture wound (Fig. 18-21) and thus cause cutaneous myiasis (Fig. 18-22). Some larvae invade and develop in living tissue; others prefer necrotic tissue, as exemplified by the surgical maggots of old, which were used to clean out wounds. However, even these maggots will feed on living tissue when the dead tissue is gone.

A large number of flesh flies (*Sarcophaga* and others) and blow flies (*Phaenicia sericata, P. cuprina, Calliphora* spp, and others) take advantage of dirty wounds or sores in warm, humid climates (common in the tropics) to provide a suitable habitat in which to lay their eggs. They are referred to as causing semiobligate myiasis. Halitosis is a siren call to such flies. Babies left out in the open in tropical climates, with running noses or sores, are frequently invaded. Many flies also lay their eggs in clothing soiled with body odor or feces. Eggs hatch from the warmth of the host's skin, and the larvae tear a hole and burrow in when the skin is tender, like that of infants.

Brought to mind is the occasion when maggots played a role in a murder case. Fly larvae that were recovered from the ear of the victim were sent to the laboratory for identification, in the hope that knowledge of the life history of the fly in question might help to determine the time of deposition of the body along the canal. More conventional techniques, however, were used to finally resolve the matter.

A number of flies, as indicated, are obligate parasites, producing obligate myiasis in man. The most notorious in the western hemisphere is *Callitroga hominivorax,* the primary screw worm. It is known to cause

Fig. 18-22. Cutaneous myiasis. **A,** Primary lesion on back of patient. Note opening to surface for posterior spiracles. **B,** Surgical removal of "maggot." **C,** Larva of *Dermatobia hominus* after removal. (Courtesy Dr. Nardo Zaias, Department of Dermatology, Mt. Sinai Medical Center, Miami Beach. Photography by Charles M. Bailey, Biomedical Communications, University of Miami School of Medicine.)

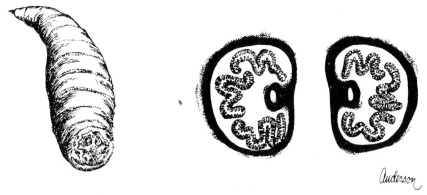

Fig. 18-23. Fly larva, or maggot. Note the stigmal plate bearing two posterior spiracles. Enlarged view of posterior spiracles of *Musca domestica* illustrate characteristic pattern of species.

a nasopharyngeal myiasis in humans. Larvae have been recovered from the mastoid cells and abscesses in the middle ear, and death has been reported in at least one known instance. The fly is strongly attracted to wounds and sores in animals. Loss of sheep, goats, cattle, and other animals in the United States, running into the millions of dollars, has been attributed to this screw worm. The larvae or maggots live only in the living flesh of warm-blooded animals. The botflies (Gasterophilidae) and warble flies (Hypodermatidae) are obligate parasites of the digestive and other body systems of many mammals. *Gasterophilus intestinalis*, a common botfly in horses, lays its eggs on the hairs of the leg primarily. The warmth of the tongue licking the area stimulates hatching of the eggs. Many larvae penetrate the mucosa of the tongue, producing lesions, while others are swallowed and develop in the intestinal tract. Eventually third-stage larvae pass out in the feces and pupation takes place in the external environment. In humans, hatched larvae wander aimlessly after skin penetration, producing a larva migrans. *Hypoderma bovis* and *H. lineata* normally lay their eggs on the hairs of cattle. The hatched larvae burrow into the skin, producing tremendous swellings on the backs of animals. Cattlemen can be seen squeezing out these large "grubs." Horses and humans are occasionally infected.

Symptomatology and pathology of myiasis will vary, depending on the location, number of maggots present, and the species involved. Fully developed or third-stage (instar) larvae, when recovered, will reveal the characteristic pattern of the two posterior spiracles on the stigmal plate which can be removed with a scalpel or razor blade and examined microscopically. Identification as to family or genus, and in some instances species, can be made, as depicted in Fig. 18-23. If live larvae are recovered, growth to the adult fly can be facilitated for morphologic study and species identification, if desired. An environment similar to that in nature can be created by putting the larvae in a jar containing meat on sand or earth. After pupation, hatching will occur, and adult flies can be studied in detail.

Mosquitoes

Of the various arthropods of medical significance the family Culicidae, or mosquitoes, are the most important, without a doubt. As pests they are well known by everyone from the temperate regions to deep into the tropics. Three genera are of major medical importance, *Anopheles*, *Aedes*, and *Culex*. Mosquitoes can be differentiated from any mosquito-like insect by the nature of the vein pattern in the wings, the third vein being unbranched and located between two branched veins, the second and fourth. The long proboscis and the scales on the veins of the wings further help to identify mosquitoes. Male mosquitoes characteristically have bushy antennae, whereas those of the females are plain. The proboscis consists of the fleshy mouth part known as the labium, which contains the structures adopted for piercing and sucking. The stylets, enclosed by the labium, contain one channel for the injection of saliva and the other for sucking. Only female mosquitoes can suck blood, since the males have shortened mouth parts adopted for feeding on plant juices.

The life cycle of the mosquito consists of the adult, egg, larva (wiggler), and pupa (tumbler). Feeding habits of various species range from some females sucking blood from nonmammalian hosts such as birds, reptiles, and amphibia to others that feed on mammalian blood or no blood at all. Flight habits also vary and play an important role in the transmission of disease agents (Fig. 18-24). Some mosquitoes overwinter in the egg stage in colder climates and hatch in the spring, whereas others hibernate as adults. One species, *Wyeomyia smithi*, spends part of its larval stage embedded in ice. All mosquitoes spend at least part of their larval stage in water and, for this reason, mosquito control leans heavily on attacking the insects during this phase as well as mass spraying against adults.

The genus *Culex* with its many species is the most common. *Culex quinquefasciatus* is one of the more important transmitters of filariasis in humans. Various species of *Culex* are important vectors of many of the viral encephalitides. *Culex tarsalis* transmits western equine encephalitis, which is widely distributed throughout the United States,

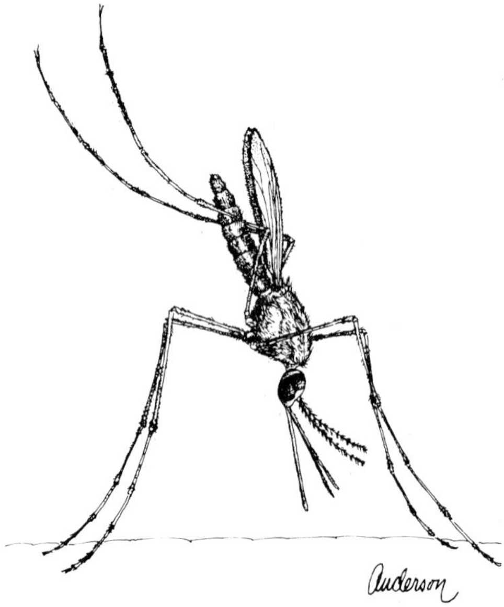

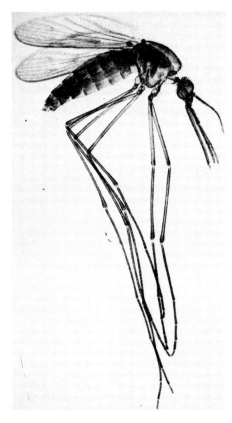

Fig. 18-24. If the lady resting on your arm is standing on her head, she is none other than the mosquito *Anopheles*, the vector of malaria.

Fig. 18-25. *Anopheles* sp ♀. Vector for malaria. (Courtesy Dr. W. Henry Leigh, Department of Biology, University of Miami.)

with human cases occurring chiefly in the West. A number of species of *Culex* transmit St. Louis encephalitis throughout the United States, wild birds being chiefly the reservoir hosts for both St. Louis and western equine. Eastern equine encephalitis, also harbored by wild birds, is found along the Atlantic and Gulf coasts and is transmitted by several species of *Aedes, Mansonia* and *Psorophora.* Venezuelan equine encephalitis, which occurs in Texas, is associated probably with species of *Aedes* and *Psorophora,* while California encephalitis, which is distributed throughout the United States, is transmitted mainly by several species of *Aedes.* Some species of the genus *Mansonia* are associated with Malayan filariasis.

Aedes aegypti is the principal vector of the arbovirus causing yellow fever. Being anthropophilic and a domestic breeder necessitates vigilant control measures for this mosquito. It is also the vector for dengue fever. Other species of *Aedes* are also involved in the transmission of various viral encephalitides.

The genus *Anopheles* is the sole vector in the cyclic transmission of the human malarias (Fig. 18-25). Species vary in their breeding place anywhere from treetops to rain puddles, wells, cisterns, and containers of various sorts. Approximately 100 species of *Anopheles* have been shown to be vectors of the malarial parasites of humans.

Mosquito control measures are dependent on the genera and species involved and their life styles. Attack is focused on the adult and larval stages chiefly, with emphasis on the breeding places of the larvae. Removal or overturning of all water-holding containers, the drainage and filling of pools, cisterns, and so on, the introduction of surface-feeding fish into large bodies of water, screening of water-barrels, and the application of light volatile oils such as nonleaded gasoline or odorless kerosene are some methods that may be used. Constant surveillance, regardless of the methods used, becomes essential for effective control.

VECTOR-BORNE DISEASES AND THEIR CONTROL

Table 16-2 lists some of the more common vector-borne diseases that affect humans. In the past the control of these has played a significant role in human settlement and agricultural development in the tropics. Even today, however, areas still exist where development is impossible because of the widespread prevalence of vector-borne disease. Trypanosomiasis and river blindness (onchocerciasis) in Africa and malaria in certain areas of Southeast Asia still constitute a serious deterrent to human habitation. Modern methods of transportation have brought the United States only a few hours away from the endemic reservoirs of these earlier scourges, so that it is just as important to maintain a vigorous control program in nonendemic areas as it is in endemic areas. Modern society is so mobile that the risk of reimportation of vector-borne disease to a normally nonendemic area is a very real one. Any of the diseases in Table 16-2 could easily be introduced into areas where both the vector and a susceptible population coexist. The possibility of a dengue fever resurgence in the United States is such an example, for in the southern states, *Aedes aegypti* is plentiful, the population is susceptible, and outbreaks of dengue in Puerto Rico and other Caribbean regions occur frequently.

As can be seen from Table 18-1, the present control strategies are primarily chemical. This is likely to remain so in the foreseeable future, but, as is discussed later, serious problems with this technology are becoming apparent. It is obvious that for future control of arthropod-related diseases, particularly malaria, alternative strategies in biologic control, hormones, genetic manipulation, and the development of new vaccines will be needed to supplement the use of chemicals.

Public health surveys in several different parts of the world have shown that the immediate concerns of present pest manage-

Table 18-1. Partial list of generic and brand names of antiparasitic drugs

Generic name	Brand name	Generic name	Brand name
Amodiaquine	Camoquin	*Nifurtimox	Lampit (Bayer, Germany)
Amophotericin B	Fungizone	†Oxamniquine	Mansil (Pfizer)
*Antimony sodium dimercaptosuccinate (stibocaptate)	Astiban (Hoffman-LaRoche, Switzerland)	*Niclosamide	Yomesan (Bayer, Germany)
Benzyl benzoate	Scabanca (Canada)	*Niridazole	Ambilhar (Ciba-Geigy, Switzerland)
*Bithionol	Bitin (Tanabe, Japan)	Paromomycin	Humatin
Chloroquine	Aralen; others	*Pentamidine	Lomidine (May & Baker, England)
Copper oleate	Cuprex		
Crotamiton	Eurax	Piperazine	Atepar; others
*Cycloguanil pamoate	Camolar (Parke, Davis)	Primaquine phosphate	Primaquine
*Dehydroemetine	Dehydroemetine (Hoffman-LaRoche, Switzerland)	Pyrantel pamoate	Antiminth
		Pyrethrins and piperonyl butoxide	Rid; A-200 Pyrinate
Diethylcarbamazine	Hetrazan	Pyrimethamine	Daraprim
Diiodohydroxyquin	Diodoquin; Floraquin; Ioquin; Moebiquin; Yodoxin	†Pyrimethamine plus sulfadoxine	Fansidar (Roche)
		Pyrvinium pamoate	Povan
*Diloxanide furoate	Furamide (Boots, England)	Quinacrine	Atabrine
Furazolidone	Furoxone	†Spiramycin	Rovamycin (Poulenc, Canada)
Gamma benzene hexachloride (lindane)	Kwell; Gamene	*Stibogluconate sodium (antimony sodium gluconate)	Pentostam (Burroughs Wellcome, England)
Mebendazole	Vermox	*Suramin	Germanin (Bayer, Germany)
*Melarsoprol	Arsobal (Rhone Poulenc, France)	Thiabendazole	Mintezol
*Metrifonate	Bilareil (Bayer, Germany)	Trimethoprim-sulfamethoxazole	Bactrim; Septra
Metronidazole	Flagyl		

*Available in the U.S.A. from the Parasitic Diseases Division, Center for Disease Control, Atlanta, Georgia 30333; telephone: 404-329-3311.

†Not available in the U.S.A.

ment strategies are because of poisonings, persistance, and resistance.

Pesticide poisoning is one of the most serious events occurring with the technology transfer in the developing countries. More than 500,000 cases are thought to occur annually and most result from the misuse of and the ignorance of the inherent toxicity of the chemicals.

Persistance is manifested by the pesticidal contamination of food, and frequently pesticide residues in a variety of foods exceed acceptable tolerances and cannot be exported. Residue contamination of food is occurring with increasing frequency in certain areas. In Central America, where 25% of the world's beef is produced, meat contamination costs the industry 1.5 million dollars. The secondary elevation of pesticide levels in the general population of the area because of incidental exposure is of special public health concern.

The third problem is the resurgence of malaria and other vector-borne diseases resulting from the increased vector resistance to each of the three major chemical group of insecticides. In most areas vector resistance has developed from the indirect selection pressures of agricultural insecticides. Anopheline mosquito resistance has been demonstrated in Indonesia, Egypt, Africa, and Central America. The resistance problem in El Salvador, where malaria rates have doubled, is so serious that, in addition to the more conventional mosquito control programs, the stocking of ponds and pools with larvivorous fish and the release of sterilized male mosquitoes have become part of innovative strategies being tested.

Problems such as these emphasize the need for alternative methods of control. In the agricultural field, high expectations exist for "integrated pest management" approaches, wherein chemical control is augmented by cultural, genetic, and biologic techniques. Pesticide management problems in developing countries are of concern to those in the agricultural and public health fields, and an interdisciplinary agromedical approach has been proposed. The attack that agriculturists have used in integrated pest control is the same that is needed for the continued control of vector-borne diseases. This agromedical partnership seems indispensible if agricultural pests and arthropod vectors of disease are to be controlled in the years ahead and a bountiful global food supply is to be ensured.

REVIEW QUESTIONS

1. What is the significance of the various types of mouthparts in insects? Explain by giving examples.
2. What diseases of medical importance, if any, are associated with the following:
   Cockroaches
   Bedbugs
   Triatomid bugs
   Sucking lice
   Fleas
3. Give examples of important dipteran flies and their reason for being medically significant.
4. Discuss myiasis. Give examples.
5. What insect is most outstanding in the class Hexapoda as a disease transmitter? Cite the diseases involved.
6. Discuss problems of modern pesticide management.

REFERENCES

Barnard, J. H. 1973. Studies of 400 Hymenoptera sting deaths in the United States. J. Allergy. Clin. Immunol. **52**:259-264.

Buxton, P. A. 1947. The louse, and account of the lice which infect man, their medical importance and control. Ed. 2. Edward Arnold (Publishers) Ltd., London.

Davies, J. E., R. F. Smith, and V. Freed. 1978. Agromedical approach to pesticide management. Ann. Rev. Entomol. **23**:353-356.

Foote, R. H., and D. R. Cook. 1959. Mosquitoes of medical importance. Agricultural Handbook no. 152, Department of Agriculture, U.S. Government Printing Office, Washington, D.C.

Frazier, C. A. 1969. Insect allergy: allergic reactions a review of 180 cases. South. Med. J. **57**:1028-1034.

Frazier, C. A. 1969. Insect allergy: Allergic reactions to bites of insects and other arthropods. Warren H. Green, Inc. St. Louis.

Horen, P. W. 1972. Insect and scorpion sting. J.A.M.A. **221**:894-898.

James, M. T. 1947. The flies that cause myiasis in man. U.S. Department of Agriculture Miscellaneous Publication no. 631, U.S. Government Printing Office, Washington, D.C.

James, M. T., and B. F. Harwood. 1969. Herms's medical entomology. Ed. 6. Macmillan Inc., New York.

Jellison, W. L. 1959. Fleas and disease. Ann. Rev. Entom. 4:389-414.

Jung, R. C., V. J. Derbes, and A. D. Burch. 1963. Skin response to a solenamine, or hemolytic component of fire ant venom. Dermatol. Trop. 2:241-244.

King, W. V., G. H. Bradley, C. N. Smith, and W. C. McDuffle. 1960. A handbook of the mosquitoes of the southeastern United States. Agriculture Handbook no. 173. Department of Agriculture, U.S. Government Printing Office, Washington, D.C.

Lavoipierre, M. M. J., G. Dickerson, and R. M. Gordon. 1959. The manner in which triatomid bugs obtain a blood meal. Am. J. Trop. Med. 53:235-250.

Pest control: an assessment of present and alternative technologies. Vol. V. Pest control and health. 1976.

The report of the Public Health Study Team, study on problems of pesticide control. Environmental Studies Board, National Research Council, National Academy of Sciences, Washington, D.C.

Roth, L. M., and E. R. Willis. 1957. Medical and veterinary importance of cockroaches. Smithsonian Publication no. 4299, U.S. Government Printing Office, Washington, D.C.

Smart, J. 1956. A handbook for the identification of insects of medical importance. British Museum, London.

Stahnke, H. L., and A. H. Dengler. 1964. The effect of morphine and related substances on the toxicity of venoms. I. *Centruriodes sculpturatus* Ewing scorpion venom. Am. J. Trop. Med. Hyg. 13:346-351.

Zumpt, F. 1965. Myiasis in man and animals in the Old World: a textbook for physicians, veterinarians and zoologists. Butterworth & Co. (Publishers) Ltd., London.

Appendixes

Solutions, stains, and procedures for examining fecal material

Neutral formalin, 5%

Na_2HPO_4	6.10 gm
NaH_2PO_4	0.15 gm
Formalin (commercial formaldehyde)	400 ml
Water	7,600 ml

Mix the formaldehyde and water. Add buffer salts and mix thoroughly. For use, mix 1 part feces in about 3 volumes of neutral formalin.

Phenol-alcohol-formaldehyde (PAF) solution

This fixative may be substituted for neutral formalin when collecting fecal specimens. It preserves protozoan cysts and trophozoites as well as helminth eggs and larvae. PAF fixed material may be examined as unstained mounts or stained with thionin or azure A. Thionin is the preferred stain.

PAF FIXATIVE

Phenol crystals (white, not old and discolored)	20 gm
Physiological saline (0.85%)	825 ml

Dissolve crystals in saline, then add:

95% ethyl alcohol	125 ml
Formaldehyde	50 ml

Mix well. If liquefied phenol is available, use 23 ml instead of 20 gm crystals.

THIONIN STAIN

Thionin powder	10 mg
Distilled H_2O	100 ml

AZURE A (OR METHYLENE AZURE A) STAIN

Azure A powder	10 mg
Distilled H_2O	80 ml

PAF fixed material may be concentrated by simple centrifugal sedimentation or by saline-ether sedimentation.

SALINE-ETHER SEDIMENTATION

1. Strain 10 to 12 ml of PAF fixed fecal suspension through wet gauze or cheesecloth into a 15 ml centrifuge tube.
2. Centrifuge at 2,000 rpm (450 to 500 g) for 3 minutes. Decant and resuspend with 0.85% saline.
3. Repeat washings until supernatant is clear.
4. Add saline to sediment up to 10 ml level, then add 1 drop 33% aqueous dilution of Triton X-100. In place of Triton, 1 drop of any one of the following may be used:

Pluronic P-75	10% aqueous solution
Irium	8% aqueous solution
Brij 35	2.5% aqueous solution

5. Mix well and let stand for 10 minutes.
6. Add 2 ml ether, stopper tube, and shake vigorously for about 30 seconds, keeping thumb on stopper.
7. Remove stopper and centrifuge at 2,000 to 2,500 rpm (500 to 650 g) for 3 minutes.
8. Four layers result: ether, plug of debris, saline, and sediment.
9. Ring plug of debris, decant top 3 layers using cotton swab to wipe inside of tube almost to sediment.
10. Transfer portion of sediment to slide, apply coverslip, and examine microscopically.
11. A drop of thionin stain may be added to stain protozoa if desired.

Alcohol-formalin-acetic acid (AFA)

This fixative is used for helminths after relaxation:

Commercial formalin	10 parts
95% ethyl alcohol	25 parts
Acetic acid (glacial)	5 parts
Glycerin	10 parts
Distilled water	50 parts

Lugol's iodine solution

Iodine (powdered crystals)	5 gm
Potassium iodide	10 gm
Distilled H_2O	100 ml

Dissolve the KI in water, then slowly add the iodine crystals. Shake thoroughly. The filtered stock solution will remain stable for months. Before use, dilute about 5 times with distilled water. Keep solutions in dark bottles.

Dobell and O'Connor's iodine solution

Iodine (powdered crystals)	1 gm
Potassium iodide	2 gm
Distilled water	100 ml

Dissolve the KI in water, then slowly add the iodine crystals. Shake thoroughly. The filtered solution is ready for use. When fading occurs, fresh iodine crystals can be added to bring back proper coloration. Filter before use to prevent overcoloration. "Rejuvenation" should be done at most only once or twice. Keep solution in a dark bottle.

Quensel's stain

1. Decant 20 ml of a saturated solution of Sudan III (in 80% ethyl alcohol).
2. Mix with 30 ml of a saturated and filtered aqueous solution of medicinal methylene blue.
3. Filter into 50 ml of 10% aqueous solution of cadmium chloride (C.P.).
4. Shake gently occasionally for 15 to 20 minutes; flocculent precipitate forms; supernatant almost colorless.
5. Filter.
6. Remove all excess liquid from the precipitate by placing the filter paper with the precipitate upon several layers of filter paper; leave overnight to dry.
7. Transfer precipitate to a fresh filter and rapidly pass through 25 to 30 ml of distilled water.
8. Dissolve washed precipitate in 250 ml of distilled water.
9. Filter in a few days to remove fine crystals of cadmium chloride.

USE OF STAIN

Quensel's stain is a supravital stain that is useful in the identification of the trophozoite stage only of the amebas. Nuclear detail is similar to that seen in iron-hematoxylin preparations. The cytoplasm stains blue.

Buffered methylene blue stain

Buffered methylene blue stain is a method of staining trophozoites of *E. histolytica* and other amebas. Acetate buffer solutions within the pH range of 3.6 to 4.8 are satisfactory.

To 46.3 ml of a 0.2 M solution of acetic acid (11.55 ml in 1,000 ml H_2O), add 3.7 ml of a 0.2 M solution of sodium acetate (16.4 gm of $C_2H_3O_2Na$ in 1,000 ml H_2O).

To this solution of pH 3.6 add a small amount of meth-

ylene blue (0.06%). A staining reaction similar to Quensel's will be obtained.

Merthiolate-iodine-formaldehyde (MIF) stain

METHOD OF PREPARATION AND USE OF DIRECT SMEAR TECHNIQUE

Lugol's iodine solution (stock)	1.00 part
Formaldehyde (U.S.P.)	1.25 parts
Tincture of Merthiolate, Lilly No. 9 (1:1,000)	7.75 parts

Place distilled water in one Kahn tube; in another tube place some MIF (freshly prepared). Put one drop of distilled water (using medicine dropper) on a glass slide and add a drop of equal size of MIF stain. To the mixture add a minute amount of feces and mix. Cover with coverslip and examine.

PREPARATION OF PRESERVED STOOL SPECIMENS

1. A stable stock "MF" (Merthiolate-formaldehyde) solution:
   - 250 ml H_2O distilled
   - 200 ml tincture of Merthiolate
   - 25 ml formaldehyde
   - 5 ml glycerin
   - 480 ml stock MF solution (store in brown bottle)
2. Fresh Lugol's solution (store in brown bottle)

Just prior to time of preservation, add 2.35 ml of MF stock solution to 0.15 ml of Lugol's stock solution. Use sufficient stain to ensure adequate fixation of stool specimen. After sedimentation, adequate supernatant should be discernible.

Polyvinyl alcohol (PVA) method for fixing and staining intestinal protozoa

PREPARATION OF FIXATIVE

PVA, powdered*	5.0 gm
Glycerol	1.5 ml
Acetic acid, glacial	5.0 ml
Schaudinn's solution	93.5 ml
(2 parts mercuric chloride [saturated aqueous solution] to 1 part ethyl alcohol [95%])	

Add the PVA to the reagents above at room temperature and heat to approximately 75° C. Keep stirring until preparation is water clear. Allow to cool and warm to 50° C before use. Add acetic acid after heating.

1. On microscopic slides
   With the aid of an applicator stick, mix 1 drop of the fecal material with 3 drops of the fixative and smear over about one third of the glass surface. To ensure thorough drying, place slides in an incubator at 37° C overnight.
2. In vials
   Mix a quantity of feces thoroughly with three or

---

*Elvanol 90-25; Delkote, Inc., Penns Grove, N.J.

more parts of fixative in a glass vial. Prepare smears on glass slides as desired and dry as above.

STAINING OF ORGANISMS IN PVA FILMS

1. The long Heidenhain iron-hematoxylin staining procedure is performed for critical staining. Staining may be interrupted at any step in the procedure except during the dehydration process.

a. 70% alcohol + I_2 (port wine color)   15 min
b. 70% alcohol   5 min
c. 50% alcohol   5 min
d. Water (tap)   5 min
e. 4% iron alum (mordant)   30 min to overnight
   (Iron alum–ferric ammonium sulfate dissolved in distilled water according to strength desired)
f. Water (several changes)   5 to 10 min
g. 0.5% aqueous hema-   30 min to overnight
   toxylin (stain)
   (Hematoxylin stain [stock solution]; hematoxylin powder, 10 gm, and ethyl alcohol [100%], 100 ml; dissolve powder in alcohol and allow to "ripen" before use; dilute with distilled water as desired)
h. Water (several changes)   5 to 10 min
i. Saturated aqueous picric acid   20 min (+)
   (destain)
j. Running tap water   Until blue
k. 50% alcohol   5 min
l. 70% alcohol   5 min
m. 95% alcohol   5 min
n. 100% alcohol   5 min each
o. 100% alcohol + xylol   5 min
   (50%-50% mixture)
p. Xylol (2 changes)   5 min
q. Mount in clarite, etc.   5 min each

2. Trichrome staining
Preparation

Chromotrope 2R   0.60 gm
Light green SF   0.15 gm
Fast green FCF   0.15 gm
Phosphotungstic acid   0.70 gm
Acetic acid (glacial)   1.00 ml
Distilled water   100 ml

Add acetic acid to dry components. Allow to ripen for 30 minutes and then add the distilled water.
Use. After fixation of slide in PVA and through drying:

Iodine alcohol (port wine color) 70%   1 min
Alcohol 70%   1 min
Alcohol 70%   1 min
Stain   2 to 8 min
Alcohol (1 drop glacial acetic   10 to 20 sec
   acid per 10 ml 95%   *or* until barely
   alcohol)   runs from
                                      smear
Alcohol 100%   Rinse twice

Preparation —cont'd
Alcohol 100%   1 min
Xylol   1 min
                                    or until refraction
                                      at the smear-
                                      xylol interface
                                      ends

Chlorazol black E stain

This is a simple procedure in which fixation and staining take place in a single solution. No destaining is necessary. Best results are obtained with fresh fecal smears. PVA fixed material is not very satisfactory.

BASIC SOLUTION

90% ethyl alcohol   170 ml
Methyl alcohol   160 ml
Glacial acetic acid   20 ml
Liquid phenol   20 ml
1% phosphotungstic acid*   12 ml
Distilled H_2O 618 ml

Add alcohols and acids to distilled H_2O and mix thoroughly.

STOCK STAIN SOLUTION

Chlorazol black E dye   5 gm
Basic solution   1,000 ml

Grind dye in mortar for at least 3 minutes. Add small amount of basic solution and grind until smooth paste is obtained. Add more solution and grind for 5 minutes. Pour off supernatant into separate dye container. Add more solution to mortar and continue grinding and mixing process until all dye appears to be in solution. Add remaining basic solution to bottle with stain and ripen for 4 to 6 weeks. Filter through Whatman no. 2 filter paper before use. Keep filtered stain in tightly stoppered bottle.

The optimal dilution and staining time must be determined for each liter of fixative stain. The following series of dilutions and staining periods are recommended.

Stain solution	Basic solution	Hours
Undiluted	—	2 to 3
1	1	2 to 4 to overnight
2	1	2 to 4
1	2	2 to overnight
1	3	4 to overnight

Trial smears should be stained with each dilution according to technique below:

Fixative-stain dilution   as indicated
95% ethyl alcohol   10 to 15 sec

---

*1 gm phosphotungstic acid crystals dissolved in 100 ml distilled H_2O.

Carbol-xylene (1:2)	5 min
or	
100% ethyl alcohol	5 min
Xylene	5 min

Mount in Permount or other suitable medium. Tissue slides after preparation by the usual histological procedures are stained as above. NOTE: Staining time is twice as long as for fecal smears.

Stains for helminths
ALUM COCHINEAL

Potassium alum	30 gm
Cochineal	30 gm
Distilled H₂O	400 ml

Boil for 1 hour. Cool and filter. Keep filtrate. Boil the filter paper in 200 ml distilled water for 30 minutes. Filter. Add second filtrate to first and boil 30 minutes. Filter and make up to 400 ml with distilled water.

DELAFIELD'S HEMATOXYLIN

Add aluminum ammonium sulfate (ammonia alum) crystals to hot distilled water, stirring continuously until saturation occurs. Let cool. Excess alum will crystallize out. Pour off supernatant or filter. Store in glass-stoppered bottle indefinitely.

Hematoxylin crystals	4 gm
95% ethyl alcohol	25 ml
Ammonium alum (saturated aqueous solution)	400 ml

Dissolve stain crystals in alcohol and add alum. Place in loosely capped container in sunlight for 2 weeks. Add mixture of:

Methyl alcohol (acetone free)	100 ml
Glycerin	100 ml

Place in glass-stoppered bottle and expose to direct sunlight for at least 1 month. Filter before use.

REYNOLD'S STAIN

Alum cochineal	3 parts
Delafield's hematoxylin	1 part
Distilled water	25 parts

Usable immediately but best after standing a few hours. Filter out fine precipitate before use.

SEMICHON'S ACETIC CARMINE

Acetic acid (glacial)	1 part
Distilled water	1 part

Add excess carmine powder to mixture in small flask and place in boiling water for 15 minutes. Cool, decant supernatant, and filter.

TECHNIQUE FOR STAINING HELMINTHS

Relaxation and extension of worms by one of the following methods:
1. Place small helminths in drop of saline on slide, coverslip for gentle pressure, and run fixative under coverslip.

2. Place helminths in bottle half filled with saline and shake vigorously for 2 to 3 minutes.
3. Place whole worms or proglottids in water and refrigerate for 30 minutes to overnight.
4. Wrap tapeworms around glass jar or slide. Then fix.
5. Strips of proglottids gently flattened and extended between paper towels are soaked in fixative, then placed between large pieces of glass or slides that are tied lightly but firmly together with string to flatten organisms. Keep moist with fixative. After relaxation, transfer to fixative.

Use of fixatives
1. Formalin 5%
Solution should be steaming hot not boiling. Pour the formalin over the worms in extended position. Pour off after several hours and add fresh, unheated 5% formalin. Can be kept indefinitely.
2. Alcohol-formalin-acetic acid (AFA)
Use cold. Worms may remain in fixative for several days but 12 to 24 hours are usually sufficient. To store, replace the AFA with 70% alcohol.

After fixation, worms are placed in 50% alcohol for 1 hour followed by 10 minutes in distilled water. From this point the organisms are ready for staining.

Stains
1. Alum-cochineal
Staining usually requires 24 to 36 hours depending on size and density of worms. Next wash organisms in water 15 to 20 minutes, followed by placement in 70% ethyl alcohol.
2. Delafield's hematoxylin
Stain for 1 hour or longer depending on size of worms. Longer periods may be used if diluted stain is used. Watch until desired point of staining is reached.
3. Reynold's stain
Stain 4 hours to overnight depending on size of worms.
4. Semichon's acetic carmine
Stain for 24 hours.

After staining
1. Place worms in 70% alcohol for 2 minutes.
2. Place in acid alcohol (1 ml concentrated HCl to 99 ml 70% ethyl alcohol) until internal structures are visible to strong transmitted light. (Omit this step usually for alum-cochineal stain.)

3. 70% alcohol	1 to 2 minutes

4. Neutralize in 70% alcohol containing lithium carbonate (several drops of lithium carbonate saturated aqueous solution to each 100 ml alcohol).

5. 95% alcohol	1 hr
6. 100% alcohol	1 hr
7. 100% alcohol	30 min
8. 100% alcohol	1 hr
9. 100% alcohol + cedarwood oil (equal parts for clearing)	½ to 1 hr

10. Cedarwood oil   1 hr
11. Mount in Permount, etc. (Do not allow drying at any stage until mounted.)

Clearing helminths without staining

This procedure is frequently adequate to reveal most structural details. Tapeworm proglottids and small worms are often handled in this manner.

1. Relax organism as previously described.
2. Fix in hot 70% alcohol or 5% formalin for several hours.
3. Put into clearing solution from choice below:
   a. Carbol-xylene (1:3)
      Clearing very rapid. Uterine branches of proglottids are easily seen by holding between two slides toward the light.
   b. Lacto-phenol (1:1)
      Equal volume of glycerin may be added. This solution is good for nematodes, but overclearing can occur with prolonged use.
   c. Beechwood creosote
      Clearing is slower but worms remain soft and pliable.
   d. Xylene
      Clearing takes place fairly quickly, but worms become brittle; it is very effective clearing for tapeworm proglottids.
   e. Glycerin
      This is fairly satisfactory for nematodes such as hookworm but shrivelling or wrinkling may occur.
   f. PVA-lacto-phenol
      Fairly good clearing and mounting medium for small nematodes.

      PVA, 15% aqueous solution   70 parts
      Lacto-phenol (1:1)   30 parts

Dehydration-clearing for permanent mounts

Pass worms up through graded ethyl alcohols 20%, 35%, 50%, 70%, 85%, 95%, and 100%. Leave in each alcohol 30 minutes to 1 hour. Mount in Permount, balsam, or other suitable mounting medium. Support coverslip on either side to prevent rocking and giving slanted surface to finished preparation.

Concentrated brine flotation method

This technique is used primarily for hookworm ova. It is effective for other helminth ova but not for operculated and schistosome eggs. Protozoan cysts are shrunken beyond recognition.

Prepare solution by stirring NaCl into hot or boiling water until excess will not go into solution. Check with hydrometer after cooling to ensure specific gravity of at least 1.20. Filter before using.

1. Mix fecal sample in vial with brine solution.
2. Fill vial to brim and superimpose 3 × 2 inch slide on top ensuring complete contact with solution.

3. Let stand 10 minutes to 1 hour. Optimum time 10 to 15 minutes.
4. Lift slide straight up without tipping, invert carefully, and examine microscopically without coverslipping.

Sedimentation

This simple technique is applicable to the recovery of all ova, larvae, and cysts and is especially suitable for operculated and schistosome ova.

1. Thoroughly comminute the feces (about 5 gm) in a small amount of tap water in a beaker (250 ml).
2. Fill the beaker with tap water and strain the suspension through cheesecloth or graded sieves into a conical-shaped flask. Let settle.
3. Decant supernatant and continue washing process until supernatant is clear.
4. Examine sediment for ova, larvae, and cysts.

Technique for hatching schistosome miracidia

This is a very effective way to demonstrate indirectly the small numbers of viable ova in the feces, which might be overlooked by other methods.

NOTE: Throughout the procedure use only chlorine-free water, which can be obtained by boiling tap water or allowing it to stand overnight.

1. Resuspend sediment (after step 3 under Sedimentation) in a 500 ml Erlenmeyer flask.
2. Fill flask almost to top with chlorine-free water and let stand for several hours or overnight.
3. Eggs will hatch, liberating miracidia, which will swim to and collect at the surface film in the neck of the flask. A hand lens is helpful in seeing the miracidia. NOTE: Care must be exercised in preventing contamination by free-living ciliates or flagellates.

Vaseline-paraffin swab technique for *Enterobius vermicularis*

A coated cotton swab is prepared by dipping cotton end into a hot mixture of 4 parts vaseline to 1 part parawax (paraffin). After cooling, place swab into a 100 × 13 mm tube and plug with cotton. For use, rub cotton swab gently over perianal surface, spreading open the perianal folds. Insert swab about ¼ inch into anal opening. Replace swab in tube and fill about one third to one half of tube with xylene (enough to cover swab). Let stand 3 to 5 minutes, then centrifuge at 2,000 rpm (500 g) for 1 minute. Remove supernatant carefully and examine sediment microscopically, without coverslipping, for eggs. Other helminth eggs may sometimes be recovered by this method.

Estimating worm burdens

Egg-counting techniques are used chiefly to estimate worm burdens in a population group in relation to control or eradication programs or to determine the efficacy of anthelminthics. This enables one to classify infections only as light, moderate, or heavy. Exact worm counts are not possible. Physicians can effectively evaluate the effectiveness of a drug regimen by comparing counts before and after treatment.

Quantitative egg-counting techniques
DIRECT EGG COUNT

Direct fecal smears made by the same technician repeatedly using the same size coverslip will usually contain about the same amount of formed feces. Assuming that the egg distribution throughout the fecal specimen is relatively constant, a means is afforded for evaluating fluctuations in worm burden following therapy.

STOLL AND HAUSHEER DILUTION
EGG COUNT

0.1 N NaOH is placed in a special graduated flask to the 56 ml mark on the neck. Feces are added to displace the solution to the 60 ml mark, thus representing 4 gm (4 ml) of feces. Several glass beads are added; the flask is stoppered, and vigorous shaking done to thoroughly comminute the feces. Repeated shakings over a several-hour period or after standing overnight may be necessary to obtain complete contamination. An aliquot of 0.075 ml is withdrawn quickly with a pipette, placed on a clean slide, coverslipped, and the egg count is made. The number of eggs of the species counted is multiplied by the factor 200 to obtain the number of eggs per gram of feces. To compensate for the consistency of the stool specimen, a correction factor must be used to convert to a formed stool basis as follows:

Mushy-formed stools	×1.5
Mush	×2.0
Mushy diarrhea	×3.0
Flowing diarrhea	×4.0
Watery	×5.0

In a gram of formed stool, approximately 44 eggs have been found to represent one female *Necator americanus*. Male and female worms are usually present in about equal numbers.

KATO THICK-SMEAR TECHNIQUE

This technique is very useful for the diagnosis of many helminth ova in extensive survey studies. Adaption for quantitative egg counts is detailed by Martin and Beaver, 1968.

1. Transfer approximately 50 mg feces to a glass slide and cover with a cellophane coverslip (22 × 30 mm) soaked in glycerin-malachite-green solution for at least 24 hours.
2. Invert the preparation onto a flat absorbent surface (thick, soft paper) and press down until the fecal mass covers an area of 20 to 25 mm in diameter.

3. Let stand for 1 hour at room temperature for clearing of the fecal specimen and examine immediately. NOTE: Overclearing may cause collapsing and loss of hookworm ova.

STANDARD SMEAR EGG COUNT

This technique involves using a light meter or photoelectric footcandle meter in preparing a fecal smear of known standard density.

1. A block about 15 mm thick, 2 to 3 inches long with a central hole 16 mm in diameter (inner surface may be coated with ink to reduce light reflection) is placed over the light meter window to produce a uniform light area.
2. Calibration or standardization is done using barium sulfate suspension as standards.
   a. 2 N Na_2SO_4 and 1 N $BaCl_2$ solutions are prepared.
   b. To each is added glycerin (2 salt : 1 glycerin). The desired concentration standard is prepared by mixing the salt-glycerin solutions in varying proportions. The most commonly used are:
      (1) One part $BaCl_2$: 3 parts Na_2SO_4, which gives a suspension for standardizing smears containing feces in the amount of 1 part per 500 ml (2 mg).
      (2) One part $BaCl_2$: 6 parts Na_2SO_4, which gives a suspension for standardizing smears containing feces in the amount of 1/1,000 ml (1 mg).
   c. The light is adjusted to a predetermined reading on the scale (for example, 200 footcandles).
   d. A clean 3 × 1 slide over the block opening covers the light meter window.
   e. With medicine dropper, place drop of standard desired on the slide and over the opening carefully spreading the suspension to *exactly* fit the opening.
   f. Read the scale.
   g. Subsequent fecal suspensions are prepared with distilled water to a density to give the same light meter reading as the standard. In preparing the fecal smear, spread the film to *exactly* fill the opening in the block. After the adjustment to light intensity is made, the slide is removed, coverslipped, and the egg count is made.
   h. To obtain eggs-per gram count, multiply the number of eggs by 1,000 if a 1 mg preparation is used or by 500 if a 2 mg preparation is used. If no eggs are found in the 2 mg preparation, report "less than 500 eggs per gram." A 3 mg or heavier sample is too thick to count eggs accurately.

Techniques for examining muscle biopsy specimen for *Trichinella spiralis*
COMPRESSION TECHNIQUE

Cut very thin slices from tissue specimen and press between two slides. Examine microscopically with low power using a drop of eosin. Light infections, however, may be missed, even after several examinations.

DIGESTION TECHNIQUE

This method should follow the compression technique if it is negative. It recovers living larvae only, however. Likewise, immature larvae as well as old calcified cysts of long standing may be destroyed.
1. Place 1 gm finely ground tissue in 20 ml digestive juice (5 gm pepsin dissolved in 1,000 ml distilled H_2O with 7 ml concentrated HCl added).
2. Incubate at $37°$ C for 18 hours or longer, stirring mixture thoroughly at half-hour intervals.
3. Add 2 to 3 volumes of H_2O heated to $37°$ to $45°$ C.
4. Pour diluted digestate into Baerman funnel, adding enough warm water to cover screen (80 mesh). Let stand 1 hour or longer to allow larvae to pass down into neck of funnel.
5. Draw off a few milliliters from neck of funnel and examine microscopically for living larvae.
6. If negative, centrifuge contents of funnel at 2,000 rpm (500 g) for 1 to 2 minutes and examine sediment for larvae.

Recovery of helminths from feces

Small worms, proglottids, and scolices may be recovered by slowly straining a well comminuted specimen of feces in water through a wire sieve. A small mesh sieve (30 to 50 mesh) is most useful. Each portion of sediment on the sieve, after being washed with running water, is carefully examined with a hand lens. Placing the strained sediment in a shallow pan with black surface is an effective way to get contrast. An applicator stick or camel's hair brush can be used to pick up the organisms.

Harada-Mori test tube culture method (modified)

1. Cut strips of filter paper about 1 inch wide (or less) and 7 inches long.
2. Smear about 0.5 gm feces (not refrigerated; about size of small pea) over one half to two thirds the length of each strip of filter paper.
3. Place each strip into a large tube containing about 3 ml of water. The lower edge of the filter paper should be in the water.
4. Cork-stopper or cotton-plug each tube and keep at room temperature (24 to $28°$ C) for 3 to 7 days. Add water if evaporation takes place.
5. Examine a drop of water after 3 days for *Strongyloides* larvae and after 5 to 7 days for hookworm larvae; also other nematode larvae.

Cultivation of intestinal protozoa
MODIFIED BOECK AND DRBOHLAV'S MEDIUM

This medium consists of solid egg base with an overlay of Locke's solution. It supports growth of most intestinal protozoa and maintains them satisfactorily. It is especially good for *Entamoeba histolytica*.

Locke's solution

Sodium chloride	8.0 gm
Calcium chloride	0.2 gm
Potassium chloride	0.2 gm
Magnesium chloride	0.01 gm
Sodium phosphate (Na_2HPO_4)	2.0 gm
Sodium bicarbonate	0.4 gm
Potassium phosphate (KH_2PO_4)	0.3 gm
Distilled water	1,000.0 ml

Add chemicals to distilled water in order given. Thoroughly dissolve, then heat 20 minutes in Arnold sterilizer at $100°$ C. Cool to room temperature and filter out precipitate. Sterilize in autoclave at 15 pounds pressure for 15 minutes, allowing temperature to reach $121.6°$ C.

Rice starch

Place about 203 gm rice starch in stoppered test tube and sterilize in dry oven at $90°$ C for 4 hours. Repeat process the next 2 days.

Procedure
1. Add 75 ml Locke's solution to 270 ml whole egg (whites and yolks beaten) and mix well with blender or egg beater.
2. Filter through one layer of surgical gauze.
3. Place filtrate under vacuum to remove all small air bubbles.
4. Dispense about 4.5 ml into 150 mm test tubes.
5. Inspissate in a slanted position in the autoclave. Close all exhaust valves and immediately run the pressure up to 15 pounds. (This procedure will entrap all air in the chamber that is necessary for proper inspissation.) Hold at 15 pounds pressure for 45 minutes and do not allow temperature to exceed $95°$ C.
6. Let pressure return to zero immediately.
7. Let slants cool to room temperature and refrigerate overnight.
8. Overlay slant with Locke's solution to desired level (about 6 ml).
9. Autoclave at 15 pounds pressure for 15 minutes with exhaust valves regulated to attain $121.6°$ C temperature.
10. Allow pressure to drop gradually.
11. Add about 30 mg sterile rice starch to each tube before use.

EGG YOLK INFUSION MEDIUM

This is an all liquid egg yolk infusion medium to which liver has been added. It is good for most intestinal protozoa. Also it can be stored for several months without deterioration. The following solutions are prepared:

Liver extract solution

Wilson's dry extract of liver (powder)	5 gm
Distilled water	1,000 ml

Heat mixture to boiling, filter, and autoclave at 15 pounds (121° C) for 20 minutes.

Buffer solution

1. Dibasic phosphate solution

K_2HPO_4	87.09 gm
Distilled water to make	500.0 ml

Dissolve K_2HPO_4 in water in 500 ml volumetric flask and add water to 500 ml mark. Store in glass-stoppered bottle.

2. Dihydrogen phosphate solution

KH_2PO_4	13.61 gm
Distilled water to make	1,000.0 ml

Dissolve KH_2PO_4 in water in 100 ml volumetric flask and add water to 100 ml mark. Store in glass-stoppered bottle.

Mix stock buffers (4.3 parts K_2HPO_4 + 0.7 parts KH_2PO_4) and dilute 1:14 with distilled water to obtain a M/15 solution.

Preparation of medium

1. Mix crumbled yolks of 4 hard-boiled eggs with 125 ml of 0.85% NaCl. Use rotary beater, blender, etc.
2. Heat mixture in top part of covered double boiler for 20 minutes after it reaches 80° C.
3. Add 20 ml distilled H_2O to compensate for evaporation.
4. Filter through Bücher funnel under reduced pressure using several layers of no. 2 Whatman filter paper or equivalent.
5. Add 0.85% NaCl to filtrate to bring volume back to 125 ml.
6. Autoclave filtrate at 15 pounds pressure for 20 minutes.
7. Cool to below 10° C and refilter out yellowish sediment through Büchner funnel.
8. Add equal volume of M/15 buffer solution to filtrate to complete yolk infusion.
9. Add 1 part liver extract to 9 parts yolk infusion.
10. Autoclave at 15 pounds pressure for 20 minutes.
11. Tube immediately in 7 to 10 ml amounts and refrigerate, or refrigerate bulk for tubing later.

LIVER INFUSION AGAR

This medium consists of a solid liver infusion agar slant with an overlay of physiological saline and fresh horse serum. It is said to give better results with *Entamoeba histolytica* than with other protozoa.

Serum saline solution (overlay)

Fresh horse serum	1 part
0.85% NaCl in distilled water	6 parts
Sterilize by filtration	

Agar solution

Dehydrated liver infusion agar (Difco)	30 gm

Disodium phosphate (Na_2HPO_4)	3 gm
Distilled water	1,000 ml

Preparation

1. Dispense agar solution into tubes to give a slant of 4 to 5 cm long without a butt.
2. Sterilize at 15 pounds pressure for 20 minutes.
3. Add overlay to slants and refrigerate until used.

CHARCOAL MEDIUM

This medium may be either diphasic (agar slant + buffered saline) or all liquid. Both are equally good for protozoa but the liquid medium is easier to prepare. Both are particularly good for isolating and maintaining *Entamoeba hartmanni* and *Dientamoeba fragilis*.

Charcoal agar slant diphasic medium

1. Solution A (M/15 KH_2PO_4)

KH_2PO_4	9.07 gm
Distilled water to make	1,000.0 ml

Store in glass-stoppered bottle.

2. Solution B (M/15 Na_2HPO_4)

Na_2HPO_4	9.46 gm
Distilled water to make	1,000.0 ml

NOTE: $Na_2HPO_4 \cdot 12H_2O$ may be substituted for anhydrous Na_2HPO_4 by using 23.88 gm per liter of solution.

3. Buffered saline overlay (0.5%, pH 7.4)

NaCl	5.0 gm
Solution A	190.0 ml
Solution B	810.0 ml

Combine Solutions A and B and add NaCl. Autoclave at 15 pounds pressure for 15 minutes. Store in refrigerator.

4. Agar slants preparation

$Na_2HPO_4 \cdot 12H_2O$	3.0 gm
KH_2PO_4	4.0 gm
Sodium citrate crystals	1.0 gm
Magnesium sulfate crystals	0.1 gm
Ferric ammonium citrate	0.1 gm
Bacto-asparagine (Difco)	2.0 gm
Bacto-tryptone (Difco)	5.0 gm
Glycerin (reagent grade)	10.0 ml
Distilled water	1,000.0 ml

Add ingredients in order listed to the water. Heat to dissolve but do not boil. Stir thoroughly, add following, stirring thoroughly after each addition:

Bacto-agar (Difco)	10.0 gm
Norite A (Charcoal)*	1.0 gm
Cholesterol in acetone 1% solution†	25.0 ml
(0.25 gm cholesterol in 25 ml acetone)	

NOTE: Keep flask away from flames when adding cholesterol-acetone.

---

*From Pfanstiehl Laboratories, Inc., 1219 Glen Rock Ave., Waukegan, Ill. 60085.

†Cholesterol, C. P., ash-free for Kline test. From Pfanstiehl Laboratories.

a. Heat the entire mixture to boiling to dissolve agar.
b. Stir frequently to keep charcoal in solution.
c. Dispense hot solution in 3.0 ml amounts into tubes and plug.
d. Autoclave at 15 pounds pressure for 15 minutes.
e. Resuspend charcoal and cool in slanted position to form short butts or no butts.
f. Add 3.0 ml sterile 0.5% buffered saline overlay to slants.
g. Check for sterility by placing in incubator overnight; then refrigerate.

Charcoal agar liquid medium

Prepare as for diphasic medium except *omit agar* and *substitute* 10 ml distilled H_2O. Bring to boil and add 1 liter of buffered 0.5% saline. Dispense in 6.0 ml amounts into tubes and autoclave at 15 pounds pressure for 15 minutes. Check for sterility by incubating overnight, then refrigerate.

NOTE: When only occasional culturing is desired, it is usually more economical and practical to purchase commercial dehydrated media. The following are available:

Bacto *Entamoeba* Medium, from Difco Laboratories, Detroit, Michigan 48232.

Charcoal Agar Modified, from BBL, Cockeysville, Maryland 21030.

Charcoal or sand culturing of helminth larvae

When either hookworms or *Strongyloides* rhabditiform larvae may be present, culturing of the feces will produce filariform larvae that can readily be identified. Hookworm culturing takes 5 to 6 days, whereas *Strongyloides* filariform larvae require only 2 to 3 days.

1. Mix large portion of feces with equal amount of finely granular wood, bone charcoal (*not powdered charcoal*) or sterilized sand.
2. Add enough water to moisten only. Place contents on filter paper or equivalent and keep moist but not too wet.
3. Keep at room temperature and examine with hand lens after 2 days (3 to 7 days). Active larvae can be readily detected. Examine small portion microscopically.
4. Recover larvae by Baerman apparatus.
   Simplified Baerman apparatus: Fill large funnel in ringstand with short rubber tubing and pinch clamp attached to neck end with warm tap water (37° C). Place culture on muslin-covered screen on top of funnel allowing water in funnel to maintain contact with culture. Let stand 30 minutes to 1 hour and then draw off a few milliliters of water from neck end into beaker. Examine microscopically.

NOTE: If soil contamination of specimen has occurred,

0.3 ml of concentrated HCl per 10 ml of tap water will kill free-living nematodes in funnel if present.

REFERENCES

Baermann, G. 1917. Eine einfache Methode Zur Auffindung von Ankylostomum-(Nematoden)—Larven in Erdproben. Meded. Geneesk. Laborat. Weltever. Feestbundel, p. 41.

Balamuth, W. 1946. Improved egg yolk infusion for cultivation of *Entamoeba histolytica* and other intestinal protozoa. Am. J. Clin. Pathol. **16**:380.

Beaver, P. C. 1949. Quantitative hookworm diagnosis by direct smear. J. Parasitol. **35**:125-135.

Beaver, P. C. 1950. The standardization of fecal smears for estimating egg production and worm burden. J. Parasitol. **36**:451-455.

Boeck, W. C., and J. Drbohlav. 1925. The cultivation of *Endamoeba histolytica*. Am. J. Hyg. **5**:371-407.

Brooke, M. M., A. W. Donaldson, and R. B. Mitchell. 1949. A method of supplying cellulose tape to physicians for diagnosis of enterobiasis. Public Health Rep. **64**:897-901.

Brooke, M. M., and M. Goldman. 1949. Polyvinyl alcohol-fixative as a preservative and adhesive for protozoa in dysenteric stools and other liquid materials. J. Lab. Clin. Med. **34**:1554-1560.

Burrows, R. B. 1969. Other surface active agents for use with the PAF sedimentation technic for intestinal parasites. Am. J. Clin. Pathol. **5**:155-156.

Cleveland, L. R., and J. Collier. 1930. Various improvements in the cultivation of *Entamoeba histolytica*. Am. J. Hyg. **12**:606-613.

Faust, E. C., and others. 1938. A critical study of clinical laboratory technics for the diagnosis of protozoan cysts and helminth eggs in feces. Am. J. Trop. Med. **18**:169-183.

Feinberg, J. G., and M. J. Whittington. 1957. A culture medium for *Trichomonas vaginalis* Donne and species of *Candida*. J. Clin. Pathol. **10**:327-329.

Garcia, L. S., and L. R. Ash. 1979. Diagnostic parasitology: clinical laboratory manual. Ed. 2. The C. V. Mosby Co. St. Louis.

Gleason, N. N., and G. R. Healy. 1965. Modification and evaluation of Kohn's one-step staining technic for intestinal protozoa in feces or tissue. Am. J. Clin. Pathol. **43**:494-496.

Graham, C. F. 1941. A device for the diagnosis of *Enterobius vermicularis*. Am. J. Trop. Med. **21**:159-161.

Harper, K., M. D. Little, and S. R. Damon. 1957. Advantages of the PVA-fixative two-bottle stool collection technic in the detection and identification of intestinal parasites. Pub. Health Lab. **15**:96.

Juniper, K., Jr., V. W. Steele, and C. L. Chester. 1958. Rectal biopsy in the diagnosis of amebic colitis. South. Med. J. **51**:545.

Kohn, J. 1960. A one stage permanent staining method

for fecal protozoa. Dapim. Refuiim Med. Q. Israel **19:**160-161.

Komiya, Y., and A. Kobayashi. 1966. Evaluation of Kato's thick smear technic with a cellophane cover for helminth eggs in feces. Jap. J. Parasitol. (English) **19:**59-64.

Kupferberg, A. B., G. Johnston, and H. Sprince. 1948. Nutritional requirements of *Trichomonas vaginalis.* Proc. Soc. Exp. Biol. Med. **67:**304-308.

Markey, R. L. 1950. A vaseline swab for the diagnosis of *Enterobius* eggs. Am. J. Clin. Pathol. **20:**493.

Martin, L. K., and P. C. Beaver. 1968. Evaluation of Kato thick-smear technique for quantitative diagnosis of helminth infections. Am. J. Trop. Med. Hyg. **17:**382-391.

McQuay, R. M. 1956. Charcoal medium for growth and maintenance of large and small races of *Entamoeba histolytica.* Am. J. Clin. Pathol. **26:**1137-1141.

Melvin, D. H., and M. M. Brooke. 1974. Laboratory procedures for the diagnosis of intestinal parasites. Center for Disease Control. Department of Health, Education, and Welfare. Publication no. 75-8282. Atlanta, Georgia.

Nair, C. P. 1953. Rapid staining of intestinal amoebae on wet mounts. Nature **172:**1051.

Nelson, E. C. 1947. Alcoholic extract medium for the diagnosis and cultivation of *Entamoeba histolytica.* Am. J. Trop. Med. **27:**525.

Norman, L., and M. M. Brooke. 1955. The use of penicillin and streptomycin in the routine cultivation of amebae from fecal specimens. Am. J. Trop. Med. Hyg. **4:**479-482.

Ottolina, C., and M. H. Atencio. 1943. Nuevos caminos para el diagnostico clínico preciso de la schistosomiasis mansoni. Rev. Policlín. Caracas **12:**348-380.

Ritchie, L. S. 1948. An ether sedimentation technique for routine stool examinations. Bull. U.S. Army Med. Dept. **8:**326.

Ritchie, L. S., and others. 1960. The possible effects of pH and specific gravity on the ether-sedimentation procedure in concentrating eggs and cysts. Am. J. Trop. Med. Hyg. **9:**444-449.

Ruff, M. D., W. S. Gallion, and J. S. Werner. 1970. Two technics for permanent staining for formalin-fixed protozoan cysts. Am. J. Clin. Pathol. **54:**864-867.

Sapero, J. J., and D. K. Lawless. 1953. The "MIF" stain-preservation technique for the identification of intestinal protozoa. Am. J. Trop. Med. Hyg. **2:**613-619.

Scholten, T. 1972. An improved technique for the recovery of intestinal protozoa. J. Parasitol. **58:**633-634.

Thompkins, V. N., and J. K. Miller. 1947. Staining intestinal protozoa with iron-hematoxylin-phosphotungstic acid. Am. J. Clin. Pathol. **17:**755-757.

Vinayak, V. K., B. N. Tandon, and O. Prakash. 1967. A comparative evaluation of formol-ether, zinc sulfate, and magnesium sulfate concentration techniques for diagnosis of helminthic ova and protozoal cysts. Indian J. Med. Res. **55:**134-138.

Weller, T. H., and G. J. Dammin. 1945. An improved method of examination of feces for diagnosis of intestinal schistosomiasis. Am. J. Clin. Pathol. **15:**496-500.

Wheatley, W. B. 1951. A rapid staining procedure for intestinal amoebae and flagellates. Am. J. Clin. Pathol. **21:**990-991.

Willis, H. H. 1921. A simple levitation method for the detection of hookworm ova. Med. J. Aust. **8:**375-376.

Solutions, stains, and procedures used in study of blood, tissue, and atrial parasites

MALARIA
Giemsa stain

Giemsa stain is the most common stain used in the study of the malaria parasite.

THICK SMEAR

1. Dip the smear for 1 second in methylene blue phosphate solution given below:

Methylene blue, medicinal	1 gm
Na_2HPO_4, anhydrous	3 gm
KH_2PO_4	1 gm

Mix well and dissolve in 250 to 300 ml of distilled water.

2. Rinse several times in buffered water:

Na_2HPO_4, anhydrous	6 gm
KH_2PO_4	5 gm

Mix well and dissolve in 1,000 ml of distilled water.

3. Place slide upside down on curved plate and flood underneath with dilute Giemsa (1 drop stain with 1 ml buffer)

Giemsa powder (certified)	0.75 gm
Methyl alcohol (pure)	35 ml
Glycerin (pure)	35 ml

4. Stain for 6 to 10 minutes.
5. Rinse in buffer, dry, and examine.

THIN SMEAR

Thin smear must be fixed in methyl alcohol before staining with Giemsa.

Wright's stain

This stain is used in hematology and may be used to stain thin and thick smears for malaria parasites.

THIN SMEAR

Since Wright's stain is not diluted when first applied, the methyl alcohol present will fix the blood film.

1. Cover the blood film with Wright's stain for about 1 minute (time varies with different batches of stain).
2. Dilute with buffered water (pH 6.8) and allow to stain for about 4 minutes (time varies with different batches of stain).
3. Float off the metallic scum with tap water; dry, and examine.

THICK SMEAR

It is necessary to dehemoglobinize the smear before staining, since Wright's stain will fix the red blood cells.

1. Dehemoglobinize the thick smear as for Giemsa stain.
2. Stain with Wright's stain as for thin smear.

Triton X-100 in Giemsa staining of blood parasites

Triton X-100, a surface-active agent, enhances the staining properties of Giemsa stain and eliminates the transfer of malaria parasites during mass staining. This method is recommended for routine staining of blood parasites, particularly malaria, trypanosomes, *Toxoplasma*, and microfilariae.

SOLUTIONS

Triton stock solution

A 10% aqueous solution is prepared and will keep indefinitely if tightly stoppered.

Stock buffers

1. Alkaline buffer: Na_2HPO_4, M/15 solution

Na_2HPO_4, anhydrous	9.5 gm
Distilled water to make	1,000.0 ml

Dissolve salt in a little water in a 1 liter volumetric flask and then add water to 1 liter mark.

2. Acid buffer: NaH_2PO_4, M/15 solution

$NaH_2PO_4 \cdot H_2O$	9.2 gm
Distilled water to make	1,000.0 ml

Prepare as for alkaline buffer, using 1 liter volumetric flask.

3. Potassium acid phosphate may be substituted for the sodium acid phosphate.

KH₂PO₄	9.07 gm
Distilled water to make	1,000.0 ml

Prepare as for alkaline buffer.

Buffered water (pH 7.0 to 7.2)

Acid buffer (NaH₂PO₄, M/15 solution	39 ml
Alkaline buffer (Na₂HPO₄, M/15 solution)	61 ml
Distilled water	900 ml

The pH *must* be in the range of 7.0 to 7.2 for satisfactory staining results. Use of an electric pH meter allows addition of Triton before determining pH whereas colorimetric standards do not.

Triton-buffered water solutions

1. For thin blood films or combination blood films, add 1 ml of stock 10% Triton solution to 1,000 ml buffered water. Concentration of Triton = 0.01%.
2. For thick blood films and tissue and exudate smears, add 10 ml of stock 10% Triton solution to 1,000 ml buffered water. Concentration of Triton = 0.1%.

Buffered water and Triton-buffered water should be fresh for best results. Check pH of buffered water that is several days old.

STAINING TECHNIQUE

Thin blood films only

1. Fix in absolute methyl alcohol 30 seconds.
2. Stain

1:50 Triton-Giemsa	45 min
(1 ml stock Giemsa to 50 ml buffered water containing 0.01% Triton X-100)	
or	
1:20 Triton-Giemsa	20 min
(1 ml stock Giemsa to 20 ml buffered water containing 0.1% Triton X-100)	

3. Wash briefly in 0.01% Triton-buffered water.
4. Let dry and examine microscopically.

Thick blood films only

1. Stain in 1:50 Triton-Giemsa   45 min
   (Use 0.1% Triton-buffered water to prepare stain.)
2. Wash for 3 to 5 minutes or longer in 0.1% Triton-buffered water.
3. Dry and examine.

Combination thick and thin film

Fix thin film first in methyl alcohol then proceed as for staining thin film only. Wash thick film portion a little longer.

Tissues and exudate smears

1. Fix in methyl alcohol   30 sec
2. Stain in 1:40 Triton-Giemsa   50 min
   (1 ml stock Giemsa to 40 buffered water containing 0.1% Triton X-100)

3. Wash in 0.1% Triton-buffered water   5 to 10 min
4. Dry and examine.

Field's rapid staining for thick blood films

SOLUTION A

Methylene blue	0.8 gm
Azure B (American stains)*	0.5 gm
Disodium phosphate (anhydrous)	5.0 gm
Potassium phosphate, monobasic (anhydrous)	6.25 gm
Distilled water	500.0 ml

SOLUTION B

Eosin	1.0 gm
Disodium phosphate (anhydrous)	5.0 gm
Potassium phosphate, monobasic (anhydrous)	6.25 gm
Distilled water	500.0 ml

Dissolve the phosphate salts before adding dyes. Azure B (granular) can be aided in dissolving by grinding in mortar with a little phosphate solution. Set solutions aside for 24 hours, then filter and use. Solutions will last many weeks without deterioration, but when solution B becomes greenish from carryover of methylene blue, discard.

STAINING TECHNIQUE

1. Dip slide in solution A 1 second.
2. Rinse film gently in clean water until stain ceases to flow from film and glass slide is free of stain.
3. Dip slide in solution B 1 second.
4. Rinse again in clean water for 2 to 3 seconds.
5. Drain, dry, and examine microscopically.

Staining reaction is similar to Giemsa.

CULTIVATION OF TRYPANOSOMES AND LEISHMANIAS

Cultures are prepared from blood, fluids, and tissue. When blood is used, 5 to 10 ml should be concentrated by fractional centrifugation using the leukocyte layer for the inoculum. Spinal fluid should be concentrated usually by centrifugation for obtaining the inoculum. Thick aspirates and solid tissue should be triturated with sterile saline prior to inoculation. Best results are obtained when cultures are maintained at 22° to 25° C. Hold all cultures at least 1 month and examine at 1, 2, and 4 week intervals by wet mounts and/or stained slides.

Offutt's medium

This medium is simple to prepare and is effective for maintaining all leishmanias, *T. cruzi*, *T. rangeli*,

---

*The German equivalent of Azur B is Azur I. If neither is available, using only methylene blue will give a satisfactory solution A.

and *T. lewisi* on 14 day transfers. Use of antibiotics increases its effectiveness. Freshly prepared slants are recommended for use.

1. Melt a flask of Bacto blood-agar base (40 gm in 1,000 ml cold distilled water) by boiling and cool to 45° to 50° C.
2. Add aseptically 10 to 20 ml fresh, sterile defibrinated blood.
3. Tube in 4 to 5 ml amounts in sterile test tube.
4. Solidify in short slants with deep butt.
5. Add 0.5 to 1 ml sterile Locke's solution or saline per tube.
6. Incubate for 24 hours at 37° C for sterility.
7. Before inoculating add 250 to 500 units penicillin and streptomycin.
8. Use rubber stoppers or screw caps to prevent evaporation.

Novy-McNeal-Nicolle (NNN) medium
MATERIALS

Bacto-agar	14 gm
NaCl	6 gm
H₂O distilled	900 ml
NaOH	0.1 N solution
Rabbit or guinea pig defibrinated blood	10 ml

PROCEDURE

1. Add the agar and NaCl to the water; bring to a boil; and neutralize with 0.1 N NaOH using litmus paper as in indicator.
2. Sterilize in autoclave for one-half hour at 12 pounds pressure. Remove and store in refrigerator.
3. For use, melt and add 10 ml defibrinated blood, mixing thoroughly.
4. Pipette into test tubes and prepare long slants. Test for sterility by incubating at 37° C for 24 hours.
5. Inoculate and culture at room temperature.

Kelser's medium

This medium was developed especially for *T. cruzi*.

MATERIALS

Bacto-beef	25.0 gm
Bacto-peptone	12.5 gm
NaCl	3.5 gm
Bacto-agar (granular)	5.0 gm
H₂O distilled	500.0 ml
NaOH	0.1 N solution
Dextrose (1% solution)	10.0 ml
Rabbit or guinea pig defibrinated blood	10.0 ml

PROCEDURE

1. Add Bacto-beef extract to water; place in water bath (55° C) for 1 hour.
2. Add Bacto-peptone and NaCl; bring water bath to

boiling point. Let stand 5 minutes, shaking several times to facilitate solution.
3. Filter twice through a thickness of absorbent cotton.
4. Neutralize with 0.1 N NaOH, using litmus paper indicator.
5. Place in boiling water bath, add Bacto-agar. Dissolve.
6. Autoclave at 12 pounds pressure for one-half hour. Store in refrigerator for use.
7. Melt in boiling water bath. Lower temperature to range of 50° to 55° C.
8. Add dextrose and defibrinated blood in a sterile fashion.
9. Pipette into test tubes and slant.
10. Paraffin the plugs; place *immediately* in refrigerator for 12 hours to obtain maximum condensation on slants.
11. Incubate at 37.5° C for 12 to 24 hours to test for sterility before use.

Weinman's medium for African trypanosomes
PREPARATION

1. Add 31 gm Difco nutrient agar and 5 gm plain agar to 1,000 ml distilled water. Heat to boiling; dissolve; cool to 45° C, and adjust pH to 7.3. Autoclave, store in refrigerator.
2. Centrifuge citrated human blood. Remove plasma and inactivate at 56° C for 30 minutes.
3. Wash RBC in sterile saline by suspension and centrifugation.
4. Melt agar base and cool to 45° C. Mix equal volumes of prewarmed inactivated plasma and washed RBC.
5. Add 1 part plasma-RBC mixture to 3 parts agar base; mix and dispense in 5 ml amounts into tubes; allow to harden in slants for several days at room temperature or overnight in refrigerator.
6. Incubate at 37° C overnight to check sterility.
7. Store in refrigerator for use. Weinman's medium is stable for at least 6 months.

USE

1. Inoculate 0.1 ml of blood onto slants or add 0.1 ml polyvinyl sulfuric acid (PVSA) to each milliliter of blood and promptly inoculate 2.0 ml of mixture to each slant. (PVSA, an anticoagulant, also inactivates complement and prevents inhibition of growth of trypanosomes.)
2. Add 0.5 mg of dihydrostreptomycin sulfate per ml of blood, or 2,000 units of penicillin per ml of blood.
3. Tilt inoculum over slant and incubate in dark at room temperature.
4. To examine: irrigate slant surface with an overlay fluid to wash down cultures. Remove drop and examine microscopically.

NOTE: Cultures rarely positive before 5 days or after 30 days.

Beemer's stain for cultural forms of hemoflagellates

This is a rapid method for effecting a temporary stain of the cultural forms of hemoflagellates. It is not as satisfactory as permanent stains.

Sodium citrate	1.1 gm
Sodium chloride	0.65 gm
Mercuric chloride (saturated aqueous solution)	0.10 ml
Brilliant cresyl blue	0.05 gm
Methylene blue	0.04 gm
Distilled water	100.0 ml

Dissolve the various components in water in the order listed. Add a drop of stain to 1 to 2 drops of culture fluid and examine microscopically. The nucleus and flagellum stain dark blue, whereas the cytoplasm stains a lighter blue.

SEROLOGIC DIAGNOSIS OF VISCERAL LEISHMANIASIS

The difficulty in obtaining organisms from patients with visceral leishmaniasis (sometimes contraindicated) supports the use of serologic methods even though the latter are nonspecific tests. Two serologic tests of value for the diagnosis of kala-azar are given. Both tests indicate an increase in the euglobulin fraction of the serum.

Napier's aldehyde test or formol-gel test

1. To 1 ml of patient's serum in small test tube, add 1 drop of commercial formalin.
2. Shake well and let stand at room temperature.

If serum becomes solid and opaque in 3 to 30 minutes, it is diagnostic of kala-azar (*L. donovani*). A delayed reaction (2 to 24 hours) is suggestive but needs confirmation. Solidification without opalescence is not diagnostic.

Chopra's antimony test

1. Place 1 ml of patient's serum (diluted 1:10 with distilled water) in a small test tube.
2. Add slowly, by capillary pipette, an equal amount of a 4% aqueous solution of urea stibamine.
3. In kala-azar a coarse flocculent precipitate forms as the serum and antimony derivative mix.

DIAGNOSIS OF BLOOD AND TISSUE PROTOZOA BY ANIMAL INOCULATION

Animal inoculation is of value in the diagnosis of suspected hemoflagellate infections and toxoplasmosis. When initial animal inoculations are negative, blind passage (subinoculation) of blood or tissue to other animals may prove successful.

Procedures

TRYPANOSOMES

Blood, lymph node aspirates, or spinal fluid are inoculated intraperitoneally into appropriate animal. Up to 2 ml may be used. Organisms may be found in the animal's blood within 1 week. If negative, examine at the end of 2 weeks and 4 weeks. Parasitemia fluctuates, and therefore smears should be made successively. Animals used:

T. b. gambiense and *T. b. rhodesiense*	Guinea pigs, white rats
T. cruzi	Guinea pigs, white mice, white rats

LEISHMANIAS

Blood, tissue, and lesion aspirates and tissue biopsy specimens, depending on the species suspected, are inoculated intraperitoneally into the hamster. Thick aspirates and biopsied tissue should be triturated with sterile saline before use. The inoculum varies from 0.5 to 1.0 ml of heavy material. The leukocyte layer of concentrated blood is used. Hamsters develop a generalized systemic infection regardless of the species. The organism can usually be demonstrated by stained spleen impressions. Wait at least 4 to 6 weeks. Animals eventually die, usually within 3 to 5 months. Animals used:

Leishmania sp	Hamsters

TOXOPLASMA

Blood, lymph gland fluid, and spinal fluid are used as inocula. Concentrated specimens are recommended. About 0.5 ml is inoculated intraperitoneally or intracerebrally. Animals are examined for ascites and general illness. Within a few days peritoneal fluid of the mouse is examined. Dab smears of the brain should be stained and examined. Blind passage of peritoneal fluid or triturated brain tissue into other mice is recommended if first mice are negatives. Animal used: White mice.

EXAMINATION OF BLOOD FOR MICROFILARIAE
Wet mount

A simple technique for demonstrating microfilariae in peripheral blood is to place a drop of whole blood on a clean slide, coverslip it, and examine microscopically for the typical thrashing movement among the red cells.

A variation is to add distilled water to whole blood in a test tube; allow to stand a few minutes to lake the RBC, then examine the sediment for active microfilariae.

CONCENTRATION PROCEDURES

Heparin method
1. Pipette 2 ml methyl alcohol into test tube. Add 10 mg heparin. Let dissolve. Evaporate alcohol by heat.
2. Add 5 ml blood to heparinized tube and mix.
3. Centrifuge at 1,000 rpm for 10 minutes.
4. Draw off "buffy coat" (middle layer of leukocyte

layer) with capillary pipette. Examine microscopically on slide under coverslip.

5. Remove some red cell sediment from bottom of tube and examine microscopically.

6. Above slides can also be dried and stained with Giemsa.

Knott's technique

1. Mix 1 ml blood with 10 ml of 2% formalin.
2. Centrifuge at 1,500 rpm for 5 minutes.
3. Pour off supernatant and transfer some sediment to a slide. Dry and stain with Giemsa.

Saponin method

The hemolysis of blood with saponin solution has not only the advantage of concentrating microfilariae in a small amount of sediment as in the Knott technique, but also the additional benefit of revealing microfilariae in an actively motile condition. The ratio of saponin to blood should not exceed much beyond 0.02 gm per 1 ml blood, if the microfilariae are to remain alive.

1. Add 1 ml blood by venipuncture to 10 ml of 0.2% saponin in physiologic saline and centrifuge at 1,500 rpm for 10 minutes.
2. Pour off supernatant and examine sediment microscopically for living microfilariae.

Plastic membrane filtration technique

Citrated blood mixed in a syringe containing physiological saline is passed through a Swinny adapter containing a commercially available membrane filter of 5 μm pore size. Several washings of saline or distilled water will remove cells and proteinaceous material, leaving the microfilariae on the filter, which can be examined microscopically for living organisms or dried, fixed, and stained as for a blood smear. Microfilariae of *Wuchereria bancrofti, Brugia malayi,* and *Loa loa* may be recovered in this manner. *Dipetalonema perstans* and *Mansonella ozzardi* microfilariae are much smaller and are not recoverable by this method.

STAINING OF MICROFILARIAE IN BLOOD

Staining reveals structures that make species identification relatively easy. Thick blood films as used for malaria are preferable to thin films because a relatively large sample of blood can be obtained. Although Giemsa stain, which is used for malarial parasites, can also be used for microfilariae, such stains as hematoxylin solutions are usually more suitable for revealing structural details.

Hematoxylin stains

BOHMER'S HEMATOXYLIN

Preparation

1. Solution A

Hematoxylin crystals	1 gm
Absolute alcohol	12 ml

2. Solution B

Alum	1 gm
Distilled water	240 ml

Solution A should be old and dark for best results. Add 2 to 3 drops of solution A to a watch glass full of solution B.

Procedure

1. Dehemoglobinize the thick film in tap water and air dry.
2. Cover with stain; heat gently until steaming occurs.
3. Rinse in distilled water.
4. Differentiate in 70% alcohol containing 2% HCl.
5. Rinse in dilute ammonia water (1:10,000) or wash thoroughly in running tap water.
6. Dehydrate in graded steps of alcohol.
7. Clear in xylol and mount in Permount or balsam.

HEMALUM

Preparation

Hematoxylin	1 gm
Water	1 liter

Dissolve, then add:

Sodium iodate (NaIO$_3$)	0.2 gm
Alum	50.0 gm

Dissolve and filter. Does not keep well. Adding 50 gm chloral hydrate and 1 gm citric (or acetic) acid will make it more stable.

Procedure

1. Dehemoglobinize dried smears in normal saline for 10 minutes.
2. Fix in 70% alcohol heated to 50° to 60° C for 15 minutes,

    or

    Gradually pass through 15%, 35%, 50%, 70%, 85%, and 95% alcohol. Allow to remain in each for 2 to 5 minutes.
3. Transfer to absolute alcohol for 10 minutes.
4. Pass backward through graded alcohols to water. If fixed in hot 70% alcohol, smears can be transferred directly to water.
5. Place slides in hemalum for 5 hours or overnight.
6. Destain in 70% alcohol containing 1% HCl for few seconds.
7. After desired differentiation, wash well in tap water.
8. Pass through graded alcohols, then clear in xylol.
9. Mount in Permount or balsam or leave unmounted.

DELAFIELD'S HEMATOXYLIN

Preparation

Hematoxylin crystals	4.0 gm
95% ethyl alcohol	25.0 ml

Mix the solution with 400 ml saturated solution of ammonium alum. Keep in loosely capped container in light, airy place for 2 weeks. Add mixture of:

Methyl alcohol (acetone free)   100 ml
Glycerin   100 ml

Bottle and expose to direct sunlight for a minimum of 1 month. Filter before use.

Procedure

1. Dehemoglobinize thick film in tap water and air dry.
2. Fix in equal parts ether and 95% alcohol for 10 minutes. Air dry.
3. Stain for 10 to 12 minutes.
4. Destain with acid water (0.5% to 0.1% HCl).
5. Wash in running water until blue color appears.
6. Mount in any neutral mounted medium or leave unmounted.

AZUR-EOSIN STAIN

Preparation

Azur II   0.1 gm
Normal saline   250.0 ml
  (Gives concentration of 1:2,500)
Eosin   0.1 gm
Normal saline   400.0 ml
  (Gives concentration of 1:4,000)

Keep stains separately in glass-stoppered bottles.

Procedure

1. Dehemoglobinize thoroughly dried thick film in normal saline for 10 minutes.
2. Place in 1:2,500 azur II–normal saline for 3 to 5 hours.
3. Differentiate and counterstain in 1:4,000 eosin–normal saline for about one-half hour.
4. Mount in eosin–saline solution under coverslip with edges sealed to prevent evaporation.
5. Correct degree of differentiation obtained from one half to 1 hour after slides are prepared.

This method is more difficult to perform but yields beautiful results in cytologic features of the microfilariae. The preparation is only temporary in nature.

METHYL GREEN-PRYONIN

Preparation

Methyl green (1% aqueous solution)   2 parts
Pyronin (1% aqueous solution)   1 part

Keep solution in separate glass-stoppered bottles. Mix before use.

Procedure

1. Dehemoglobinize dry smear in normal saline for 10 minutes.
2. Transfer directly to stain for 5 to 15 hours.
3. Quickly pass through graded alcohols:

70%	5 sec
85%	10 sec
95%	15 sec
100%	20 sec
100% (second change)	1 to 3 min
Xylol	5 min

4. Mount in Permount, balsam, or cedar oil ringed with balsam.

This technique is simple, definite, good, and lasts at least 1 year.

Commercial media

Dehydrated commercial media, more economical and certainly more practical when only occasional culturing is desired, can be obtained. The following are available:

Bacto *Entamoeba* Medium, from Difco Lab., Detroit, Michigan 48232.

Charcoal Agar Modified, from BBL, Cockeysville, Maryland 21030.

CULTURE MEDIA FOR *TRICHOMONAS VAGINALIS*
Feinber's medium

Panmede	12.5 gm
NaCl	3.3 gm
Dextrose	2.5 gm
Horse serum (inactivate at 57° C for 25 minutes)	40.0 ml
Distilled water	500.0 ml
Penicillin	500,000 units
Streptomycin	250,000 units

Adjust pH to 6.5 with NaOH. Filter through Seitz filter and dispense into small 100×13 mm screw-cap tubes about half full. Store in refrigerator. Incubate inoculated tubes at 37° C. Examine at 24 and 48 hours. If negative, examine again at 72 hours. Subculture at 48 hours if *Candida* growth is excessive.

Trypticase serum medium

Trypticase (BBL)	20.0 gm
Cystine monohydrochloride	1.5 gm
Maltose	1.0 gm
Bacto-agar (Difco)	1.0 gm
Distilled water	950.0 ml

Adjust pH to 6.0, heat to boiling in water bath until agar is completely dissolved, and filter while hot through porous Reeve-Angel filter paper no. 845. If desired, an indicator, 0.6 ml of 0.5% aqueous methylene blue, may be added. Cool to 45° C, adjust pH to 6.0 if required, and restore volume to 950 ml with distilled water. Cool and add 0.5 ml human serum sterilized by filtration to each tube. Refrigerate. At time of inoculation add 1,000 units penicillin and 500 units streptomycin per ml of medium. Incubate inoculated tubes at 37° C. Examine at 24 and 48 hours. If negative, examine again at 72 hours. Subculture at 48 hours if *Candida* growth is excessive.

REFERENCES

Beemer, A. M. 1947. Supravital staining of amoebae and some observations on laboratory diagnosis. S. Afr. Med. J. **21**:550-552.

Brooke, M. M., and A. W. Donaldson. 1948. Transfer of malarial parasites between blood films during mass staining procedures. Public Health Rep. 63:991-1004.

Brooke, M. M., and A. W. Donaldson. 1950. Use of a surface-active agent to prevent transfer of malarial parasites between blood films during mass staining procedures. J. Parasitol. 36:84.

Brooke, M. M., and A. J. Sulzer. 1955. Directions for performing Sabin-Feldman cytoplasm-modifying (methylene blue dye) test for toxoplasmosis. Public Health Lab. 13:136-147.

Chopra, R. N., J. C. Das Gupta, and J. C. David. 1927. The antimony test in the diagnosis of kala azar. Indian Med. Gas. 62:688-691.

Donaldson, A. W., and M. M. Brooke. 1950. Effects of various modifications of a mass staining procedure on the transfer of malarial parasites between blood films. J. Natl. Mal. Soc. 9:239-247.

Kershaw, W. E., B. O. L. Duke, and F. H. Budden. 1954. Distribution of microfilariae of *O. volvulus* in the skin. Br. Med. J. 2:724-729.

Mazzotti, L. 1951. Observations based on cutaneous biopsies in onchocerciasis. Am. J. Trop. Med. 31:624-627.

Melvin, D. M., and M. M. Brooke. 1955. Triton X-100 in Giemsa staining of blood parasites. Stain Technol. 30:269-275.

Nakamura, M. 1967. An autoclaved medium for routine cultivation of *Trypanosoma cruzi*. Trans R. Soc. Trop. Med. Hyg. 61:792-794.

Napier, L. E. 1921. Kala-azar. Indian Med. Gaz. 56:401-404.

Roger, F. C., and J. A. C. Brown. 1957. Assessment of the density of infection with onchocerciasis and the probable level of safety from its ocular complications. Trans. R. Soc. Trop. Med. Hyg. 51:271-282.

Russell, P. F., and others. 1965. Practical malariology. Ed. 2. Oxford University Press, London., 750 pp.

Shute, P. G., and M. E. Maryon. 1966. Laboratory technique for the study of malaria. Ed. 2. J. & A. Churchill Ltd., London.

Trigg, P. I. 1968. A new continuous perfusion technique for the cultivation of malaria parasites *in vitro*. Trans. R. Soc. Trop. Med. Hyg. 62:371-378.

Walker, A. J. 1963. Manual for the microscopic diagnosis of malaria. Ed. 2. Pan American Health Organization Scientific Publication no. 87. U.S. Government Printing Office, Washington, D.C.

Wilcox, A. 1960. Manual for the microscopic diagnosis of malaria in man. Public Health Service Publication no. 796, Washington, D.C.

Young, C. W., and H. Van Sant. 1923. *Leishmania donovani* in the peripheral blood. J. Exp. Med. 38:233.

APPENDIX C

Collection and preservation of arthropods

Because of the enormous numbers of species of arthropods, identification can best be accomplished by a specialist trained in a particular group. Usually the biology department of the nearest university can give help either with the specific identification or by directing you to a specialist.

MOSQUITOES

An aspirator is prepared consisting of a heavy glass tube about 18 inches long with a bore of about one-fourth inch. Over one end a piece of fine mesh cloth or netting is pasted so that one end of rubber tubing of any desired length can be slipped over it and held securely. The other end of the rubber tubing is placed in the mouth, and the glass tubing placed gently over the resting mosquito. A quick inhalation will draw the insect into the tube. A dozen or more can be picked up in this manner and quickly killed by gently blowing them into a killing bottle. Any small, delicate insect difficult to handle can be collected by this method. The killing bottle is prepared by placing a half inch of cut rubber bands or other rubber scraps in the bottom of a large shell vial or test tube saturated with chloroform and covered with a plug of crumpled paper or cotton. A circle of cardboard or stiff paper is placed on top of the cotton or crumpled paper. The vial is stoppered and ready for use.

Captured adults may be mounted on pins by conventional methods or preserved unmounted between layers of cleansing tissue in pill boxes or other containers.

Mosquito larvae and eggs can be removed from the surface of water by skimming with a dipper or spoon. Before mounting, larvae can be killed by dipping in hot (not boiling) water for 15 to 20 seconds. For storing, run through 50% alcohol, then into 70% alcohol.

Different media and techniques for mounting mosquito larvae as well as many other small arthropods on slides for microscopy are available.

Modified Berelese's medium

This all-purpose chloral-gum medium will serve to kill, fix, and preserve many specimens. No dehydration in alcohol is necessary.

Gum acacia	8 gm
Water (distilled)	8 ml
Glycerin	5 ml
Chloral hydrate	70 gm
Glacial acetic acid	3 ml

Polyvinyl alcohol–phenol–lactic acid medium

Clearing and dehydration in alcohols are also not necessary with this medium

Polyvinyl alcohol stock solution	56%
Phenol	22%
Lactic acid	22%

The stock solution is prepared by dissolving the powdered PVA in water until the solution becomes viscous, like thick molasses. On standing, clearing takes place. It can be hastened by placing the solution in a hot water bath.

Mounting

For specimens using xylol as a solvent, dehydration through 50%, 70%, and 95% alcohols is necessary. Clearing is done in clove oil, carbol-xylol (3 parts xylol to 1 part melted phenol crystals), or absolute alcohol followed by xylol. Specimens should remain 15 to 20 minutes in the various changes. Mounting in balsam or clarite will take several days for hardening of the medium, whereas in isobutyl methacrylate, drying is rapid and the slides can be used in a few hours. Ringing or sealing is not necessary.

MITES

For temporary mounts, cover with a drop of 50% alcohol and gently heat. Clearing and extension of the specimen occur, and details are discernible.

For permanent mounts, specimens can be prepared

335

directly from life by placing in a drop of chloral-gum medium (see below), covered and gently heated until bubbling begins, then set aside for use. Alcohol-preserved specimens must first be washed in distilled water or lactic acid to remove the alcohol.

The following modification of chloral-gum medium is recommended for mites:

Water (distilled)	35 ml
Chloral hydrate	30 gm
Gum arabic	20 gm
Glycerin	12 ml
Glucose syrup	3 ml

FLEAS

Specimens may be preserved in 70% alcohol or mounted on slides for identification by using the following procedure:

1. Drop living fleas or preserved specimens into 10% KOH and let remain for few days until cleared sufficiently.
2. Transfer to watch glass containing water with few drops HCl for 30 minutes.
3. Dehydrate through 50% alcohol for 30 minutes.
4. Dehydrate through 95% alcohol for 30 minutes.
5. Clear in beechwood creosote for 1 hour to run through several changes of absolute alcohol and clear in clove oil or xylol.
6. Mount on slides in balsam, isobutyl methacrylate, or clarite.

TICKS

Specimens may be preserved in 70% alcohol or cleared and mounted on slides. Ticks can be fixed in an extended position by pressing gently between two glass slides while killing by immersion in hot water. Clearing in KOH, dehydration in alcohols, and mounting in balsam, clarite, or isobutyl methacrylate are accomplished using the procedure described for fleas.

MISCELLANEOUS ARTHROPODS

Spiders, scorpions, centipedes, lice, bedbugs, maggots, and other larvae, nymphs, and soft-bodied insects may be preserved in 70% alcohol containing a small amount of glycerin to prevent drying and shrinking. Coating the corks with paraffin will prevent loss by evaporation. Larger, hard-bodied insects may be pinned, labeled, and stored in boxes containing naphthalene flakes or paradichlorobenzene to prevent mold and damage from living insects.

REFERENCES

Brues, C. T., A. L. Melander, and F. M. Caprenter. 1954. Classification of insects. Ed. 2. Harvard Museum, Cambridge, 917 pp.

Doetschman, W. H. 1944. Some suggestions in microtechnique particularly useful in microentomology and parasitology. Trans. Am. Microsc. Soc. 63:175-178.

Gordon, R. M., and M. M. J. Laviopierre. 1962. Entomology for students of medicine. Blackwell Scientific Publications, Ltd., London.

Grubb, H. R. 1929. Laboratory technics of collecting, dissecting breeding, preserving and mounting arthropods. Pages 706-735. In W. S. Patton and A. M. Evans, Editors. Insects, ticks, mites and venomous animals of medical and veterinary importance. Croydon, England.

Horsfall, W. R. 1962. Medical entomology. The Ronald Press Co., New York, 467 pp.

James, M. T., and R. F. Harwood. 1969. Herms' medical entomology. Ed. 6. The Macmillan Co., New York, 484 pp.

Matheson, R. 1950. Medical entomology. Ed. 2. Comstock Publishing Co., Ithaca, New York. Chapter 20. Collecting, preserving and mounting insects, pp. 586-599.

Ribeiro, H. 1967. A solidifiable formic acid PVA solution for transporting, preserving and mounting mosquito larvae and pupae. Stain Technol. 42:159-160.

Rohlf, F. J. 1957. A new technique in the preserving of soft-bodied insects and spiders. Turtox News 1957, pp. 226-229.

Smart, J. 1965. A handbook for the identification of insects of medical importance. Ed. 4. British Museum of Natural History, London, 303 pp.

List of drugs available from Center for Disease Control

Drug	Disease or organism effective against	Drug	Disease or organism effective against
Pentamidine Pentamidine isethionate Lomidine	*Pneumocystis carinii* Interstitial plasma cell pneumonia *Trypanosoma b. gambiense* Gambian trypanosomiasis	Bithionol Lorothidol	Paragonimiasis Pulmonary Subcutaneous Cerebral Endemic hemoptysis
Astiban Sodium antimony dimercaptosuccinate	Schistosomiasis Bilharziasis *Schistosoma japonicum* *Schistosoma haematobium* Urinary-vesical schistosomi- asis *Schistosoma mansoni* Visceral schistosomiasis	Suramin Fourneau 309 Bayer 205 Germanin Moranyl Belganyl Naphuride Antrypol	*Trypanosoma b. gambiense* Gambian trypanosomiasis *Trypanosoma b. rhodesiense* Rhodesian trypanosomiasis
BAY 2502 Lampit	Chagas' disease Megaesophagus Megacolon	Mel B Melarsoprol Arsobal	Gambian trypanosomiasis Rhodesian trypanosomiasis
Pentostam Sodium antimony gluco- nate Sodium stibogluconate	Leishmaniasis Kala-azar Espundia ulcer	Furamide Diloxanide furoate	Asymptomatic cyst passers of *Entamoeba histolytica*
Yomesan Niclosamide	*Taenia saginata* *Taenia solium* *Diphyllobothrium latum* *Hymenolepis nana* *Hymenolepis diminuta* *Dipylidium caninum*	Aralen Chloroquine Dehydroemetine	Malaria Amebiasis Amebic dysentery
Ambilhar Niridazole	Schistosomiasis Dracunculiasis Guinea worm	Quinine dihydrochloride	Malaria

From Center for Disease Control, Parasitic Disease Drug Service, Atlanta, Georgia. Telephone: 404-329-3670 (day); 404-329-3644 (night).

Index